THE MAGIC PILL

THE MAGIC PILL

Your Prescription for a Longer, Healthier, and Happier Life

MATT O'BRIEN

iUniverse, Inc.
Bloomington

The Magic Pill
Your Prescription for a Longer, Healthier, and Happier Life

You should not undertake any diet/exercise regimen recommended in this book before consulting your personal physician. Neither the author nor the publisher shall be responsible or liable for any loss or damage allegedly arising as a consequence of your use or application of any information or suggestions contained in this book.

iUniverse books may be ordered through booksellers or by contacting:

iUniverse
1663 Liberty Drive
Bloomington, IN 47403
www.iuniverse.com
1-800-Authors (1-800-288-4677)

Because of the dynamic nature of the Internet, any web addresses or links contained in this book may have changed since publication and may no longer be valid. The views expressed in this work are solely those of the author and do not necessarily reflect the views of the publisher, and the publisher hereby disclaims any responsibility for them.

Any people depicted in stock imagery provided by Thinkstock are models, and such images are being used for illustrative purposes only.

Certain stock imagery © Thinkstock.

ISBN: 978-1-4502-8280-2 (sc)
ISBN: 978-1-4502-8282-6 (dj)
ISBN: 978-1-4502-8281-9 (ebk)

Printed in the United States of America

iUniverse rev. date: 02/21/2011

For all those who have struggled to find the motivation to change. You are my inspiration because I am you.

CONTENTS

Introduction: The Magic Pill 1
How to use this book. 9

PART ONE
MOTIVATION: *Get the Facts*

1. ***The Fountain of Youth*** 13
   Can We Really Turn Back the Clock on Aging?

2. ***Preventive Medicine*** 52
   An Ounce of Prevention is Worth More than a Pound of Cure

3. ***Better than Prozac*** 97
   Improve your Mood and Alleviate Anxiety

PART TWO
EDUCATION: *The Knowledge*

4. ***Invest in Yourself*** 111
   The Costs of Exercise and the Costs if You Don't Exercise

5. ***Exert Yourself*** 123
   Commit Yourself to Exercise

6. ***Motivate Yourself*** 166
   Are You Lost in Love or in Love to be Lost?
   A Labor of Love

7. ***Nourish Yourself*** 185
   Do you Eat to Live or Live to Eat?
   The Nutritional Road Map to Dietary Success

8. ***Reduce Yourself*** 231
   The Time Tested Strategies of Losing Weight

9. ***Supplement Yourself*** 273
   Live Longer and Perform Better

PART THREE
ACTION: *The Path to Success*

10. *Moderate Yourself* 291
Matt's Moderation Mantra

11. *Assist Yourself* 301
Getting Some Help: Hire a Personal Trainer!

12. *Empower Yourself* 316
The Power of the Mind

13. *Direct Yourself* 340
Action Leads the Way to Your Destiny

HELPFUL TOOLS AND TABLES

Age Defying Benefits of Exercise 16
Calculate Your Body Mass Index (BMI) .72
Exercise Recommendations for Diabetics .81
Exercise Guidelines for Adults 131
Exercise Guidelines for Children 134
Calculate Your Target (Training) Heart Rate 143
Walking Program Chart 151
The Menu Workout 156
Daily Caloric Intake Worksheet 200
The Ten Commandments of Nutrition 202
The Five Critical Steps of Weight Loss 254
The Nutrition Traffic Light 264
The Supplement Trilogy 277
Goal Setting Worksheet 342

Acknowledgements 357
Selected References and Further Reading 361

INTRODUCTION

The Magic Pill

Imagine for a minute I was your personal doctor and during a routine check-up I told you there was a pill with seemingly magical powers now available to everyone and I was incredibly excited (bouncing off the walls, jumping up and down, shouting from the mountain tops) to tell you about it. So excited, in fact, I believe the whole world should be taking it, every doctor should prescribe it to their patients and it is now up to me and a few select others in the know, to get the word out starting with you right now!

I'm telling you as sure as you are now reading these words, this pill does exist. Some doctors have already branded it the true "Fountain of Youth." This magic pill has been scientifically proven to lengthen your natural lifespan, improve your self-esteem, increase your energy level, decrease your body fat, improve your skin tone, increase the natural production of your body's youthful hormones, improve your sex drive, increase your bone density, and improve your memory.

At this point you're probably thinking out loud... *"Wow 'Doc' that's truly amazing! There's really a pill for that?"*

Yes there is, but this pill does so much more. Taken just once a day, it significantly reduces high blood pressure, improves the flow of blood

1

throughout the body, lowers your bad cholesterol and also raises your good cholesterol. The magic pill can reduce your risk of getting cancer by 55%, reduce your risk of having a heart attack by 50%, and reduce your risk of having a stroke by over 40%. Scientific research has also discovered it can help prevent type 2 diabetes because it controls blood sugar, decreases insulin resistance and improves metabolism.

"Okay, okay already," you say, "what is this 'magic pill,' where can I get it, and how much is it going to cost me?"

All excellent questions, but before I tell you, I must let you know about some of the side effects. But because this truly is a magic pill, the side effects are good, not bad. When you start taking it, you may notice it will improve your posture, increase your strength and muscle tone, improve your mood, improve the quality of your sleep, release the tension in your body, decrease your appetite, and even reduce your anxiety.

"Come on now, you're killing me! Let the cat out of the bag so I can get my hands on this pill. It sounds like a true miracle... the elusive Magic Pill."

Alright, it may surprise you to learn this pill does exist, is already available to everyone and at the most, might cost you one to two dollars a day. The "Magic Pill" which we should all be taking is a daily dose of exercise, pure and simple. Thousands upon thousands of scientific studies have proven the undeniable and almost countless benefits of exercise and we are learning about more and more benefits each day as new studies are conducted and published. Exercise is the ultimate preventive medicine because it will improve your overall health, fitness, and well-being, while also helping to prevent or decrease the probability of getting many illnesses, reduce your likelihood of getting sick, and likely keep you out of the hospital during most of the days of your life.

Every successful journey begins with a single step

Congratulations! If you are reading this now, you have taken the first step on your journey to a healthier and happier life. You have made a decision to make your life better. My job is to illuminate your journey with helpful signs to guide you in the right direction. These signs will motivate, educate, and inspire you to take positive action, eliminate your fears, and forget about any guilt from past failures.

All of our time on earth is priceless. Time is hearing the emotion-provoking sounds of beautiful music, seeing the majesty of an eagle in flight, tasting the savory flavor of your favorite foods, and feeling the warmth and security of true love. Time is the precious moments we have with our family, loved ones, and closest friends. I want to give you more of this time and all it takes is a little effort on your part. We are going to take this walk together and our destination is a younger, healthier, and happier you.

For most of my life, I have been searching for a way to help people with their health and happiness. I want people to feel the way I feel and experience the positive, life-altering benefits I've experienced from exercise. Initially I was thinking a career in medicine might be the best approach to achieve this goal. But I was convinced by people I respect and my own internal voice, this might not be the best way for me. Instead, I decided to become a practitioner of the ultimate preventive medicine, which I'm convinced is exercise. I'm convinced not only because of the overwhelming preponderance of scientific evidence and the hundreds of people I have personally seen improve their lives with exercise, but primarily because of the influence exercise has had in my own life.

Let me briefly tell you a little about my story and why I am here today. I realized at an early age that I was lazy and I also really loved food — I mean I liked to eat! I always felt like I could eat a whole cow when we sat down at the dinner table and I think on some occasions I came pretty close. Growing up on a farm as the oldest of two brothers and two sisters, I exercised my "king of the jungle" sibling birthright when it came to the leftovers at mealtimes. We were very lucky because we had a hard-working father providing for us and a loving mother who did anything and everything for us. We were never without food in the pantry, milk and eggs in the fridge, and plenty of meat and fish in the freezer. I definitely took advantage of the convenience of this "food proximity" and the bounty we had to choose from. My only saving grace was how highly active my parents kept us working on the farm, doing chores, and playing sports year round. Sitting around the house was not an option at the O'Brien house and this is what probably saved me from childhood obesity because I'm sure I ate enough to get me close.

Even so, I still accumulated a great deal of pudge on my bulky frame and my mom shopped for most of my clothes in the "Husky" section. I'm not sure if it still exists today, but back when I was an adolescent, I thought husky meant big and bulky like a football player. I later realized this was a polite, ego-stroking way of putting overweight kids into clothes that fit. To think I used to strut around proudly displaying the Husky logo like it was a right of passage to a future NFL career is hilarious to me today.

The outward signs of my love of food first became apparent around the age of seven and by the time I was 12, the embarrassing rolls of good eating were unmistakably displayed on my waistline. These rolls, which today would earn you the nickname "muffin top," coupled with a matching pair of "man boobs" were the kind of liabilities you want written off your physical balance sheet when you are about to enter high school. Throw in a first name that rhymes with "fat" and I'm sure you can imagine the nickname quickly bestowed upon me. I will always credit my wonderful mother for getting me through those awkward developmental years without a lifetime of psychological damage. But the pain, verbal suffering, and humiliation were certainly real at the time and definitely had a lasting impact on my self-esteem.

Thank God for what happened next in my life. I was introduced to weight training and professionally designed exercise programs. If you are not familiar with high school football in the "Sunshine State" of Florida, well let me tell you that it is taken very seriously. As a freshman at Pine Forest High School, I learned to lift weights three to four days a week with the skill and enthusiasm of an Olympic athlete getting ready to break a world record. This changed my body and it changed my life.

Within the first three months of this training, I already looked better and felt a lot better about myself. My dad recognized the change and my passion for exercise and signed me up for a membership at a local health club. While he and my brother were taking karate classes, I would lift weights and ride the exercise bikes. By the time I was a sophomore, I was a different person, changed on the inside and out. Despite relocating to the intimidating hustle and bustle of New York City, a new, confident persona began to emerge.

I walked on the football team at Stuyvesant High School in Manhattan. I continued to get stronger, faster, and happier with the way I looked. This culminated with a senior season as team captain and selection as the most valuable player. Besides other distinguished awards, I was offered the chance to play football at a number of colleges who recruited me. The most important benefit of this self-transformation was the opportunity I received to go to the US Air Force Academy, fulfilling a dream I had since I was in seventh grade.

If you have never been to the US Air Force Academy campus in Colorado Springs, Colorado, and especially if you have young children, you owe it to yourself to visit... like my Dad did with our family when I was 12 years old. While I was standing there on one of the many scenic overlooks peering down on the stunning architecture of the Cadet Chapel, the amazing monuments, airplane displays, proud cadets marching in formation, and unparalleled athletic fields and facilities, I made it my goal to attend this wonderful institution when I graduated high school. Without the confidence in myself I gained from athletics and exercise, I'm convinced this dream would have been a fading reality and would not have been a part of my life today.

The day I received my acceptance letter, which is called an "Appointment" by the Academy admissions office, was probably the proudest day of my life. In hindsight, it is certainly the most significant. Besides getting an unbelievable academic education, I learned incredibly valuable leadership skills and discipline which I have used throughout my career and lifetime relationships. Having achieved my first big dream with the mental and physical changes that exercise brought to my life, I decided to study the science behind it. I majored in Biology and took every class possible on exercise physiology, biomechanics, sports psychology, and human anatomy. I wanted to learn how this stuff works and why it works, so I could "pay it forward" to other people someday down the road.

I continued to study exercise science after graduation by reading everything I could get my hands on. I continue this practice to this very day. After six and half years of military service for the Air Force, I soon put this knowledge and my own personal experience to work as a personal trainer in New York City and eventually, here in Tampa, Florida, where I reside today. Despite the long workdays and tremendous physical energy it requires, being a personal trainer is the most rewarding occupation I could ever imagine. On a daily basis, I have the privilege of helping people change their bodies, mind, and spirit, and ultimately improve their lives, the same way I did for myself years ago.

Over the past twenty years, I have had the great fortune to be mentored by some of the best exercise, nutrition, and self-help gurus. I've attended hundreds of scientific lectures, read almost every current book published on diet and exercise, and reviewed thousands of scientific studies related to health, nutrition, exercise, and nutritional supplementation. Like Tony Robbins would say: I tell you this not to impress you, but to impress upon you the

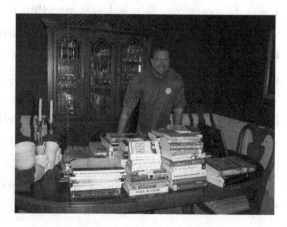

validity and credibility of the information I will present to you. While I may not have completely captured all of the information and research I reviewed for this book, please be assured that I tried my best to summarize the essence of it throughout the book. For more information on selected topics, I have included a references list in the appendices.

In *The Magic Pill*, I hope to educate you on the substantial benefits of exercise, inform you on the latest research and guidelines on cardiovascular and resistance training, and motivate you to begin and maintain a consistent exercise program that meets the current exercise guidelines recommended by the US Department of Health and Human Services, the American College of Sports Medicine and the American Heart Association. I will help you with goal setting, recommend useful tools for accountability, take you through my systematic approach to designing a progressive exercise program, and teach you about nutrition and supplementation. Most importantly and above all else, I want you to attain the lasting health, energy, and self-worth you deserve.

> *The mediocre teacher yells.*
> *The good teacher explains.*
> *The superior teacher demonstrates.*
> *The great teacher inspires.*
> William Arthur Ward

Inspiration is a powerful force that can launch us closer to our hopes and dreams. The Merriam-Webster's online dictionary defines the word inspiration as "a divine influence or action on a person believed to qualify him or her to communicate sacred revelation." Nothing inspires me more than helping people achieve their goals. Everyday I get to share in the joy and sense of accomplishment my clients and friends feel as they experience all the benefits exercise has to offer. I've been fortunate enough to see people lose 40, 50, 60, and even 100 pounds in less than 12 months with consistent effort. These are real people with real jobs, real kids and real problems, living in the real world.

I have worked with people of all ages, race, ethnicity, and any other demographic you can think of which is why I call exercise the universal law of health. Besides the visibly obvious cosmetic benefits of exercise, the changes that happen on the inside, in the heart, soul, and spirit are even more beautiful to see. When you see someone regain their sense of hope, self-confidence and self-esteem after living without it for years, it can move you emotionally. Quite frankly, this highly rewarding aspect of my profession keeps my motivational flame burning and served as the inspiration for writing this book. I want you to be inspired too. So throughout this book I have included the stories, results, and photos of everyday people who incorporated *The Magic Pill* prescription into their lives. For many people "seeing is believing" so I hope their testimonies will serve as convincing evidence to inspire you whenever you need it.

Your commitment, discipline, and achievement will motivate others to follow in your footsteps too! People tend to model the behaviors and attributes of the people they are around the most. I have had many clients whose success inspired others to make positive changes in their own lives. The secret to accomplishing this is by focusing on you. Let your results be the beacon of light that illuminates the pathway to success. Others will follow. If you have children, parents, friends, brothers, sisters, or anyone you care about, keep this in mind. Your actions (not your words, best intentions, suggestions, or nagging) will always be the best example of positive leadership.

I wish you good luck on your journey, but I have a feeling you will not need luck. You have asked for the *Magic Pill* and that decision, coupled with your desire and determination, will steer you in the right direction. You are already on your way!

HOW TO USE THIS BOOK

I f you are like many people I know, you may not have a lot of spare time for reading but still want to increase your knowledge and improve your motivational skills. I encourage you to invest the time to read this one book, because it is like reading 20 books. *The Magic Pill* is truly an executive summary or cliffsnotes on many fitness related topics including: anti-aging, preventive medicine, exercise, diet and nutrition, weight loss, and supplementation. It goes even further and includes self-help topics like: how to join a health club, how to live in moderation, how to hire a personal trainer, how to empower yourself, and how to set and achieve goals. Your knowledge, motivation, health, and longevity can only be improved by reading the content that follows.

That being said, the book is written and arranged like a collection of short stories where each chapter can stand on its own. But as a body of work, I believe it will serve its greatest purpose. There is something for everyone and I would recommend you explore what interests you the most. Use the table of contents to find the chapter that covers a topic you want more information about. If you get bogged down reading the scientific details, just move on to the next section or next chapter. There are also many helpful tools and tables located throughout the book. I have listed their respective page numbers for your reference at the end of the table of contents.

I sincerely hope this book will have a positive impact on your life and help change the course of obesity in America. If you benefit from the information, please share it with others and pay it forward. Individually we can change ourselves, but together we can change the future health and prosperity of our great nation.

PART ONE:

MOTIVATION
Get the Facts

CHAPTER ONE:

The Fountain of Youth

"Exercise is the closest thing we have to the fountain of youth."
Dr Linn Goldberg and Dr Diane Elliot
(Authors of *The Healing Power of Exercise*)

Can We Really Turn Back the Clock on Aging?

Thousands of studies have illustrated the countless benefits and biological clock-reversing power of exercise. Even with all the advances in medicine, bioengineering of "superfoods," and high-tech supplements, nothing surpasses exercise in its ability to keep us young and help us live longer. Gerontologists who research and study aging have come up with dozens of theories and four schools of thought on what causes aging, but have universally concluded that exercise is the closest thing we have to an anti-aging pill. By revitalizing the biological processes involved in

AVERAGE LIFE SPANS	
1796	25 Years
1896	48 Years
1996	80 Years

aging, exercise increases lifespan and dramatically improves the quality of life during our later years. We can't overlook the impact of science and medicine in giving us vaccines, antibiotics, trauma surgery, drug therapies, psychotherapies, and life saving treatments, all which have contributed to our significantly longer life spans. In spite of all the medical breakthroughs though, and the fact that the average human lifespan has increased by 50 years during the past two centuries, many health experts agree that *children being born today have a shorter expected life span then their parents.*

Why is this? Simple answer: Because of the ever-increasing prevalence of sedentary lifestyles and poor nutritional habits. Now more than ever, American adults and their children are sitting on their collective butts and eating surplus calories from highly processed, low nutrient foods. We are at the golden age of medicine as biomedical information doubles every three and half years, genes are being decoded, and scientific research unmasks the microscopic processes which make life possible. Allopathic medicine will gladly continue to research and develop more and more drugs to treat the symptoms and discomforts resulting from our poor choices. *Exercise treats the underlying cause!* I ask you this: Is it better to treat the symptoms or cure the disease itself? Exercise is like a vaccine to old age.

It is amazing to look back just over 100 years ago and see that the three leading causes of death were influenza, diarrhea, and pneumonia. Today's leading causes of death are heart disease, cancer, and stroke. But the tide is turning again as diabetes and downstream diseases related to obesity are working their way to the top. Medicine helps us live longer, but exercise helps us live longer *and* better. As I've been advocating for the past 15 years to anyone willing to listen, exercise is the best preventive medicine there is and the true fountain of youth. You can quote me on this... *An ounce of prevention is worth more than a pound of cure!*

We can reform health care with prevention

According to the Budget of the US Government (Fiscal Year 2009), our government spent over 600 billion dollars on health care in 2008 and the US Department of Health and Human Services projects health care expenditures to double over the next 20 years. In his first State of the Union address to Congress, President Barack Obama declared health care is "one of the largest and fastest-growing parts of our budget." In a 2009 public address on health care reform, President Obama said the United States spends one dollar out of every six on health care. The true cost of our poor health is close to 700 billion dollars when you factor in lost wages, impact to our gross domestic product (GDP) from lost productivity, uninsured medical expenses covered by hospitals nationwide, and all government-backed programs related to the treatment and prevention of disease.

The best impact on health care costs we can make collectively as Americans is to focus on prevention. In fact, I don't think it is appropriate to consider aging normal anymore because for 98% of the people in our country, the rate of aging and probability of developing most diseases are a choice. Scientific research has conclusively proven the ability of exercise to dramatically slow the aging process and to significantly reduce the risk of getting almost every disease. With that in mind, I want to coin the term *"sedentary aging"* to differentiate the rate of inactive aging from "healthy aging." The difference between the two can be profound. Over 250 thousand deaths each year are attributable to a sedentary lifestyle. With 48 million Americans currently being classified as sedentary, something must be done to get America moving again.

How we age is a choice!

It is never too late to start exercising. Granted, the benefits are more pronounced the earlier you start, but studies have proven the anti-aging benefits of exercise even in ninety-six-year-olds. Studies involving feeble, elderly nursing home residents proved that this fast-growing segment of our population could park their wheelchairs, ditch their walkers, and drop their canes with the addition of a little strength training exercise. Other studies have shown we have the ability to restore 75 percent of the muscle mass lost from decades of inactivity with just twelve weeks of training. Like I said, it is never too late to get started and you can see and feel the benefits almost immediately.

When I turn 85 later down the road of life, I want to be more than alive and kicking. I want to be able to "chuck the rock" and hit grounders with my future great grandkids in the backyard. I want to continue traveling without special accommodations or any limitations on when or where I can go. I want to be able to go for a run on the beach and dive into the cool ocean waves. I want to be able to go to the gym and knock out some reps of squats with 200 pounds on my back. Science and history says I can.

Look at Jack LaLanne, arguably the "Godfather of Fitness," who in his seventies and eighties was performing incredible feats of strength and endurance. Do you remember him at 70 years of age towing 70 boats loaded with 70 people for one and a half miles in the murky waters of San Francisco Bay while shackled and handcuffed? I sure do. I had the pleasure of meeting Jack last year and at 94 years young, he looked fantastic and still had the passion for exercise.

We have a young lady running around our gym named Ellen. At 93, she can run through our agility ladder, balance on one foot and simultaneously lift a five pound dumbbell over her head, stand on a balance board and still crack a decent joke. She credits her health and vigor

Age Defying Benefits of Exercise

- **Boosts energy production and increases metabolism**
- **Increases muscular strength and endurance**
- **Controls blood sugar and improves insulin sensitivity**
- **Decreases inflammation and free radical damage**
- **Decreases illness by boosting immune function**
- **Improves circulation (capillarization & vasodilation)**
- **Strengthens bones by increasing bone mineral density**
- **Protects joints from degenerative disease**
- **Improves length and quality of sleep**
- **Prevents muscle loss and decreases body fat**
- **Increases flexibility**
- **Improves reflexes and coordination**
- **Lowers blood pressure**
- **Lowers total and LDL (bad) cholesterol**
- **Improves mood and sense of well-being**

to a lifetime of physical activity. Speaking of health and vigor, Chuck is another living testimony to the benefits of daily exercise. At 94 years of age, he drives himself to the gym six days out of each week to complete his two hour routine that includes walking on the treadmill, lifting weights, and stretching. If you stop him to say hi you better be prepared to avoid his shadow-boxing hands and obligatory pat on the butt when you turn to leave. We have another member at our health club named Mildred who just celebrated her 101st birthday. Thanks to decades of her daily exercise routine, she looks like she is 70 and she still has all her faculties, competently drives her own car, plays golf, and does volunteer work. Ellen, Chuck, and Mildred are all wonderful testimonies to the benefits of exercise and for some of you I hope their example will help you believe in the anti-aging power of exercise. *Seeing is believing!*

Chronological age verses calendar age. How old are you?

At 40 years of age plus, I can do everything (and more) I could do when I was 18. I want to increase awareness of the anti-aging benefits of exercise and show people how to slow down the biological clock. Personally, I have reaped tremendous benefits by keeping exercise as an important part of my life since I was 13 years old. According to my doctor, I am in "excellent health" and he gave my blood work an "A+" when we met last year. It gives me tremendous piece of mind and reassurance knowing I'm proactively taking care of my health.

For my 40th birthday in 2008 I decided to celebrate what I call "The New 40" with a workout for the ages. I wanted to prove to myself and others that I could do more at the age of 40 than I could do at the age of 20. I set out with an initial goal to lift over 40 cumulative tons of weight in 40 minutes but ended up lifting over 52 tons — that's 104,000 pounds of workload volume! Because I am intensely passionate about proving my point (and was inspired by Dean Kanares in his book *Ultramarathon Man*), I decided to follow-up this intense weight training session with a little 8 hour, 40 mile jaunt on the treadmill. Although I was very sore the next day, I was still amazed at the God-given capabilities we possess. If you are a glutton for punishment or are crazy enough to try, I challenge you to give this combined workout (40 tons in 40 minutes and then 40 miles) a test drive.

In the book *YOU, The Owner's Manual*, authors Michael F. Roizen, M.D. and Mehmet C. Oz, M.D. discuss their RealAge® Test. They devised a system to determine our biological age, which they consider to be far more important than our chronological (calendar) age. Having experienced the benefits of exercise for over 25 years and comparing myself to those of the same age who don't workout, I completely agree. Personally following the guidelines of this book, my biological age or "RealAge®" is 29.2 years! I'm not saying I'm Dick Clark or an anti-aging phenom, but I still get regularly ID'd at bars and restaurants. Usually the waitress or bartender apologizes when they see the 1968 birthdate, but I thank them anyway for the unintentional compliment. Just the other day, my wife and I were talking to a pair of fifty-somethings and the man said "You young kids have no idea what it was like when I was your age." When I revealed to him that I was probably a lot closer to his age than he thought, he was astonished and probably a little embarrassed because of the stark differences in our appearance.

I'm sharing these stories with you not because I want you to think I'm anything special. Honestly, I want you to experience what I have for yourself. Don't bury yourself prematurely because there is so much great life to live. We really can buy more time with a little effort. I encourage you to take the "Real Age" test too at www.RealAge.com and see where your biological age is right now. If you exercise, eat a reasonably nutritious diet with the appropriate amount of calories and take the right nutritional supplements, you can expect to be ten to twenty years younger biologically than if you are sedentary, eat whatever you want (and in excess), and avoid taking your daily multivitamin. After you follow this program for a few months, go back and check again. Watch the real age clock go backwards and enjoy reaping the benefits of your newfound youth!

Some anti-aging experts have gone as far as saying exercise equals immortality because you can live free of mental and physical disease and degeneration for 20 additional years. In their very comprehensive 500+ page book *The New Anti-Aging Revolution*, authors Dr Ronald Klatz and

Dr Robert Goldman thoroughly reviewed all of the current anti-aging science and medicine and concluded: *"Exercise at least 30 minutes daily. It is your number-one defense against the infirmities of old age."* Age-related declines in metabolism, muscular strength and physical capacity have been proven reversible with strength training exercise and can no longer be blamed as the inevitable consequence of aging.

> The American Cancer Society conducted a twenty year study on over one million men and women and concluded: *"Physical exercise lengthens life and wards off heart disease and stroke."*

How do we age?

Let's take a brief look at how we age and what we can do about it. I'll try to keep the techno-jargon and scientific mumbo jumbo to a minimum, but it's important to have a basic understanding of the science of aging so I can properly illustrate the relevance, benefits and importance of exercise. There are four schools of thoughts on the aging process:

1. Programmed Aging: We have an internal biological clock which is programmed or set at birth for various changes like bone loss, hearing loss, muscle loss, and vision loss. As we pass 40 years of age, the body starts breaking down to get rid of us on earth and make way for the next generation. (*Exercise has been proven to prevent, reverse, or delay all of these processes.*)

2. Accidental Aging: We get older from a series of random events during our lifetimes – free radical damage of our DNA, wear and tear of body parts, exposure to chemical toxins and our environmental conditions. (*Exercise mitigates these random events by enabling the body to deal with stressors, improve immune function, and improve circulation and removal of toxic waste products of our metabolism and environmental exposure.*)

3. <u>Developmental Aging</u>: Aging is developed from the choices we make in life and is not chronological. The rate of aging can be controlled with lifestyle intervention, dietary choices, and stress management. (*This explains why a 65-year-old who exercises, eats right, and keeps stress to a minimum can be physiologically younger than a sedentary, stressed out 50-year-old with a donut addiction.*)

4. <u>Pathological aging</u>: Aging is caused by diseases that ravage the body's tissues, attack our immune system, harden our arteries, destroy our livers, and mutate our genes causing cancer, diabetes, and other complications which shorten our lives. (*Almost every disease we can experience is preventable before it happens with an exercising lifestyle and some are even reversible with the addition of exercise.*)

Why do we age?

Scientific research has led to dozens of theories on how and why the body ages. Following are some of the most common theories on the specific ways we age and ultimately die:

<u>Wear and tear theory</u>: Postulated by Dr August Weismann in 1882, our cells, tissues and organs become damaged by overuse and abuse. Repetitious use of our joints; excess consumption of sugar, fat, alcohol, nicotine, caffeine, and prescription and non-prescription drugs; as well as exposure to environmental toxins all speed aging according to this theory. (*Exercise has been proven to extend the body's ability to repair and maintain its organs, tissues and cells. By speeding removal of aging cells, exercise keeps a newer body of cells at the ready and decreases the likelihood older cells will be around to mutate.*)

<u>Neuroendocrine theory</u>: Credited to Dr Vladimir Dilman, our youth hormones of testosterone, growth hormone, thyroid hormones, and

IGF-1 all decline with sedentary aging. According to this theory, these biochemical messengers are regulated by our hypothalamus and after we have passed our productive and reproductive age, they are programmed to decline. (*Resistance exercise has been proven to elevate all of these youth hormones as we age, extending our productive life span and vigor.*)

Genetic control theory: This is also called the planned-obsolescence theory; our DNA is programmed like a biological time bomb to go off when our time is up. Essentially, the body self-destructs, ages, and dies. (*Studies on identical twins growing up in different environments have largely countered this thinking by showing how lifestyle choices like exercise can dramatically affect appearance, weight and the rate of aging. The MacArthur Study of Aging in America found that lifestyle trumps genetics when it comes to getting old and the quality of life.*)

Hayflick Limit Theory: Dr Leonard Hayflick author of *How and Why We Age* and his colleague Dr Paul Moorehead demonstrated the senescence (aging) of cultured human cells in 1961. They postulated that lung, skin, muscle, and heart cells divide approximately 50 times then die and thus "limit" human longevity to a maximum of 125 years. (*Lifestyle factors and nutrition can affect the rate of division -- overfed cells divide faster and thus, die faster and underfed cells divide slower allowing them to live longer.*)

Death Hormone Theory: Former Harvard University endocrinologist, Dr Donner Denckle describes that, as we age, the pituitary gland in the brain starts releasing DECO (decreasing oxygen consumption hormone) which inhibits cellular use of a metabolic hormone produced by the thyroid gland called thyroxine. This slows our basal metabolism, inhibits conversion of food to energy, and thereby accelerates aging. (*Exercise elevates metabolism by preventing muscle wasting from disuse and by slowing the declining production of metabolic hormones.*)

<u>Thymic-Stimulating Theory</u>: Dr Alan Goldstein, chairman of the Biochemistry Department at George Washington University, discovered the size of the thymus gland is 200-250 grams at birth and only about three grams by the age of 60. Some scientists believe thymic hormones are the pacemaker of aging and regulate immune function. As the gland diminishes in size, fewer hormones are produced and immune function deteriorates. (*Exercise in the right quantities has been proven to boost immune function at any age which can compensate for the biological losses from thymic hormones.*)

<u>Mitochondrial Theory</u>: The mitochondria are the energy producers of our cells and produce metabolic waste products from burning fuel like the exhaust from a combustion engine. These metabolic waste products produce free radicals which target the unprotected mitochondria. This causes DNA damage and reduces the total energy production in our cells and accelerates aging. (*Exercise facilitates the removal of metabolic waste products via increased circulation, perspiration (sweat), and expiration (breathing) and improves the efficiency of free radical neutralization, thereby reducing aging associated with free radical damage. Exercise also offsets the decrease in energy production by increasing the number of mitochondria making more energy conversion possible throughout the body.*)

<u>Cross-Linkage Theory</u>: In 1941, Dr Johan Bjorksten proved that proteins can cross-link with neighboring proteins, forming a flexible mesh. As we age, more and more of these cross-links form, decreasing the elasticity of proteins and making nutrient flow in and waste product flow out slower and more difficult. Damaged proteins are normally broken down by enzymes called proteases, and the presence of cross-linkages inhibits the activity of proteases. The excess presence of glucose increases these cross-links. (*Exercise and good nutrition work hand-in-hand to increase circulation and nutrient flow throughout the body to delay or inhibit the cross-linking process. Exercise also lowers glucose levels in the bloodstream by burning it for fuel in the active muscle cells.*)

<u>Caloric Restriction Theory</u>: Gerontologist Dr Roy Walford of UCLA Medical School, pioneered research which showed caloric restriction, coupled with high nutrient supplementation and exercise correlates to maximum health and life span. The body will settle to a weight of metabolic efficiency, maximizing health and life span. (*Dr Walford stressed the importance of exercise in retarding the functional and chronological aging process.*)

<u>Telomerase Theory</u>: Originally discovered by scientists at the Geron Corporation, telomeres shorten each time a cell divides. Telomeres are sequences of nucleic acids on the ends of chromosomes. As telomeres shorten, it is believed the cell is less able to duplicate itself correctly ultimately leading to cellular damage, susceptibility to mutations, and eventually cell death. (*Exercise increases cellular turnover speeding the renewal of the body's cells. Exercise and hormone introduction may possibly enhance the action of telomerase which has been shown to repair and replace telomeres and thus help to recycle the clock that regulates life-span.*)

<u>Free Radical Theory</u>: Introduced by Rebeca Gerschman in 1954 and subsequently developed by Dr Denham Harman of the University of Nebraska, the theory proposed that a free radical is any molecule that possesses a free electron. The electron carries a negative electric charge causing it to react with neighboring molecules in volatile and destructive ways. Free radicals are like promiscuous gigolos because they go around looking to break up the happy marriages of molecules to steel an electron partner. Free radical damage begins at birth and continues until we die. When we are young, the body's compensatory mechanisms of repair and replacement are working at peak efficiency. With sedentary aging and overeating, this process begins to slow down allowing free radicals to accumulate in the body and take their toll. Free radicals are credited with creating mutant cells that lead to cancer. Free radicals attack the collagen and elastin which keep our skin smooth, flexible, and elastic. Long term exposure to free radicals produces the visible wrinkles on

our face and hands. (*Exercise is your best defense because it keeps the free radical filters working at peak efficiency, delaying and minimizing free radical damage. Supplementation with a cross-section of antioxidants like vitamin C, vitamin E, and beta carotene can help neutralize oxidative damage of free radicals.*)

Okay, enough of the theories describing how we deteriorate because my head is about to explode and I fear you may be losing interest. Let's review how the various systems and composition of our bodies are affected as we get older and how exercise positively impacts each one. This is truly exciting stuff and once you understand the breadth and thorough benefits of exercise, you will have the motivational edge to get started and continue exercising throughout your lifetime. While we may not be able to live to be 150, we can definitely extend our time on earth and ensure a better quality of life during the years we are blessed with.

Nervous System and Cognitive Function

As we age, worries of losing our mental edge or our ability to remember things begin to seep into our consciousness. For some people, fear of getting Parkinson's, Alzheimer's, and dementia can invade and takeover their predominant thoughts. The brain is a complicated mesh of neurons, synapses, and neurotransmitters that all work together to give us thought, memory, sensations of smell, touch, taste, sound, and sight, as well as our emotions of fear, sadness, anger, loneliness, happiness, and love. The brain also controls our movements, heartbeat, breathing, balance, voice, and regulates all the functions in our bodies necessary for life.

Research has concluded that novel tasks and movements create new synapses in the brain. Synapses are essentially the wiring pattern of the brain. Neurons are connected in a specific pattern and sequence to represent a thought or memory. The more something is repeated, the more hardwired the connection. If you write with your right hand, the complicated and precise movement patterns required have been hardwired into your brain from the time you started writing one inch letters in kindergarten. Try writing with your non-dominant hand and you will instantly see the difference that years of brain conditioning can make. The anatomy and physiology of your non-dominant side are no different, other than the control signals they receive from the brain.

An aging brain gets smaller and has less capacity to control movement. Reaction times slow down significantly. And life's sounds, sights, and tastes seem less vivid. Studies have concluded the importance of performing new tasks, new challenges, new trades, new hobbies, and new physical activities to prolong brain development, essentially keeping it younger. Exercises that require muscular coordination, balance, agility, hand-eye coordination, and performing novel movements will help you keep a young brain.

Exercise can at the very least slow down the process of brain aging and research has even shown it can reverse the effects of age-related mental decline. At the 2008 American College of Sports Medicine Annual Meeting, I saw promising new research on the benefits of incorporating exercise into the treatment of Parkinson's disease. One of the researchers I spoke with hypothesized that because exercise positively alters the brain chemistry (serotonin and dopamine levels) it can counteract some of the deterioration associated with this disease.

Our nervous system is organized into the central nervous system, consisting of our brain and spinal cord and the peripheral nervous system, consisting of the thousands of miles of afferent and efferent nerve fibers, and the sensory and motor neurons. Combined as a system, they electrochemically route the command directives of the brain to their intended muscles and organs, as well as bringing the sensory impulses of taste, touch, sight, smell, and hearing to the brain where they are translated and interpreted. It is an amazing system which the most powerful and advanced computers on earth can't even come close to replicating.

Our cognitive ability or 'brain power' (in other words), normally decreases with age. This negatively affects memory recall, thoughts, functions controlled by the brain, and speed of information processing (reaction times). Studies have shown that you can prevent this age-related cognitive decline with an active, exercising lifestyle, coupled with using your noggin on a daily basis. Get on a treadmill with a crossword puzzle (attempt to solve it and stay on the treadmill — that's no small feat) and you knock out two birds with one stone. My wife likes to solve Sudoku puzzles while she is on the elliptical doing her cardio.

With sedentary aging, the motor neurons which innervate our muscle fibers and give us the ability to lift hundreds of pounds or control the precise tip of a pen when we write begin to die off in a classic case of *"use it or lose it."* With fewer motor neurons, we lose the speed, precision, and coordination of our movements, have less proprioception, and easily lose our balance. This combination increases the likelihood of falls, which in turn, increases the likelihood of fractures and all of the associated complications of broken hips, wrists, and vertebrae. *More women die of complications related to hip fractures each year than breast cancer*, yet you don't see any colored-ribbon-wearing celebrities promoting "Hip Fracture Walks" because it's not as glamorous and the cure is simple: exercise!

Our touch, taste, smell, sight, and hearing (our sensory system) all decrease in acuity and sensitivity with sedentary aging which dramatically decreases the quality of life. When you can no longer taste the sweet acidity and herbal vibrance of a fresh marinara sauce or the subtle and complex flavors and tannins of a great California cabernet, then life gets a little duller. When you can no longer hear the laughter of children playing, smell the intoxicating scent of your favorite perfume, see the changing colors of the autumn leaves in Vermont, or feel the intensity of a sensuous stroke on your cheek, are you truly living the quality of life you deserve and are capable of? Of course not!

Exercise, coupled with sound nutrition and nutrient supplementation can prevent or slow the rate of deterioration in our senses. It keeps your sensory functions working properly by maintaining the neural network connecting the sensory cells in the skin, taste buds, nose, eyes, and ears to the interpreting brain. Exercise also prevents some of the circulatory problems which can dull our senses, particularly our eyesight. High blood pressure and poor circulation can damage vital parts of our eye leading to glaucoma and macular degeneration.

Your Brain on Fitness

An impressive body of recent research has concluded that there is a positive correlation between exercise and cognitive function of the brain in both adults and children. Recent studies have proven that aerobically fit adults have better cognitive abilities than their sedentary peers. Exercise increases circulation to the brain and keeps the neurotransmitters cranked up. One study demonstrated consistent exercise improved mental efficiency by 15%. Another one found people who exercise five times per week improved their mental acuity from 10 to 29%, making them more efficient and productive at work. Want to keep your brain working? It's time to get your body moving.

Research has also linked declines in spatial memory with declines in growth hormone levels. Exercise increases growth hormone levels (see Endocrine System later in this chapter) and makes it less likely you will forget where the keys are or where you were on your last anniversary when your wife asks. There are countless other benefits of exercise on the brain, particularly on brain biochemistry, which I will discuss in more detail in Chapter 3. Suffice it to say, exercise positively alters dopamine, serotonin, and endorphin levels in the brain which collectively help govern our feelings of happiness, satisfaction, motivation, and mood.

I often wonder at what point in the aging process the brain says: "Hey, it's ok to wear black dress socks with white slip-on sneakers and plaid Bermuda shorts." And we can't forget the luminescent polyester pants or the black shades that cover 85% of the face either. Our city governments should employ fashion police to arrest this criminal symptom of aging. Unless of course this applies to you, in which case, I meant the guy next to you. Even if you are that guy, the benefits of exercise will ensure that you are as sharp as you can be — shades, slippers, socks, shorts, and all!

Muscular System and Body Composition

A 1995 research study conducted at the Baltimore Veterans Affairs Medical Center concluded that modifying lifestyle factors with weekly exercise reduced fat accumulation from 17% per decade to only 3% per decade in men and from 26% to just 5% per decade in women. Let's put some numbers on this so we can better understand the impact this can have. Pretend you're a typical five foot, nine inch 200 pound male in his mid-forties carrying around 50 pounds of total bodyfat. Without exercise, by the time you are 55 you will be hauling around an additional 8.5 pounds of fat. By the time you are 65, you will add another ten pounds of fat to your proud and ever-expanding belly, giving you a total fat mass of 68 and a half pounds. This puts you at close to 220 pounds with a bodyfat percentage of around 31% and a waist measurement well over 40 inches. With a waist measurement over 40 inches for males and 35 inches for females, you are now at a much higher risk for a myocardial infarction (that's a heart attack ladies and gentlemen).

Now let's start over and go back to your mid-forties but now you incorporate exercise into your lifestyle. When you reach 55 years of age this time, you will have only added 1.75 pounds of fat and by 65, only another 1.8 pounds. This would put you at a bodyfat percentage of 26%: that's *26% versus 31%!* This is just doing the minimum. Factor in a little more exercise and some nutritional intervention and you would be losing your accumulated fat and be on your way to a healthy and long life.

Besides the subcutaneous fat we can see all over our bodies, we also have the non-visible, visceral fat which surrounds our organs and serves to protect and insulate them. If you have too much, however, your risk of heart disease, stroke, and diabetes increases, along with your distended belly. Your doctor can help you determine if you have too much visceral fat by testing for a blood protein called RBP4. A study published in the *Journal of Cellular Metabolism* concluded the best treatment for excessive visceral fat is exercise.

If you ever need some motivation to start exercising, get a picture of an enlarged fatty heart and take a good look at it. It is gross! Imagine a raw ribeye steak molded into the size and shape of a volleyball and you would be pretty close. An obese heart is crammed with epicardial fat and can barely function like it was designed to. It would be like cramming yourself into a straight jacket three sizes too small and then try to get through a normal day. It just wouldn't work very well, would it? If you are extremely overweight, it is imperative you begin a medically supervised diet and exercise program (immediately!!!) because it is only a matter of time before the disease levy breaks and the flood of health problems begins.

Do you want to lose weight to look great? Whether we like it or not, we live in a very cosmetic society. Television, magazines, billboards, internet spam, and popular culture have filled our heads with idealistic images (and often digitally enhanced) of what we are supposed to look like. The constant barrage of attractive celebrities and skinny "supermodels" we are exposed to every day has driven into our DNA the desire to look good. In my personal training business, nine out of ten people I work with were initially motivated to exercise because they wanted to look better. As my client Kate put it when she started: "I just want to fit in my clothes." While I am not promising you will be the next movie star or fashion model, I can promise you that regular, consistent exercise (paired up with a calorie-correct nutrition program) will help you lose your extra (unnecessary) weight and then help you maintain your new healthy weight.

Exercise helps the body lose excess weight by utilizing the calories we eat and raising the metabolic rate. Think of the muscles you have as an engine like the one in your car. The faster and further you go, the more fuel you burn right? Sitting on the couch is like leaving your car in the driveway idling. A tank of fuel will last a long, long time. The body is the same. If you want to lose weight, you have to get the car out of the driveway everyday and take it for a good spin around town. Keep in mind, the faster and farther you go, the more fuel you will burn.

Like the fuel in your car, the calories we eat supply the body with the energy necessary to move, think, and breathe. The body needs a minimum supply of energy to maintain itself in idle. Idle for the body would be considered a sedentary lifestyle, meaning there is very little activity other than sleeping, eating, and sitting around the house. For most people, it only takes about 800 to 1,400 calories to maintain the body in idle. This is called the basal metabolic rate (BMR). Weight gain occurs when we consume more calories than we collectively burn with our BMR and daily activity. Since Americans are becoming more and more sedentary, the "daily activity" calories burned aren't much. This is a problem we can do something about.

If you are trying to lose weight, the basic formula is simple: $C_{out} >$ C_{in} If you're like me and not good with math or formulas, this simply means: *Move more and Eat less!* Calories out (C_{out}), the calories you burn through metabolism and daily activity must be greater than (>) Calories in (C_{in}), the calories from the food and beverages you put in your mouth and swallow. This book is going to help you do both and show you how to increase your BMR too!

By following a progressive strength training program, you can essentially build a bigger engine by increasing the amount of lean muscle tissue you have. A six cylinder car burns more gas (typically) than a four cylinder model, right? This is one example where bigger *is* better. Later in the book, I will show you how to build a bigger engine and also help you determine the appropriate amount of calories to take in to help you feel great and get to a healthy weight.

Personally, I have used exercise over the years to build the metabolic equivalent of a big SUV engine. According to a metabolism measuring device called the BodyGem (indirect calorimeter by MicroLifeUSA), I have a metabolic rate that is over 2,300 calories a day. That means when I add a 600 calorie workout and my substantial daily activity training clients, I can eat a whopping 3,300 calories and not gain weight. Since I love to eat, this is a good thing and I get to enjoy more of the healthy foods I love. So can you! Most of my clients witness this effect after a few months of consistent exercise. They say: "Wow, I can eat more than I used to and still lose weight!" Want a more extreme example? Look at Michael Phelps during his historic, record-breaking swims in the 2008 Bejiing Olympics. According to reported estimates, he was able to consume around 10,000 calories a day and still stay a lean, mean, record-breaking machine. His highly-trained physique burned fuel like a Formula One race car — lots of it!

Energize yourself! Exercise increases your stamina and natural energy levels. Because exercise demands more energy, with routine exercise habits, the body eventually adapts by increasing the number of cellular mitochondria. Mitochondria are specialized, energy-producing generators located in the cells throughout our body. When you first start an exercise program, it can leave you feeling a little tired when you finish your 30 minutes. This is your body telling you "I'm not used to this!" Over time, however, with improved circulation, more oxygen traveling in your blood, a stronger heart, a higher mitochondrial density, and more mood-boosting chemicals pumping in your brain, you start to find some of the vigor and energy you thought you lost in your youth. Most of the people I start on exercise programs notice an energy and mood boost within the first two weeks. Your body tackles every day activities with ease and is more prepared to deal with any obstacles put in your path.

If you recall the previous car in the driveway analogy, with regular exercise, your body will have a faster idle speed, will produce more horsepower and will look better on the inside and out. It's time to trade in your model T for a newer, fuel-injected super car!

Skeletal System

Exercise prevents "shrinking-man" and "shrinking-woman" syndrome. Sedentary aging causes loss of bone mineral density, decreased elasticity and resilience of connective tissue, and degeneration of the intervertebral disks in our spines. Collectively they contribute to the loss of height as we age, but as you hopefully are beginning to realize, these changes are largely preventable with strength training and other forms of weight-bearing exercise.

Let's take a brief look at some exercise physics and biomechanics. Our muscles, bones, and connective tissue function as a mechanical system (lever, fulcrum, axis of rotation) much like the hydraulic system on a backhoe or front-end loader does. When you lift a weight against the force of gravity, you generate a mechanical load on the body. The resultant force of this load causes compression and strain on the bones of our structural (appendicular) skeleton. Wow, that was a mouthful. I'm glad I was paying attention in my biomechanics class. But I digress.

These forces, if strong enough, provide a stimulus, which signals the bone-building cells, called osteoblasts, to strengthen the bones in a process called bone modeling. The osteoblasts secrete matrix proteins (primarily collagen) which eventually become mineralized. This added bone mineral density is what most people would consider the hard bone. The higher the bone mineral density the stronger the bone is. Weight-bearing exercises such as walking and lifting weights have been proven to increase the bone mineral density of the structural bones in our bodies and increase collagen metabolism in our joints. This is in contrast to most osteoporosis medications which attempt to chemically interfere with the natural process of bone modeling and degradation.

When you walk briskly or run, the impact of the heel on the ground causes an opposing force load to go through the bones of the foot, shin, leg, hip, and spine. For people who aren't accustomed to exercise, this force is typically significant enough to cause a small bend in these weight-bearing bones. This deformation of the involved bone surfaces is called the minimum essential strain (MES) and it signals the body to build stronger, denser bones in an attempt to prevent this bending in the future. Without this deformation stimulus from exercise and activity as we age, the mineral content in our bones starts to decrease and the bones, cartilage, and collagen get more brittle and less resilient. Stronger bones are less brittle and less prone to fracture.

It is estimated that over 80% of the hip fractures in the elderly could be prevented with exercise. This is far better than the percentage of hip fractures which prescription osteoporosis drugs purport to prevent. Three of my elderly clients (76+ years of age) have fallen for various reasons (getting a foot caught in their pajama pants; stepping on a slick, algae-covered surface; and catching a foot on the curb of the sidewalk) and I am proud to say they all fared well on their tumbles to the ground. From the three serious falls I am aware of, the only negative outcome was one broken wrist (unless you count a bruised ego). This is far better than any broken hips, backs, or shoulders. The body is very efficient at keeping only what it needs so consider it your job to provide the necessary stimulus to maintain strong bones throughout your lifetime.

The skeletal benefits don't stop there either. Regular exercise also takes the creak out of arthritis by stimulating specialized cells in your joints to release synovial fluid. Synovial fluid lubricates our joints like motor oil lubricates the mechanical parts of an engine. When you don't exercise regularly, less of it is secreted resulting in more joint friction and pain. If this continues on a long-term, frequent basis (those of you stuck on the couch), your joints will wear down faster (like a motor without oil or one with lots of cold starts) which could lead to arthritis or even more severe joint problems.

In addition to keeping our joints lubricated, muscle-building exercises keep our joint capsules tight and stable. This ensures the proper mechanical function of the hinge-like joints (knee and elbow) and the ball and socket joints (shoulder and hip). With less room for the articulating surfaces to move around the joint capsules, there is less overall friction which results in less wear and tear. So if you want your body to function like a well-oiled machine, you must continue exercising regularly.

Endocrine System

Hormones are the body's chemical messengers which are manufactured, stored and released into the bloodstream by the endocrine glands. The endocrine glands are regulated by both chemical and neural signals and help the body maintain homeostasis and respond to the situations we encounter each day. Hormones play many critical roles in the body including regulating reproduction, energy production, muscular development, and growth of bodily structures and tissues. Think of hormones like a recipe in a cook book. They provide the body specific instructions on how to make a cake, which in this case is a physiological response.

Beginning in our 30's, our anabolic "fountain of youth" hormones testosterone, estrogen (in women), growth hormone, dehydroepiandrosterone (DHEA) and insulin-like growth factors (IGF-1) naturally start to decline. These hormones regulate and influence our strength, vigor, stamina, body fat, skin elasticity, connective tissue, bone development and ability to recover from intense exercise. Without any "exercise intervention," by the time we reach retirement age in our 60's and 70's, the circulating levels of each of these powerful, body altering hormones are significantly reduced. Less of these anabolic hormones cause our muscles to shrink, skin to sag, and libidos to disappear like a white bunny in a magic show. Following a regular exercise program constantly stimulates the body to release more of these youthful hormones and prevent a lot of what we formally considered to be normal aging.

During high-intensity exercise, the concentrations of these anabolic hormones can be amplified 10 to 20 times over resting levels. By choosing not to exercise, you are essentially deactivating this muscle-building hormone injector and depriving your body of the youthful effects they have. According to Henry S. Lodge M.D., who coauthored the book *Younger Next Year* with Chris Crowley, adults who exercise regularly throughout their adulthood, are up to 14 "biological" years younger than their peers of the same age who did not. Much of this anti-aging benefit can be attributed to the acute increases and chronic maintenance of youth hormones associated with exercise.

Growth hormone is a naturally produced polypeptide hormone. Injectable and ingestible versions of growth hormone have gained popularity in athletes and aging men because of their ability to build muscle, reduce bodyfat, and speed recovery from exercise and healing from injury. Some athletes have gained recent notoriety by turning to the needle to get a synthetic version of this hormone and many aging adults have sought expensive (but legal) interventions from anti-aging clinics. The good news is that you can use resistance exercise (force-produced stress on the body) to stimulate the anterior portion of pituitary gland to secrete a healthy dose of growth hormone free of charge and free of public scrutiny. Just think of your trip to the gym as a means to get a free injection of this powerful hormone and by performing compound weight-bearing exercises two to three times a week, you can maintain high circulating amounts of this growth hormone and reap all of its muscle-building and fat-burning benefits.

Similarly, testosterone which is produced in the testes in males and ovaries in females; parathyroid hormone produced by the parathyroid glands; IGF-1 produced by the liver; thyroxine produced by the thyroid gland; beta-endorphin produced in the anterior pituitary gland; and the adrenal hormones epinephrine and norepinephrine all can be naturally increased with the appropriate exercise stimuli. Individually, they are all powerful hormones with significant effects on the body. Together, they can be manipulated favorably to produce the anti-aging benefits of increased: muscle mass, strength, energy, stamina, concentration, pleasure, bone formation, cardiac output, fat metabolism, and libido. The following table provides a summary of these and some other endocrine hormones and their roles in the body:

Hormone	Physiological Function
Growth hormone	Increases protein synthesis, metabolism, and growth
Testosterone	Increases energy, protein synthesis, libido, and red blood cells
Insulin-like growth factors (IGF-1)	Increases protein synthesis
Dehydroepiandrosterone (DHEA)	Improves immune function, increases energy, decreases bodyfat
Luteinizing hormone	Increases secretion of the sex hormones listed above
Thyroid-stimulating hormone (TSH)	Increases thyroid hormone synthesis and secretion
Thyroxine	Increases oxidative metabolism and cell growth
Parathyroid	Increases blood calcium and bone formation
Cortisol	Maintains normal blood sugar levels and regulates use of fat
Beta-endorphin	Decreases ability to feel pain (analgesia)
Epinephrine	Increases cardiac output, glycogen breakdown, and fat metabolism
Norepinephrine	Similar to epinephrine; also constricts blood vessels
Peptide F	Increases immune cell function and decreases pain (analgesia)

Who wouldn't want frequent doses of this powerful hormone cocktail? If you are not exercising now, you are missing out. If you are addicted to exercise and always wondered why – well now you know. The magnitude of the hormonal response is directly proportional to the amount of tissue stimulated by the exercise and the intensity with which it is stimulated. This is why I always advocate whole-body resistance exercise. Strength training programs like the one I outline in Chapter 5 will provide the stimulus package you need to get the life-extending waters flowing in your personal fountain of youth.

Don't pause in life, keep going!

Andropause: This is the fairly recent name given to the natural decline of male sex hormones and associated declines in muscle mass (sarcopenia) and libido (erectus nolongeris). Ok, I'm joking about some of my Latin nomenclature, but research has proven that testosterone declines by 50% in men from their late forties to their early seventies (Yikes!). Lower testosterone levels in males equates to higher body fat, less muscle, less libido, more erectile dysfunction, and less brain power. Many studies have shown that strength training can prevent or reverse this hormonal decline in men. If you drew a male's testosterone level as a line on a graph, it would look like a gradual declining slope from around the age of 35 to the early 60's then it would drop off like a cliff. With resistance-based exercise like weight lifting, the gradual declining slope is much more gradual and starts from a higher point on the graph. Most importantly, the cliff would look more like a hill or a slide at the pool. Do you want to slide down into your 70's and 80's or do you want to jump off the cliff? It is your choice.

Menopause: Typically between the ages of 45 and 55, a woman's body starts to decrease the production of estrogen and progesterone, ultimately leading to the time when her menstrual periods cease, called menopause. It is often referred to as the "change of life" because of the vast amount of changes these hormonal fluctuations have on the female body including the infamous hot flashes, as well as mood swings, irritability, increased LDL (bad) cholesterol, lowered HDL (good) cholesterol, trouble sleeping, hair loss, and bone loss.

Exercise has been proven to counter most of these changes and it comes without the increased risk of heart attack, stroke, breast cancer, and blood clots found with hormone replacement therapy (HRT) during the Women's Health Initiative (WHI) study. The WHI study began in 1991 and studied over 161,000 postmenopausal women for fifteen years through 2006. Because of the findings of the study, the FDA currently recommends not using HRT or taking the lowest dosage possible for the shortest time possible. To be fair, the increased 'absolute' risks were small (38 cardiac episodes per 10,000 with HRT versus 30 without) but if you're one of the eight, it would be very significant. If you want more information on this study, I would encourage you to visit the WHI website at www.womenshealth.gov. Although exercise can't prevent menopause, it can certainly lessen most, if not all, of the symptoms. If menopause was a poison, exercise would be the perfect antidote.

Symptoms of Menopause	How Exercise Helps
• Hot flashes	• Hot flashes are less common
• Increased risk of heart disease	• Decreases risk of heart disease
• Increased LDL cholesterol	• Decreases LDL cholesterol
• Lowered HDL cholesterol	• Increases HDL cholesterol
• Increased bodyfat	• Decreased bodyfat
• Decreased muscle mass	• Increased muscle mass
• Mood swings and irritability	• Improves positive feelings
• Poor sleep quality	• Improves sleep quality
• Loss in bone density	• Maintains bone density

Immune System

When I was in eighth grade, I entered a regional science fair with a project on the immune system I titled: "White Blood Cells: Friend or Foe?" The essence of my juvenile, but enthusiastic, research compared the necessity of white blood cells in fighting disease to the self-attacking autoimmune diseases like leukemia during which the immune system goes haywire. It's similar to the cliché: "Men, can't live with 'em, can't live without 'em." Or maybe you prefer: "Can't shoot 'em" if you're in a one-sided relationship.

All kidding aside, the point is this: we want our immune system to work like the external walls and roof of a well-built house (acting as a solid barrier to keep the bogeyman out) and a good handyman who fixes the things that are broken, disposes of the trash that he can't fix, and unleashes your guard dog to attack any prowlers trying to get into your house. And no, my science project didn't win first prize, in case you were wondering. I guess it lacked the entertainment value of the simulated tornado machines or the colorful amusement of the erupting volcanoes. But all is fair in love and war...and science fairs too.

The immune system is composed of two functional divisions: innate immunity (system we are born with) and acquired immunity (immunological response and memory of specific invaders). Both divisions working together act as our external and internal defense mechanism designed to protect against, destroy, and eliminate foreign invaders in our bodies. It is analogous to a city under attack, with the city walls (like our skin and mucous membranes) keeping the enemy out and various white blood cells (neutrophils, macrophages, and T and B lymphocytes) acting as the city's emergency response team to deal with the invaders who get in. The neutrophils, like the police and firefighters, serve as the first responders. The macrophages are the ambulances staged throughout the body ready to rush in and pick-up the wounded, while the killer T cells are the body's S.W.A.T. team. The killer T cells shoot deadly cytokine into the enemy invaders, effectively killing them in their tracks. The helper T cells (serving as the on-scene command and control center) dispatch and coordinate other T cells. The B cells secrete antibodies (acting like military smart bombs) which seek out and destroy specific targets and the suppressor T cells act as the political "cease fire" switch.

The entire system is regulated primarily by the thymus gland which is located in the chest and reaches its largest size at puberty when our immune system is at its peak. As we age, the thymus gland shrinks (by involution) significantly by the time we reach our 40th birthday and by our 60th, it is so small, it is hard to find. A disappearing thymus gland has a direct link to our disappearing immune function. Scientists now know the thymus gland, even late in life, acts in the role of immunological surveillance and it continues to secrete hormones and T cells. Research has shown how an acute or immediate stress on the body can rapidly shrink the thymus gland.

Fortunately, scientists have proven a positive correlation between human growth hormone (hGH) and the size of the thymus gland. I already discussed how exercise positively amplifies our endocrinology earlier in the chapter, but specifically, resistance exercise has been shown to elevate hGH secretions (by 200 - 400%) which can delay or reverse some of this shrinkage. In fact, a 2001 study published in the Journal of Clinical Endocrinology and Metabolism stated: "Exercise is a potent stimulus for hGH secretion." The researchers also concluded that obesity and the lack of fitness negatively affect growth hormone output.

Now I realize I am dramatically simplifying the research and applying

> ### Exercise your immune system
>
> When I was at the Air Force Academy many moons ago, we had a salmonella outbreak from improperly washed lettuce at our dining hall (kind of like the salmonella outbreak linked to tomatoes we had in 2008). Any cadet who ate the tuna salad that day was exposed and over 900 cadets were hospitalized and I credit the medical staff with their ability to deal with the situation. I ate the tuna salad that day and besides an undefeatable mindset and a little stomach discomfort, I can only attribute my lack of illness to my hyper-drive immune system.
>
> My good friend and classmate, Ed Stack and I used to always joke about building immunities anytime we ate something off the floor. You don't have to resort to "floor-food" snacking -- keep your immune system in hyper-drive too by exercising regularly and minimizing your exposure to processed foods, toxins like alcohol, and environmental pollutants.

some of my own conjecture, but I want to make the following point: If we can keep more of our thymus gland (the master gland of immunity) around with exercise, then we can boost our immune function throughout our lifetimes, which will in turn, decrease the frequency and severity of illnesses we will experience. The Florida and California orange growers associations have pounded the health and immune system benefits of orange juice into our heads, but it would be better to consider exercise our daily "glass of juice" because its benefits are more pronounced and conclusive.

The President's Council on Physical Fitness and Sports published a report in 2001 about the immune-boosting benefits of exercise. The report's authors concluded that "people who exercise report fewer colds than their sedentary peers" and "near-daily physical activity reduces the number of days with sickness." In addition to exercise, the report recommends eating a well-balanced diet, keeping life stresses to a minimum, avoiding chronic fatigue, and obtaining adequate sleep to maintain good immune function.

More recent research has discovered an immediate and positive change in immune function with each bout of exercise. This is an acute, "use it or lose it," response to exercise so you must keep it up routinely to keep the benefits. Think of your immune system as a cell phone battery and your daily calls are the stresses of life which drain the charge. When you exercise, it's like a jump-start boost to your immune system battery, giving it more energy to do its job.

Cardiovascular System

The cardiovascular system consists of the heart and circulatory system and serves primarily to transport nutrients, hormones, and oxygen to our living cells and also to remove the metabolic waste products generated from these same cells. If the body was a modern building with the nervous system acting as the electrical wiring of the body, then we can conclude the heart would be the central pumping station, the lungs would be the air handler, and the circulatory system (composed of the arterial and venous systems) would be the plumbing and air ducts.

In this analogy, the arterial system acts like the water pipes and fresh air ducts, transporting fresh water and clean air to all the rooms and offices (our cells) in the building via arteries, arterioles, and capillaries. The arterial system is also the food delivery service, bringing essential nutrients to all the living cells. The venous system, consisting of veins and venules, would be considered the sewage system and air returns of the building. It collects the waste and stale air and brings it to the proper location for removal.

Exercise plays a vital role in maintaining the functionality and efficiency of our cardiovascular system. Poor exercise and nutritional habits are largely to blame for the cardiovascular problems suffered by many Americans including hypertension, heart attack, stroke, angina, high cholesterol levels, and atherosclerosis. Exercise in sufficient quantity and intensity can keep all of these problems in check. It will also help the cardiovascular system become more efficient and have more capacity to serve the body in the roles I described previously. In fact, recent studies have determined that older adults who have maintained a high level of physical activity will experience a 50% less decline in aerobic capacity compared to their sedentary peers.

Exercise has been proven to improve the output capacity of the heart called logically, cardiac output. Cardiac output is determined by multiplying the amount of blood pumped from the heart's left ventricle with each heartbeat (called stroke volume) with the heart rate in beats per minute (BPM). With repetitive cardiovascular exercise, neuromuscular changes to the heart allow it to beat faster and pump more blood with each beat. In other words, maximal heart rate and stroke volume will both increase yielding a higher cardiac output.

Ever wonder how Lance Armstrong won seven Tours de France? Both his stroke volume and heart rate were off the charts compared to normal human beings. He could get his heart rate up to 204 BPM, sustain it well above 185 BPM, and his heart (and stroke volume) was much larger than average. You can estimate your own maximum heart rate by subtracting your age in years from 220 ($220 - age = HR_{max}$). Lance was in his 30's when he won and a normal 35 year old person would have an estimated maximum heart rate of 185 ($220 - 35 = 185$). Obviously, as far as his cardiovascular system goes, Lance had a distinct advantage but it is one he largely earned by intense training.

You can take advantage of the improvements to your own heart with consistent exercise. I have documented my own heart rate into the high 190's. When I was 38 (two years ago at the time I'm writing this) I witnessed my heart rate climb to 195 when I was running up 41 stories in the Tampa Bay Stair Climb challenge. I would have to say that was as close to my max as I'll ever want to be because the pain in my lungs and chest was definitely intense. But knowing I have the heart of a much younger man (from consistent and intense exercise) gave me supreme satisfaction too. I'm not suggesting you should strive to break heart rate records, but one of the distinct advantages of exercise is the physiological changes to the heart and its capacity to pump blood.

According to some anti-aging proponents, you can determine the biological age of your heart by reverse engineering the maximum heart rate formula with your actual maximum heart rate. Using my max heart rate during the stair climbing insanity will help illustrate an example.

Estimated maximum heart rate formula: $220 - Age = HR_{max}$

Biological age of heart formula: $Age = 220 - HR_{max}$ (actual)

My "stair-climbing" heart: $Age = 220 - 195$

$Age = 25$

Now as much as I'd like to believe my heart is 25, it may be a stretch. But I can say this though: I have trained with people half my age, both in and out of the gym, and I can at least keep up with them. So maybe there is some truth to this formula. I'll let you be the judge.

Besides the benefits to the heart, exercise can affect positive changes to the circulatory system too. When you exercise and force the body to increase blood flow throughout the body, it is like cleaning out the plumbing pipes in our building analogy. If you flush your pipes often enough with regular exercise, there is less likelihood that plaque and other "gunk" will build-up in your arteries and veins. Less artery-clogging gunk means better circulation and less chance of blood-flow stopping completely. When blood-flow stops to your heart you have a heart attack (myocardial infarction). When blood-flow stops to your brain you have a stroke. Exercise has been proven to dramatically reduce the risk of both which I will be discussing in Chapter 2.

Exercise also helps maintain the elasticity and resilience of your blood vessels, improves peripheral blood-flow by increasing the density of the capillary network, and through complicated interactions with nitric oxide, relaxes the smooth muscles of the vessel walls causing vasodilation. When you combine these circulatory benefits, exercise improves circulation of nutrients to our skin (promoting healthy skin tone), improves erectile function (who says Viagra has cornered the market?), lowers blood pressure, speeds healing of injured tissues, decreases headaches and muscular tension, improves eyesight (by nourishing the retina, rods, cones and other parts of our eyes), and more quickly removes metabolic waste products giving them less time to cause damage to the body. I would say these are all compelling reasons to exercise.

Digestive System

If the love of money is considered "the root of all evil," then the love of food should be called "the root of all obesity" because all the calorie-laden, sugary, salty, and fattty processed foods causing the obesity epidemic must at first, enter our mouths. The mouth, with its teeth, tongue, and salivary glands serves as the entranceway for food and drink to our digestive system. This vital system consisting primarily of the mouth, stomach, small intestine, and large intestine takes the energy produced by the sun and nature (plants, animals, fungi) and converts it into useable energy for our body to function properly. Ideally, we should put in just enough energy to meet the cellular fuel demands of each day.

Unfortunately, most people knowingly and sometimes unknowingly, put in far too much energy into the system creating a surplus. With money, a surplus is a good thing but with food, a surplus is a bad thing unless you're a bear in the woods preparing to hibernate for the winter when food is scarce. Extra food energy, measured in kilocalories (shortened to "calories" on food labels), is ultimately stored in the form of fat. This is a primitive survival mechanism now being abused because of the ever-present abundance of food in modern society. If you have ever bought a larger pair of pants or went up a dress size, than most likely you are storing some surplus calories.

Either we get a hold of ourselves and learn to properly budget the calories we consume with the calories we burn or we will continue to build our waistlines and fund all the various businesses that thrive on our collective lack of willpower. From bariatric surgical procedures like gastric bypass and lap-band to the miracle pills promising to transform your body into a lean and toned Adonis virtually overnight, the multi-billion dollar weight-loss industry is growing along with our waistlines. Exercise (coupled with proper nutrition) is a low-cost solution to the problem and if more people learn to incorporate it into their lives, we may be able to turn the tide and start blowing the winds of change in the right direction.

Besides the outside-in benefits of exercise on the digestive system, exercise can have inside-out benefits as well. *Keep those bowels moving!* Regular exercise is a great way to keep things moving along in your intestines and to prevent constipation. A study published in *Medicine and Science in Sports and Exercise* proved resistance training accelerates movement of food through the intestines by a whopping 56%. The study also concluded people who live a sedentary lifestyle are 50% more likely to suffer from constipation than people who exercise regularly. When food moves properly through the digestive tract, nutrients are properly absorbed and food has less time to ferment in the bowels resulting in less gas and irritation. So, in other words, if you want to keep things moving (and avoid offending your downwind friends), get yourself moving.

Functional Health

If you still aren't convinced, consider the fact that exercise can help you stay active and maintain your independence as you get older. This is undeniably the best long-term benefit of exercise. No one wants to be a burden to others or themselves, although some people you know may convince you otherwise. For most of us, however, we want to be able to enjoy the freedom and flexibility of being mobile and capable of getting ourselves around.

Modern medicine can definitely help us feel better, reduce pain and suffering, repair damaged tissue, and live longer with surgical procedures and drug therapies. But surgery leaves scars and drugs have side effects. Without exercise, medicine is essentially extending the quantity of suffering in my opinion and does very little for the quality of life. If you lose the ability to do and enjoy everyday activities, then you've lost what I call your "functional health." Why have quantity of life without the quality of life so easily attained with a little sweat and exertion?

Exercise is the best insurance policy for maintaining or even improving your ability to do functional things like: gardening, pushing a lawn mower, getting in and out of a car, cleaning the house, lifting a box, walking, climbing stairs, swinging a golf club, throwing a ball, putting on your clothes, picking up a toddler, tying your shoes, pushing your grandson on a swing, and I could go on ad infinitum. Experts in the field of aging tell us how exercise can extend this functional health well into our 80's and even longer for the most diligent people. Dr Ronald Klatz, President of the American Academy of Anti-Aging Medicine, says it succinctly: "Aging is not inevitable. By systematically revitalizing the biological processes involved in aging, the human lifespan can be increased while the quality of life is maintained or improved."

Think about your body and health in this fundamentally simple way: *"Use it or lose it!"* Your muscles, nerves, bones, joints, connective tissue, and brain will all degenerate without constant use and stimulation. You can prevent this functional atrophy by following the guidance outlined in this book. Press on amigo! The fastest growing segment of the population is those over the age of 85 and it is estimated that there were 70,000 centenarians (100+ years) in 1996, 140,000 in 2005, and will be over 1 million by 2050. Unless we collectively start exercising, they better start building a lot more nursing homes.

Exercise serves as anti-aging medicine because it delays the onset of the aging process and leads to more functional and productive years throughout a lifetime. In the book *Successful Aging*, the authors Dr John Rowe and Robert Kahn suggest three things to improve our longevity:

1. Avoid illness
2. Maintain mental and physical abilities
3. Stay engaged with life

Exercise positively affects all three suggestions by increasing our resistance to infection, increasing our mental and physical capacities, and affords the opportunity to join a fitness group or club, which will help you stay engaged with life. In my community, a major health insurance company sponsors a seniors-oriented fitness program called Silver Sneakers. It brings people together for physical activity five times a week and let me tell you, these are social folks. It is refreshing for me to see the smiles on their faces as they make their daily trek into the fitness room, greeting their fellow exercising friends. If you find yourself home alone or need some companionship, and who doesn't, I can't think of a better way to stay healthy and engaged with people. Most communities and health clubs offer similar programs, so get out there and get involved. You will be thanking me and more importantly, yourself.

As we age, our nervous system loses some of its sensitivity and ability to recruit muscle fibers to contract. This affects our ability to balance, move, and react to stimuli...all of the things necessary for daily living and even driving ourselves around in our cars. The *"use it or lose it"* principle applies here as well. It can't prevent vehicular accidents but certainly can improve our reaction times and our sensory mechanisms, making one less likely.

Exercise helps maintain your mobility. With regular and appropriate exercise, our body builds lean muscle tissue, stronger bones, and more elastic connective tissue. Together these comprise the machine which allows us to move, stand up, lift things, bend down, turn around, and drive a car. It is currently estimated by aging experts that regular exercise can maintain our functional mobility well into our 80's with only a marginal decrease in capability. Because of the people I've met, I'm convinced that it can be into the 90's if we start early with the right exercises and stay consistent.

Exercise will also help improve and maintain our balance. Like a modern skyscraper, our bodies have thousands and thousands of miles of electrical wiring, a main fuse box, and a central processing center. The motor and sensory neurons, spinal cord, and brain make up the central nervous system which provides the electrical and chemical messages allowing us to feel, smell, taste, see, and hear things, as well as move our bodies by directing the muscles to contract and relax. Exercises that incorporate novel tasks, balance, and movement in all three planes of motion will keep your nervous system firing properly.

Neal
Age: 76
Retired Pharmacist

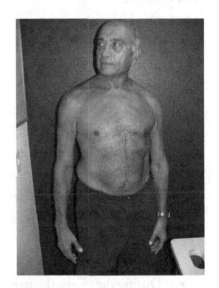

THE FACTS:
In three months…
- Lost over 9 pounds of body fat
- Gained 4.5 pounds of muscle
- Lowered his body fat by 5%
- Improved strength, stamina, and balance

"Working out with proper guidance has made a world of difference in my life. I have less back pain, got rid of my sciatica, and improved my balance. Exercising in the gym has helped me with my flexibility too. I can move my body again without pain and I can even touch my toes.

At 76 years old, I am actually improving my golf game and I'm able to hit the ball further and more consistently. I regularly score birdies now where previously I was happy getting a par."

When compared to the rest, Exercise is best!

Exercise along with a healthy diet will help you recapture your youthful vitality by slowing or reversing the physiological changes associated with aging. Thousands of studies have confirmed the protective role of exercise. In a 2002 landmark study of 6,200 men published in the *New England Journal of Medicine*, researchers concluded that physical fitness was a more important longevity factor than high blood pressure, cholesterol levels, and even smoking. Physical activity has a greater impact on your mortality risk (risk of death) than all risk factors for heart disease. Confused? Let me translate the results of this study with a few examples:

- A smoker who exercises regularly will live longer than a non-smoker who doesn't exercise.

- Two people have high blood pressure – one exercises regularly and one doesn't. The person who exercised during the study had a 50% less risk of death than the non-exerciser.

- A physically fit person with high cholesterol can expect to live longer than a sedentary person with normal cholesterol levels.

- During the study, the participants who did not exercise were four times more likely to die than the fit participants.

Get me on a treadmill quick! The evidence is simply overwhelming and conclusive and it only takes about twelve weeks of regular exercise to become fit and begin enjoying the anti-aging benefits. But the immediate (acute) benefits of exercise start with your first brisk walk. Studies have shown a six to eight hour blood-pressure-lowering effect from each bout of exercise. Blood sugar and triglycerides are immediately lowered from each exercise session, as well. As you consistently exercise day after day, the chronic benefits of exercise kick in: lower LDL (bad) and higher HDL (good) cholesterol levels; increased insulin sensitivity; mood improvement; strength, flexibility, and balance improvement; sleep improvement in quality and length; improvement in creativity; immune function improvement...and many, many more.

The Magic Pill at Work

These benefits and others collectively represent what I call preventive medicine and it is the title and subject of the next chapter. But before you read on, let's look at a real world example of exercise working to turn back the clock on one of my clients. Dennis came to me in June of 2005 to shed a few pounds to impress a beautiful lady he was dating at the time.

Dennis' story

Dennis is in his 60's and has an intense work schedule. While interviewing him about his health history, he told me his last two annual physicals had revealed an elevated blood pressure. During the most recent check-up, his doctor warned him to get his blood pressure down or she would put him on blood pressure medication. She gave him two months.

Dennis had no desire to start taking prescriptions and he believed if he conceded to taking one, an avalanche of others would soon follow. He asked me if there was anything he could do to get his blood pressure down naturally. After hitting him on the head with a tack hammer (not literally people), I assured Dennis that in addition to the strength training we would do and a little dietary intervention (no more fries and chips), 30 minutes of cardiovascular exercise, three times a week would help serve this purpose. He followed this plan with vigilance and he was rewarded for his efforts. Within six weeks, his blood pressure (a ten measurement average) dropped from 170 over 105 to 137 over 76! Dennis was like a kid in a candy store. With his new average in hand, he went to his follow-up appointment with his doctor. She told him he was "in the clear" and to keep the exercise program going. Dennis also lost ten pounds in the process and gained tremendous energy to get through his hectic days managing a large construction project.

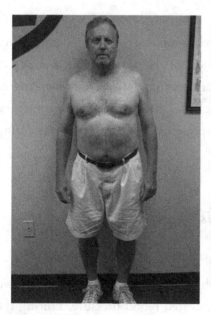 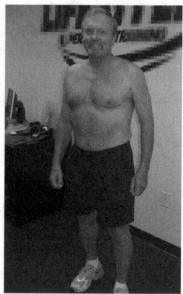

I can't claim the credit, but I firmly believe and know in my heart Dennis' transformation and newfound confidence helped him successfully land a senior VP position as Director of Construction with an international hotel chain. It never fails, when you change the body with exercise and willpower, you change the mind, and when you change the mind, you change the spirit. When you change the spirit, your confidence, self-esteem, and positive energy shine bright for all to see. I will never forget when he took me out to celebrate his reclaimed health and work promotion. Dennis said: "Look what you did for me. I can't believe it." To which I replied: "No, you did it! You are the captain of your ship. I am just the navigator helping you get to where you want to go."

"Matt has been a great inspiration for me and has helped me both mentally and physically. He has taught me to eat right, exercise right, and sleep right. In just a couple on months, I was able to lose 14 pounds of bodyfat, gain four pounds of lean muscle, and most importantly, lower my blood pressure by over 30 points. I have more energy now than ever and I have more focus on the job. Who would have known that exercising just three days a week could have such a dramatic impact. Everything has improved in my life!"

- Dennis Jones

CHAPTER TWO:

Preventive Medicine

> *"Better to hunt in fields for health unbought;*
> *Than fee the doctor for a nauseous drought.*
> *The wise, for cure, on exercise depend;*
> *God never made his work for man to mend."*
>
> John Dryden
> (1631 - 1700)

An Ounce of Prevention is Worth More than a Pound of Cure

The next step in your success journey is to educate yourself about the countless and undeniable health benefits of exercise. Physical activity, in all its forms, triggers a remarkable cascade of hormonal, enzymatic, biochemical, and physiological changes in the body which will serve you better than any drug you can put in your mouth or surgical procedure you can have done. People who exercise on a regular basis dramatically reduce their risk factors for disease by decreasing their cholesterol and triglyceride levels, improving the elasticity of their blood vessels, improving blood sugar control by increasing insulin sensitivity, lowering their blood pressure, and increasing the strength of their muscles and bones. Exercise truly is preventive medicine.

Even the once skeptical medical community (and the industry with the most to lose if more people begin to exercise) is embracing the practicality and benefits of exercise for disease treatment and prevention. Thanks largely to the pioneering efforts of exercise and lifestyle modification advocates like Dr Dean Ornish, Dr Caldwell Esselstein Jr., Dr Neal Barnard, Dr Michael Roizen, Dr Mehmet Oz, Dr Linn Goldberg, Dr Diane Elliot, and Dr John McDougall, and recent initiatives by the U.S. Surgeon General's office, American College of Sports Medicine, American Heart Association and many other people and organizations, the overwhelming wealth of scientific evidence is being spread to the masses. Having a thorough knowledge of these benefits may serve as your arsenal of motivational weapons to fight off the dark forces of the energy-consuming couch in your living room. It may also help you convince someone you love to get moving with you.

Like the tidal wave of medical and scientific information has changed the way we think about smoking today versus thirty years ago, the tide is also turning with exercise (or technically the lack of exercise). Culturally, smoking was pervasive from the 1930's through the 1970's. Movie stars delivered their lines between puffs on a cigarette and smoking ads even featured medical doctors lighting up in their offices while examining patients. It was once cool and socially acceptable to smoke, but now, unless you were living under a rock for the past twenty years, you know smoking is one of the worst things you can do for your health. In fact, the top two mortality risk factors are smoking and lack of exercise.

Within the next ten years, I firmly believe *not exercising* will carry the same social stigma as smoking does today. In fact, choosing not to exercise is a similar risk factor for heart disease as smoking a pack of cigarettes a day. If you are not already exercising regularly, I plead with you now to begin an exercise program so you can reap all the benefits of *The Magic Pill* prescription. You don't need to deal with the snooty, ostracizing eyes of John and Jane Q. Public who will likely turn up their ever-present judgmental noses when you walk by. There will be no patches to wear or drugs to take. You have to help yourself and take the first step which was largely the motivation for me to right this book. I want to help you and the people you care about.

Exercise is the ultimate preventive medicine against the ravages of disease, infirmity, and illness. In May of 2008, I had the pleasure of meeting the acting U.S. Surgeon General, Rear Admiral Steven K Galson and the President of the American College of Sports Medicine, Dr Robert Sallis as they jointly launched the Exercise is Medicine initiative to promote the ever-increasing, scientifically-proven benefits of exercise (www.ExerciseisMedicine.org). Speaking the following year at the 2009 ACSM Health and Fitness Summit, Dr Sallis stated: "The obesity epidemic gets all the press but the inactivity epidemic is what we need to focus on." He continued by saying: "There is irrefutable evidence proving the benefits of regular physical activity on both the primary and secondary prevention of diabetes, hypertension, cancer (particularly breast and colon), depression, osteoporosis, and dementia."

In October of 2008, the U.S. Department of Health and Human Services released the first-ever Physical Activity Guidelines for Americans advocating exercise for all adults, seniors, and children. The American Heart Association (AHA), the American College of Sports Medicine (ACSM), the Centers for Disease Control and Prevention (CDC), and the National Institutes of Health (NIH) all advocate 30 minutes or more of moderate to intense physical activity on most days of the week. According to renowned facilities like the Mayo Clinic and the Cooper Institute in Dallas, 30 minutes of regularly scheduled aerobic exercise just three to four days a week can prevent certain diseases, manage others, and help you live a longer, healthier life.

Do you want to feel better too? Who wouldn't? Exercise helps relieve chronic muscle pain and fibromyalgia. Studies have shown that regular exercise can reduce chronic muscle pain more effectively than both over the counter and prescription pain relievers. Regular exercise stimulates the body to grow more tiny blood vessels, called capillaries, in the muscle tissues. This helps get more oxygen, nutrients, and antioxidants to the muscles and also helps get rid of the metabolic waste products that build up from cellular metabolism. With more good stuff flowing in and more bad stuff flowing out, muscle pain is substantially reduced.

Cardiovascular exercise specifically, improves this circulatory benefit. My clients who fit in their cardio are always a lot less sore than the ones who don't and I say "let the punishment fit the crime!"

Are you tired of getting sick? Unless you are a glutton for punishment, I'm sure you hate being sick. On the rare occasions when I get a cold I always realize how much we take feeling good for granted. Well the good news is exercise helps boost our immune function, allowing the body to better fight off infection. It has been proven that people who exercise are less likely to get sick from viral illnesses like colds and flu. If you're like me, I'm sure you want your immune system to be a high octane, supercharged, cold-fighting machine.

Additionally, the preventive medicine of exercise can:

- Reduce your risk of coronary artery disease
- Reduce your risk of having a heart attack or stroke
- Reduce your risk of developing breast, colon, and prostate cancer
- Reduce your risk of developing type 2 diabetes
- Reduce your risk of developing high blood pressure (hypertension)
- Reduce LDL cholesterol and triglyceride levels
- Reduce your risk of osteopenia and osteoporosis

A nutritionist would say: "An apple a day keeps the doctor away," but I would say: 30 minutes of exercise a day keeps the doctor away! I hope I can present you with a sufficient and convincing summary of the numerous health benefits of the ultimate preventive medicine which is exercise.

The "Big Three" – Heart Disease, Cancer, and Stroke

Heart disease, cancer, and stroke combined cause 61% of all American deaths each year and this is why I call them the "Big Three." Collectively, they account for 50 percent of the ever-increasing, multi-billion dollar U.S. health care budget and unless we reform our waistlines along with reforming health care in general, we will continue to suffer physically and financially as a nation.

In 2004, heart disease was responsible for 652,486 deaths (31.4% of all deaths) making it America's number one killer. Every minute of every day three Americans have a heart attack and it may surprise you that more women die of heart disease in America than men. Cancer takes second place in the Big Three causing over 552,000 deaths (23.3%) and arguably produces the most fear in our society because of all its different permutations. You would be hard-pressed to find anyone who doesn't know of someone who has suffered from lung, breast, colon, pancreatic, prostate, ovarian, or some other type of cancer. Strokes are the heart attack of the brain and are the third leading health-related cause of death (6.9%) in America. Affecting one out of every 250 people, strokes, if not fatal, can lead to permanent disabilities and complete dependence on others. Research has proven a definitive correlation between exercise and lowering the risk of getting any of these diseases.

Heart Disease and Stroke

Heart disease (and its many relatives with more technical names like coronary artery disease, cardiovascular disease, coronary heart disease, coronary atherosclerosis, and coronary arteriosclerosis) is the result of many years of dietary abuse and exercise neglect and is the number one killer of men and women in the United States. For the most part, it is completely preventable with a healthy lifestyle which includes exercise and sound nutrition. Countless studies have proven a significant risk reduction for heart disease and stroke in people of all ages who add moderate physical activity into their daily routine. In other world populations where physical activity is an every day part of life, heart disease is virtually nonexistent.

In his New York Times bestselling book titled *Dr Dean Ornish's Program for Reversing Heart Disease*, Dr Ornish proved that heart disease can even be *reversed* without drugs or surgery with stress management, nutrition, and exercise. If heart disease is a serious concern for you or a loved one, I highly encourage you to read his book and talk to your doctor as soon as possible. We have to be proactive about our health and not sit around waiting for lightning to strike. Because most heart attacks and strokes are caused by the same physiological mechanism and have similar risk factors, I will address them together.

If you were to visit your doctor today and ask: "Am I at risk for heart disease and stroke?" He or she may want to hook you up with wires to run an electrocardiogram (EKG) and run advanced blood tests to check your levels of C-reactive protein (CRP), homocysteine, and apoprotein B, or have you scheduled for an angiogram or PET scan to get a look inside your body to visually see if there are any blockages in the arteries leading to your heart and brain. But more than likely, they will want to know your smoking history, total blood cholesterol levels and blood pressure, which collectively are still considered the medical "gold standard" for assessing risk for heart disease and stroke.

Because of the health-risk-lowering effects of exercise, many exercise advocates in the medical field are also pushing to add physical activity levels as a new "vital sign" to be determined by all physicians during every patient visit. It won't be long before you will start hearing the "exercise question" from your doctor, so I would highly recommend you become an early adopter if you aren't already exercising now. Initially, all it takes is one little percent of your available time each week to get most, if not all, of the health benefits. I call this the 1% Principle and I will be discussing it in detail in Chapter 6.

Medical research has determined both the cause and cure of heart disease and stroke. By eating the typical Western diet consisting of highly processed, calorie-dense foods, coupled with stress and a lack of exercise, we increase our blood pressure and build up the low-density lipoproteins (LDL cholesterol) in our blood. Like sludge in a drain pipe, this causes problems with our internal plumbing by impeding the flow of the blood and increasing the pressure the heart has to pump against. LDL cholesterol is a white, waxy substance found only in animals and is an important component of our sex hormones and cell membranes. Let's take a quick look at this process.

Whenever you eat food or drink a calorie-containing beverage, the macronutrients (proteins, carbohydrates, and fats) are broken down and enter the bloodstream. Both fatty and high-glycemic carbohydrate foods cause an immediate elevation in the triglycerides circulating in our blood. A triglyceride consists of three molecules of fatty acid combined with a molecule of glycerol and serves as the backbone of many types of lipids (fats). When triglycerides and low-density lipoproteins (cholesterol) are constantly elevated from poor eating habits and lack of exercise, they can lead to the formation of plaques in our arteries. As more plaques accumulate, they collectively reduce the internal size of the blood pipes. This restricts the flow of blood which in turn, decreases the amount of oxygen and nutrients delivered to tissues served downstream from the blockage. If this happens in an artery leading to the heart, called a coronary artery, it will cause chest pain (angina) as the heart muscle screams for more oxygen and toxic amounts of metabolic waste build up.

Heart attacks and strokes are typically the result of plaque build-up in the arteries leading to the heart and brain, respectively. Just like a clogged pipe, plaque can slow or stop the blood flow to these vital organs and without oxygen, the tissue dies. After tracking the health and lifestyle habits of three generations of Massachusetts residents beginning in 1948 and continuing still today, the Framingham Heart Study defined the risk factors for heart disease which include high blood pressure, elevated blood cholesterol levels, smoking, obesity, diabetes, and physical inactivity. High blood pressure and physical inactivity are also the most significant risk factor for strokes. On their website, www. americanheart.org, the American Heart Association takes the "Scientific Position" that physical inactivity is a major risk factor for heart disease and stroke and regular physical activity plays a role in the primary and secondary prevention of cardiovascular disease. The U.S. Surgeon General's Report on Physical Activity (way back in 1996) made the case that active people have a lower risk for stroke.

A cautionary note: *If you are so motivated now and feel the urge to rush out to start exercising and you have any of the risk factors I listed in the previous paragraph, make sure you talk to your doctor first. If you are* *exercising and experience any chest pain, feel faint or lightheaded, or become extremely out of breath, stop immediately and get medical attention.*

If you decide not to heed the advice I (and countless others) am giving you and unless you are a plant-eating, marathon-running, stress-free monk with great genetics and no family history of disease, you at some point in your life will encounter some form of heart disease. With enough time, abuse, and neglect, coronary plaques will build up and can eventually rupture. Like any other wound, the body will try to heal it and blood platelets are rushed in to clot the injured area.

Normally this is a good thing like when you cut your finger, but in a coronary artery it can be deadly. When a clot forms in an artery leading to the heart, it can shut off blood flow completely (like a greasy hairball in the drain pipe of your kitchen sink) and within a few minutes, the heart muscle served by it will essentially starve to death. This is what a heart attack is. A portion of the heart dies (myocardial infarction) and if the amount of dead heart tissue is large enough or not treated immediately, it can result in death as the rest of the body becomes oxygen and nutrient deprived when the body's blood pump seizes up.

If you are fortunate, you will get a warning sign before the volcano blows and you can get in line for some surgical intervention like a $10,000 angioplasty, a $30,000 coronary bypass operation, or in extreme circumstances a $100,000 heart transplant. These are only temporary fixes (although the scar on your chest will be permanent), because despite the best efforts of even the most competent surgeon, if you don't change your lifestyle and exercise habits, you will be in line again. As Tom Hanks famously said in his Oscar-winning title role as Forest Gump, "Stupid is as stupid does." If this is hitting close to home, please let me or someone else help you ASAP! We don't need another statistic when the cure is obvious, proven, available, and for the most part, free of charge. Read on my friend.

Obviously, when it comes to your heart and heart disease (and your brain and stroke), the best treatment is prevention and I'm sure you would agree that we owe it to ourselves to do everything in our power to keep our arterial pipes clean. The good news, according to the U.S. Center for Disease Control and Prevention (CDC), is that our consumption of cholesterol-containing and cholesterol-elevating foods is down and coupled with more effective drug therapies like statins, Americans now have lower cholesterol levels overall. The bad news (yes, there always seems to be bad news) is that obesity is on the rise and we are still having heart attacks and strokes. Exercise has been proven to help prevent and even reverse heart disease and stroke by: lowering the level of circulating bad, sticky, artery-clogging cholesterol called low-density lipoproteins (LDL); raising the level of good, artery-clearing cholesterol called high-density lipoproteins (HDL); lowering blood pressure; and increasing the diameter and elasticity of our blood pipes (coronary, carotid, and cranial arteries).

By combining these exercise benefits, the arterial walls will have less plaque build-up, allowing blood to flow more freely and without unnecessary impedance. Like Drano˙ for your arterial drain pipes, exercise will help improve your blood flow and clear out the clogs along the way. Even a small reduction in the size of an arterial plaque will dramatically improve blood flow. The clogs take years to build so don't expect them to disappear overnight. You have to be consistent with your exercise, nutrition, and stress management.

Medical researchers have now shifted their focus to other blood markers like triglycerides and apoprotein b (Apo B). Recent studies have determined that fit people clear post-meal triglycerides from their blood much faster than unfit people — an average of five hours faster. So if I decide to enjoy a sugary candy bar with caramel and peanuts (and yes I'm assuming I'm fit) causing my triglycerides to climb to over 300ng/dL, within two hours or so, they will be back down to my normal range of 105. Compare this response with an unfit person who doesn't exercise and eats the same candy bar. Their triglycerides may climb to 450 (or higher if they are really out of shape) and will stay elevated for seven or eight hours. This increases their dangerous exposure time to this fatty sludge in the bloodstream and by repeating this exposure meal after meal, their long-term risk of heart disease and stroke will skyrocket.

How does exercise help clear the fats from our blood? Besides using up more energy (including sugars and fats), exercise stimulates activation of an enzyme called lipoprotein lipase (LPL). LPL has a central role in fat metabolism because it speeds the breakdown of the fatty acid molecules in the blood. The more LPL we can activate with exercise, the faster the triglycerides will be cleared from the blood. Think of lipoprotein lipase like a fat sponge in the bloodstream. Deficiencies and abnormal functioning of this enzyme have been associated with heart disease, diabetes, obesity, and even Alzheimer's disease.

At the American College of Sports Medicine (ACSM) 2009 Health and Fitness Summit, Clinical Lipid Specialist Ralph LaForge equated the muscular contractions involved in brisk walking to a lipoprotein lipase activator. He pointed out very eloquently that this effect is most significant about 8 to 12 hours after exercise and is directly correlated with the total caloric volume of exercise, independent of any caloric restriction from dieting. In other words, if you know you are going to have a high fat meal in the evening, you better get a good dose of exercise that morning to maximize the cardio-protective, lipid-lowering effect of exercise.

High blood pressure, also called hypertension, is considered by most medical researchers to be the most significant risk factor for cardiovascular disease. When you go in for a check-up or anytime you are admitted to the hospital, the medical staff will most likely check your blood pressure and pulse. These are called vital signs and give medical professionals information about our well-being and state of health. Besides cardiovascular disease and stroke, high blood pressure is also linked with peripheral arterial disease, renal insufficiency (kidneys), and retinopathy (eyes).

According to the National Institutes of Health (NIH) guidelines published in the Seventh Report of the Joint National Committee on Prevention, Detection, Evaluation, and Treatment of High Blood

Pressure (JNC 7), normal blood pressure is when systolic (top number) pressure is less than 120 mmHg (millibars of mercury) and diastolic pressure (bottom number) is less than 80 mmHg. If your systolic pressure ranges from 120 to 139mmHg or your diastolic pressure ranges from 80 to 89mmHg, then you would be considered prehypertensive. Anything higher than these numbers and you would be diagnosed with hypertension (Stage 1 or Stage 2). If this does apply to you, you should definitely be under the care, treatment, and monitoring of a good physician.

As outlined in the American College of Sports Medicine 2004 Position Stand on Exercise and Hypertension, it is estimated that 58.4 million American adults (28.7% of the population) have high blood pressure and "exercise remains a cornerstone therapy for the primary prevention, treatment, and control of hypertension." Epidemiological studies in both the United States and Finland have determined that the lower your level of fitness, the higher your risk of getting high blood pressure. Medical research has determined that exercise has both an immediate (acute) and long-term (chronic) effect on blood pressure. Each single exercise session can lower your blood pressure for hours afterward and routine exercise over weeks and months will lower your average (round the clock) blood pressure. How much you ask?

One study found that walking just 30 minutes every other day can lower systolic pressure by 11 points and diastolic pressure by 8 points. This change alone would reduce your stroke risk by 25 percent! It is important to note that aerobic (walking, bicycling) and resistance (weight training) type physical activities have blood-pressure-lowering benefits and are both recommended in all current exercise guidelines. In a recent meta-analysis of several studies on exercise's effects on blood pressure, resistance exercise was found to cause a "statistically significant" decrease of 3mmHg in resting systolic and diastolic pressure. This is enough to lower your risk of heart disease by 5 to 9%! Imagine the blood pressure lowering power if you put both cardiovascular and strength training into a routine exercise program.

Regular exercise can also strengthen the cardiac muscle over time allowing the heart to pump blood more efficiently. With a stronger heart, the amount of blood the heart circulates with each beat, called stroke volume, actually increases. With a higher stroke volume, the heart can circulate more blood with each beat and therefore, meet the oxygen requirements of the body's tissues more efficiently (in fewer beats). This is why highly-conditioned athletes have such low resting heart rates and why you can expect to see your own resting heart rate go down if you follow the exercise prescription outlined in this book. Having a low resting heart rate (less than 70 beats per minute) is a primary indicator of fitness and can even help predict how long you will live. A study in the *New England Journal of Medicine* found that men whose resting heart rates were above 75 beats per minute (bpm) were three times more likely to die of a heart attack than those with lower rates.

Exercise has so many other benefits related to heart and circulatory function. It improves the elasticity of our blood vessels (arteries, arterioles, capillaries, veins, and venules) making them more pliable and their inner lining less likely to tear, decreases peripheral resistance which reduces blood pressure, and improves endothelial function. Endo what you ask? The inner lining of our blood vessels have specialized endothelial cells which play a crucial role in the elasticity of our arteries. Research has determined that as sedentary people age, their blood vessels ability to expand will decrease. Exercise counters this aging effect. A more elastic artery can dilate properly, which opens up the pipe for blood to flow with less resistance and under lower pressure. Poiseuille's Law (as related to arterial blood flow) states that as the radius of an artery increases, the flow resistance and fluid pressure will decrease. Therefore, to keep blood pressure normal, it is critical for our blood vessels to have the ability to dilate.

In his book titled *Prevent and Reverse Heart Disease*, Dr Caldwell Esselstyn Jr of the Cleveland Clinic makes the bold statement: "My message is clear and absolute: Coronary artery disease need not exist, and if it does, it need not progress." He discusses the role of the endothelial cells and explains that even a single meal can have a toxic effect on endothelial function. The endothelial cells produce nitric oxide, which signals the smooth muscle cells within the artery to relax. When these smooth muscle cells relax it causes vasodilation. Eating a high fat meal like the typical American lunch of a cheeseburger and french fries interrupts this process. Downing some fried chicken wings smothered in ranch dressing, or a tub of lard for that matter, will essentially paralyze the ability of your blood vessels to dilate normally for up to six hours. If you experience a stressful event during this six hour period, your body won't be able to deal with increased blood flow demands properly and a heart attack is more likely. So if you have trouble avoiding the culinary temptations of your local sports bar or have a penchant for Paula Dean's delicious home cooking recipes, then exercise will be your guardian angel.

Exercise and physical activity signals our endothelial cells to produce nitric oxide which dilates the coronary arteries and increases blood flow to the heart. Nitric oxide or NO for short, has many other helpful functions including prevention of white blood cells and blood platelets from becoming sticky or viscous, prevention of smooth muscle cells from growing plaques, and may even help diminish vascular plaques that are already formed. Most people are at least familiar with sildenafil citrate. It is the compound found in the popular prescription drug Viagra. When in the bloodstream, sildenafil citrate signals the specific cells of the male anatomy to dilate thus reducing erectile dysfunction. With this type of dilation I guess you could say things are looking up. Likewise, we want all of our arteries and veins to dilate to keep our blood pressure down, improve blood flow, and keep our blood less thick and sticky. Think of exercise as Viagra for our whole body.

Science has proven conclusively that lifestyle changes, nutritional intervention, and exercise can prevent and reverse heart disease and stroke. If you found out a terrible drug gang with a well-established reputation for deadly violence had moved into your neighborhood, would you stay and take the risk of you and your family being hurt or even killed. Would you take precautions to protect yourself? Or better yet, would you move to a safe neighborhood? Heart disease is the drug gang and exercise is the steel fortress around your house or the moving truck in your front yard. It will protect you from the inevitable confrontation with the evil drug lords.

For more information on heart disease and stroke prevention and treatment, go to:

American Heart Association	www.americanheart.org
American Heart Association Start!	www.mystartonline.org
Centers for Disease Control and Prevention	www.cdc.gov/heartdisease
National Institutes of Health	www.nlm.nih.gov/medlineplus/ heartdiseasesprevention.html
WebMD	www.webmd.com/heart-disease/guide

Cancer

Cancer is the second leading cause of death for Americans and claims 1,500 lives each day on average. Technically called a malignant neoplasm, cancer is best explained as an uncontrolled growth of cells that can invade vital tissues, disrupting their function, and then spread like a wild fire (metastasize) throughout the body via the bloodstream or lymphatic system. This tendency of cancer to stampede our body and spread like a herd of raging bulls on the loose, differentiates cancer from a benign tumor which would be more like the raging bulls being locked up in a small, confined area. As long as you are outside the bullpen and the bullpen isn't getting larger, generally you are fine. In current cancer treatment, surgeons attempt to remove the bulls and the entire bullpen before the bulls cause anymore problems.

Cancer is like 200 different diseases because of all its different manifestations and finding a cure still eludes our nation's top researchers and oncologists. Most cancers are caused by a genetic defect or mutation triggered by repeated exposure to carcinogens like tobacco smoke, chemicals, radiation, and infectious germs called pathogens. One in four Americans will experience some form of cancer in their lifetimes and one in seven will die from it.

The good news, according to the National Institutes of Health is that the five-year survival rate for all cancers has improved by 15% since the 1970's. This is largely attributed to improvements in cancer treatment protocols which can include surgery, combination chemotherapy, refined radiation techniques, hormone therapy, and vaccines. Currently, the most common forms of cancer and their respective five-year survival rates are: breast cancer - 90%; colon cancer - 65%; lung cancer - 16%; prostate cancer - 100%; and rectal cancer - 65%. If you are a bettin' man, you're best bet with this hand of cancers, in terms of survivability, would be prostate cancer and the worse bet would be lung cancer. If you don't understand what these survival rates mean, let me explain it this way. If 100 people were diagnosed with lung cancer today, only 16 of them would still be alive five years from now. If it was breast cancer, 90 of the 100 people would survive for at least five years. I hope that makes sense.

There are many other forms of cancer (and more being discovered each year) including leukemia, pancreatic cancer, cervical cancer, testicular cancer, skin cancer, Hodgkin's disease, brain cancer, and liver cancer. Cancer has a unique stigma among diseases and puts fear into our hearts and minds because of its tendency to spread. I previously likened cancer to a wild fire and like Smokey the Bear would say: "Only you can prevent forest fires, only you." Prevention is the key and exercise has been proven to reduce the risk of all forms of cancer — that's great news!

Routine exercise improves our genetic fingerprint, so to speak, and researchers believe this reduces the likelihood of the mutations that lead to cancer. Although they aren't yet positive and more research is being done, epidemiological studies provide strong evidence of the cancer protective and preventive effect of exercise. An analysis of 50 separate bowel cancer studies done by the Cancer Research Campaign and Scottish Cancer Foundation in the United Kingdom (and reported by the BBC), yielded the following conclusion: People who exercise regularly were 50% less likely to develop the disease. Likewise, a study on women and ovarian cancer (reported in the *International Journal of Cancer*) found that women with a high level of physical activity cut their risk of ovarian cancer in half. Want some more proof? A study led by Alpa Patel of the American Cancer Society found that very active American women cut their risk of breast cancer by 30%. Another cancer study (published in the *American Journal of Epidemiology*) found that men and women who exercised vigorously five or more hours a week lowered their risk of colorectal cancer by 40 to 50%.

I could provide more scientific evidence, but I hope I have made the point. Exercise regularly and you substantially reduce your risk of developing cancer. Whether it's 30% or 50%, I like the odds. Applied knowledge is power. If you are at risk for cancer (and who isn't?), I would say it's time to pack your gym bag. With more and more carcinogens creeping into our lives and who knows what else science will find in the coming years, doesn't it make sense to put a little insurance on your bet? I already told you your risk for cancer is one in four. Reduce that by 50% and now your risk is one in eight if my math is correct (and it probably isn't). You now have the knowledge and it is up to you to apply it. And if you already are…more power to you!

So I've made the prevention argument, but what about those people who do get cancer despite their best intentions? If you are unfortunate enough to get cancer at some point in your life or are already dealing with it now, you have my complete sympathy, and I am happy to share with you some new hope. Exercise is considered by many cancer clinicians to be the perfect antidote to the symptoms of cancer treatment. Many of the current cancer treatments ravage the body and its tissues in order to get rid of the bad guys causing all the problems.

Chemotherapy and radiation therapy (to a lesser degree) are double-edged swords. While destroying the bad cancer cells, they also can wreak havoc on our good cells. This can reduce red blood cells counts, damage heart muscle (reducing stroke volume), decrease skeletal muscle tissue, disrupt nerve function (reducing strength), cause painful swelling (lymphedema), decrease the oxygen carrying hemoglobin in the blood (causing fatigue), decrease our immune function (making it easier to get sick), and cause nausea. As if this wasn't enough to deal with, cancer treatment leaves many people feeling hopeless, anxious, and depressed too.

Exercise, by its pure nature and effects on the body's functions, counters these negative outcomes of cancer treatment. In studies done with cancer survivors, exercise has been shown to raise red blood cell counts, strengthen the heart muscle called myocardium (improving heart function and increasing stroke volume), improve muscular strength, reduce swelling, increase hemoglobin in the blood, increase Natural Killer Cell Activity (NKCA) improving immune function, and decrease nausea. Most importantly, the positive, immediate and noticeable benefits of exercise give cancer survivors hope and new life. This has been demonstrated to improve their quality of life, reduce depression, and alleviate most of their anxiety.

In May of 2008, I had the good fortune of meeting and listening to some great men and women who are using exercise in their cancer treatment protocols and they were unanimous in recommending it to all clinicians dealing with cancer patients. Dr Alejandro Lucia (MD, PhD), who works with children cancer survivors put it succinctly: *"Cancer exercise rehabilitation is critical for cancer survivors."* The Lance Armstrong Foundation and YMCA are currently conducting a pilot study to develop exercise programs and protocols for cancer survivors and hope to roll it out nationwide. Both aerobic and resistance type exercise are important but it would seem strength training is slightly more important due to its ability to counter the most pronounced effect of cancer treatment which is muscle-wasting.

For more information on cancer, cancer treatment, or getting involved in the fight for the cure I recommend:

American Cancer Society — www.cancer.org
The Lance Armstrong Foundation — www.livestrong.org
Susan G. Komen for the Cure — www.komen.org

The Iceberg Diseases

Obesity and diabetes are commonly referred to as the "Iceberg Diseases" and since they are usually joined at the hip, modern medicine has coined the term *diabesity* to refer to them collectively. Not only do they account for over $250 billion of combined health care costs to Americans each year, but the high blood sugar levels associated with diabetes and the large amounts of visible fat in obese individuals are just the "tip of the iceberg" when it comes to their health risks. Downstream complications of these conditions (what you don't see below the surface) are high blood pressure, high cholesterol, heart disease, stroke, some cancers, sleep apnea, glucose intolerance, arthritis, blindness, circulatory problems, gallbladder disease, colon cancer, and most importantly, premature death.

Because of the current trends of physical inactivity and poor nutritional habits, about two out of every three American adults are obese or overweight and one out of every three American children being born today will have diabetes sometime during their lifetime. Our current generation of children is the first generation in history to have a shorter life expectancy than their parents! We have to break the chain now (!!!) and remove the shackles of inactivity and poor food choices we are putting on ourselves and our children's health. The future of our great nation depends on it.

Obesity

No one is born obese. Obesity occurs over time. As a result, obesity is the condition when your weight is associated with significant health problems and is typically defined as a factor of height versus weight called the body mass index (BMI). Depending on which statistics you go by, between 30% and 50% of the American population is now classified as obese. The health implications and lifestyle complications of obesity are enormous, to use a bad pun. The short list... high blood pressure, insulin resistance, higher cancer risk, metabolic syndrome, cardiovascular disease, joint stress, enlarged heart, reduced self-esteem, discomfort when traveling, requiring special accommodations, requiring special clothes, and the list, like our waistlines, keeps growing. Being overweight doubles your risk of heart disease, triples your risk of high blood pressure, and more than quadruples your risk of developing type 2 diabetes.

Obesity is estimated to be directly and indirectly responsible for 15-20% of all deaths in the United States and has an annual economic cost of $117 Billion. According to the National Institutes of Health (NIH), obesity in America has been steadily increasing since 1960 and is now climbing like a set of crampons on an ice face – up, up, up! Health care officials have called it an epidemic. The data from the National Health and Nutrition Examination Survey (NHANES) published on the CDC website at www.CDC.gov , show Americans went from an obesity rate of 15% (adults ages 20 to 74) in 1980 to a staggering 32.9% in 2004. The obesity rate in children is equally discouraging; going from 6.5% of children ages 6 to 11 to an unconscionable 18.8% in 2004.

Fortunately, there is some good news. According to International Health, Racquet, and Sportclub Association (IHRSA) statistics, health club attendance is on the rise. Members going to the gym for over 100 days per year increased from 5.3 million in 1987 to 17.6 million in 2005. Likewise, many of the initiatives of the National Institutes of Health and Center for Disease Control have begun to pay off — illustrated by the slowing adult obesity trends in recent surveys. Unfortunately, child and adolescent obesity rates are still climbing in epidemic proportions.

In 2008, the American College of Sports Medicine (ACSM) and the U.S. Surgeon General jointly launched an initiative called Exercise is Medicine™ with a stated goal of having every physician prescribe exercise to their patients. The scientific evidence of the benefits of exercise is mounting at a rapid pace and it won't be long when exercise will be prescribed as treatment (and hopefully paid for by health insurance) for many health complications in lieu of or in addition to drugs or surgery. Making the choice to exercise is the single best thing you can do for your health. Mortality data shows that an overweight person who exercises will live longer, on average, than a normal weight person who doesn't exercise. Enough said!

Exercise helps prevent or treat obesity by increasing lean muscle mass, improving the rate and efficiency we convert food energy to fuel, and raising our overall metabolic rate. This combination is like stoking a furnace to burn fuel faster, hotter, and more completely. The fuel for our metabolic furnace is the calories we eat and have stored as fat. When you are clinically obese, you have enough stored energy to burn the furnace for a long time and it will require persistent effort to get through all the surplus fuel. Cardiovascular exercise helps speed the rate calories are burned and strength training will build you a bigger furnace and therefore, both are essential to body fat loss.

Are you overweight or obese?

There are several ways to determine whether you are considered overweight or obese, although the mirror and good old-fashioned common sense can give you the short answer. Wayne Westcott said it best at the 2009 ACSM Health and Fitness Summit. His advice was simple: When you get out of the shower in the morning, stand in front of a full-length mirror with nothing on but your birthday suit and jump once. If everything jiggles when you land then you have fat on your body, no scale or charts necessary.

If you want to take a more technical approach, then I would recommend getting your body composition analyzed. For decades, exercise physiologists have used hydrodensitometry (underwater weighing) as the gold standard for determining estimated body composition. It is based on Archimedes' principle: a body immersed in water will be buoyed by a counterforce equal to the weight of the water displaced. If you have access to an exercise physiology lab that has the special equipment needed, knock yourself out. For most of us, this isn't a realistic possibility and other methods have been developed.

Most gyms offer either calorimetry with skinfold calipers (which determines estimated body composition by using skinfold measurements from various sites on the body and an associated chart) or electromagnetic impedance (EMI), which utilizes an electronic device to measure your body's resistance to a current passed between two or four points. Studies have shown these devices to be somewhat accurate (within 5 to 7%) and provide a convenient way to measure yourself and keep track of your progress. More recently, plethysmography (BodPod.), which measures body volume with air displacement and dual energy x-ray absorptiometry (DEXA), which uses low energy x-ray technology, have been increasingly used to get more accurate measurements. Most major metropolitan areas will have either or both of these devices available if you want to get a good objective measure of your body composition.

Many people don't realize they are overweight because they truly have an altered sense of self-perception called body dysmorphia. I want to help you determine objectively where you are right now. The most common criterion for rating body composition is the body mass index or BMI. You will simply need your height in inches and weight in pounds. Go ahead and do it right now. Get out a pen or pencil and a calculator. The formula for calculating BMI is provided below, along with an actual example and a space to determine yours.

Calculating Body Mass Index	*Calculating Your Body Mass Index*
BMI = [weight(lbs) / height2(in)] x 703	**Enter your values**
	weight (lbs) = _____
Example: *193lb male at 5' 8" (68 inches)*	height (inches) = _____
	height^2 =
BMI = [193 / 68^2] x 703	_____ *height x height*
[193 / 4,624] x 703	**Divide weight by height^2**
[.042] x 703	_____ / _____ =
29.53	*weight (lbs)* *height squared* *A*
	Multiply A by 703 =
	_____
	Your BMI

Now that you know your BMI, you can use this number to determine whether you are classified as overweight or obese and also your risk classification for health problems associated with obesity.

Generally speaking, a BMI over 25 classifies someone as overweight and over 30 as obese. If your BMI is higher than 30, your risk of high blood pressure, heart disease, high cholesterol, and premature death are greatly increased. The major criticism of BMI is that it does not distinguish between bone mass, muscle mass, and bodyfat. If you are athletic and have a higher amount of muscle mass and denser, heavier bones, your BMI may be high even though your body fat is low. On the other side of the coin, weight gain (without exercise) usually underestimates fat gains by 50% because it doesn't account for losses in muscle mass associated with sedentary aging. In other words, if you gained 30 pounds on the scale since you graduated high school twenty years back, you may have actually gained 45 pounds of fat and lost 15 pounds of muscle.

So determining your body fat percentage may be a better way to go or use Dr Westcott's mirror test I described earlier. At the 2008 American College of Sports Medicine Annual Meeting, several studies were presented on the efficacy of BMI as a reliable indicator of body composition; the consensus of the research scientists I spoke with was that it has some major flaws. The example I used above is actually my own measurements. According to my BMI, I would be classified as overweight and hovering close to obesity. I am a fitness professional who exercises for a living. I want to spare some of you the frustration of discovering that you too have a high BMI. If you exercise regularly and calculated that you have a high BMI, I would encourage you to get a bodyfat test. This will differentiate your lean mass (muscle, skin, organs, and bone) from your fat mass and give you a better idea of how you measure up. At 193 pounds, I measure: between 11% and 13% bodyfat with electromagnetic impedance, 13% using 4-site skinfold caliper testing, and 18% with a DEXA scan I had done in March of 2008.

Using any of these body composition measurements, even the highest of 18% body fat with DEXA, I would be classified in excellent health by most healthcare practitioners despite having a very high BMI. The moral of this story is: take your BMI measurement with a grain of salt. But if your BMI is high *and* you have a waist measurement higher than 35 inches for females and 39.5 inches for males, you definitely have some work to do and need to be seriously concerned. By taking into account your waist measurement, the truth will be told. Use the BMI you previously calculated and your waist circumference (waist circumference is measured at the navel a.k.a. "belly button") with the table below to get an estimate of where you are classified and your associated health risk.

BMI	Classification	Health Risk	Waist (inches) Females	Males
< 18.5	Underweight	Possibly elevated	< 28.5	< 31.5
18.5 - 24.9	Normal	Very Low	28.5 - 31.0	31.5 - 35.0
25.0 - 29.9	Overweight	Increased	31.5 - 35.0	35.5 - 39.0
30.0 - 34.9	Obesity I	High	35.1 - 39.0	39.5 - 43.0
35.0 - 39.9	Obesity II	Very High	39.5 - 43.0	43.5 - 47.0
≥ 40	Obesity III	Extremely High	> 43.0	> 47.0

If you have been overweight for a considerable amount of time, you will need to be patient with your progressive weight-loss. The hypothalmus is a region in the brain which regulates our set point, called homeostasis. The longer you remain at a certain weight and bodyfat percentage (high or low), the more your body wants to keep you there. It is going to take some hard work and persistence to get the weight-loss ball rolling. I tell my clients: "the weight didn't get there overnight and it's not going to disappear overnight either." A program which combines some form of calorie restriction with exercising five or more days a week represents a two-pronged attack and will be more likely to break the internal set point and allow weight to start evaporating off your body. Like gravity pulls objects to the earth, the set point pulls pounds onto our bodies. Exercise lowers the gravitational pull of calories to the waistline.

Our genetics can influence our appetite, satiation from food, metabolism, rate we gain or lose weight, and our set point range, but they don't control us. Some of you may have to work a little harder; so what? Don't use it as an excuse. It just means you can praise yourself more for your accomplishment. If you are morbidly obese and/or have type 2 diabetes, then you have to take action and do something about it pronto. Like life-saving surgery, you are going to require medical intervention and monitoring. Whether it is a low-calorie, medically supervised diet, gastric bypass surgery, lap band surgery, or something else, any of these options would be the lesser of two evils, trust me — unless dying a premature death appeals to you.

Are there risks? Yes there are risks associated with obesity treatment, but not getting help is analogous to not getting in an ambulance after a severe trauma because you fear you will be in an accident on the way to the emergency room. Would you refuse a ride in a Life Flight helicopter if you were shot in the stomach because there is the possibility it would crash? It would be ridiculous not to get in because your chance of dying from the wound is far greater than the risk of crashing.

Obesity treatment is the same. If you are moderately overweight, you can get to a healthy weight with lifestyle changes, a good nutrition plan, and the help of a good personal trainer or a committed workout buddy. If you are severely or morbidly obese, you are going to need medical help and a drastic change in your every day environment. You have to do this right now! Get help! Your life is on the line and time is running out. Carrying around the extra weight is just the tip of the iceberg and it is only a matter of time before all the inevitable health complications rise to the surface. If you aren't selfish enough to do this for yourself, take a selfless pill and do it for someone else... your spouse, your friends, or your kids who will eventually have to bear the financial burden of your medical bills and inability to take care of yourself. If this doesn't apply to you but it does apply to someone you know, please help them or pass on these words. At least you can know in your heart that you tried.

Exercise in all its many forms is undoubtedly the best way to prevent or reverse obesity. The relationship between physical activity and weight is straight forward – the more active you are the less you will weigh. I will be discussing exercise in Chapter Five and nutrition and weight loss in Chapters 7 and 8 respectively, but the benefits related to obesity are simple and straight forward. Do more movement-based exercise like walking, cycling, and playing enjoyable sports to burn more calories and also do strength and muscle-building exercises like lifting weights to build muscle and increase your metabolism. Couple this with a sound nutrition plan and you will create a caloric deficit which will force the body to tap into its energy stores. Do this consistently week in and week out and the weight will come off.

If you have ever watched the NBC show *The Biggest Loser*, you have seen what is possible with complete focus, support, and dedication. By immersing themselves in a healthy environment, contestants have lost 60, 70, and even over 100 pounds in less than twelve weeks. More importantly, many of them come off the obesity drugs they were on prior to the show. Since thrusting yourself into a 24-hour-a-day weight loss program isn't realistic for most people because of commitments like jobs, family, sleep, and a lack of eight hours a day to devote to exercise, let's take a look at success in the real world.

The National Weight Control Registry tracks over 5,000 people who have successfully lost weight (over 66 pounds on average) and kept it off for at least five years. It lists the following success factors and their relative participation from their collective surveys: 78% eat breakfast, 75% weigh themselves at least once per week, 62% watch less than 10 hours of television per week, and a whopping 90% exercise for at least one hour per day. You can see the most obvious common denominator in their success is exercise. On average, exercising for 45 minutes everyday will maintain a bodyweight that is about 15 pounds lighter than it would otherwise be. Since the number of obese Americans just recently surpassed the number considered just overweight, we have plenty of excess weight to get rid of. According to the CDC, less than 5% of Americans are active for 30 minutes a day, five days a week. My pledge is to reverse these trends and help stop the obesity epidemic before it's too late.

Diabetes

Diabetes is the other iceberg disease and since 1958, the number of Americans with diabetes has increased by over 600%! Currently over 21 million Americans are estimated to have diabetes (one million with type 1 and 20 million with type 2) and over 800,000 new cases of type 2 diabetes are being diagnosed each year. Twenty percent of all Americans over the age of 65 have some form of diabetes and over 47 million Americans are estimated to have prediabetes, a condition called metabolic syndrome, insulin resistance syndrome, and syndrome x depending on who you ask.

This is a serious issue because of its epidemic spread among American adults and now even to our children. The health care costs associated with diabetes have skyrocketed, exceeding $132 billion each year since 2002 and the costs continue to increase. According to the American Diabetes Association, having diabetes doubles the risk of heart disease in men and quadruples it in women. Diabetes claims 178,000 American lives each year and it is the leading cause of blindness. Other complications of diabetes include high blood pressure, high triglycerides, high LDL (bad) cholesterol, retinopathy (eye problems), circulatory problems, nervous system problems, central fat accumulation, obesity, heart degeneration, kidney failure, and skin problems. The National Institutes of Health (NIH) allocates over one billion dollars of its budget to diabetes research each year and the future for diabetics looks a lot more promising.

Diabetes comes from the Greek word meaning to "run through" as glucose runs through the body of diabetics. Without appropriate treatment, the unutilized glucose ends up in the urine. Normally, when blood sugar levels rise, insulin is produced by the pancreatic cells in the islets of Langerhans. These specialized beta cells release insulin into the bloodstream which facilitates the transport of glucose molecules directly into our cells. Glucose is the energy which fuels every living cell in our bodies. It can be used for immediate energy, stored for short bursts of energy (glycogen in muscle and liver cells), or converted to fat and stored for long-term energy. Without this system working properly, blood sugar levels begin to rise and once they are above 180-200 milligrams per deciliter, the kidneys begin to excrete glucose into the urine. This is why undiagnosed insulin-dependent diabetes is characterized by great thirst and increased urination as the body attempts to wash out the unmetabolized blood sugar.

There are two types of diabetes, type 1 and type 2, as well as gestational diabetes which occurs during pregnancy in some women. Type 1 is chiefly hereditary and affects about one million Americans. It is diagnosed when you have a fasting blood sugar level of greater than or equal to 126 milligrams per deciliter and greater than or equal to 200 milligrams per deciliter at two hours during a glucose tolerance test. It is caused by a partial or complete failure of the body to produce insulin and usually begins before the age of 30. Treatment, lifestyle modification, and proper monitoring of type 1 diabetes are essential or the condition will become fatal.

Fortunately type 1 diabetics can control their blood sugar levels with insulin therapy. Rudimentary insulin therapy was first discovered by Canadian researchers Frederick Grant Banting and Charles Herbert Best in 1922. Today, type 1 diabetics use combinations of rapid, intermediate, and long-acting insulin, as well as insulin pumps, to more precisely control their blood sugar levels than they could in the past. Artificial pancreas devices (closed-loop systems which automatically sense blood glucose levels and dispense insulin) and islet cell transplants are being tested in clinical studies and may be viable treatment options in the not too distant future. Human genome research is being conducted to identify genetic determinants of the condition in hopes of preventing the autoimmune destruction of insulin-producing cells before it happens. In the interim, constant monitoring of blood glucose levels and management with insulin therapy, combined with an active lifestyle and good nutritional habits are the recommended interventions.

Type 2 diabetes currently affects over 20 million Americans and the diagnosis rates in adults and children are climbing like the space shuttle leaving its launch pad. Something must be done immediately! It is a condition we bring upon ourselves by repeatedly overstressing the body with highly refined carbohydrates and doing little to no physical activity. This combination essentially wears the insulin system out. Many of the complications lie below the surface, doing damage to bodily systems and tissues before the disease is diagnosed. Researchers have determined that age-related environmental factors, specifically diet quality and less physical activity are common causes that hasten changes in insulin resistance. In other words, eating junk food and not exercising makes insulin less effective in doing its job. Because it has become epidemic in the United States, glucose testing is more common and prediabetic conditions like metabolic syndrome have been identified to get a jump start on treatment.

Metabolic syndrome, also called syndrome x or insulin resistance syndrome, has been identified as a means of surfacing the warning signs of full-fledged diabetes. It was originally theorized by Stanford endocrinologist Gerald Reaven in 1988 that central obesity will lead to impaired glucose tolerance and insulin resistance. Knowing this correlation gives health practitioners a means for earlier intervention to hopefully prevent the onset of diabetes. If you determined yourself to have a high BMI when we calculated it a few pages back, you need to be on the lookout for metabolic syndrome and discuss it with your doctor.

Conditions of Metabolic Syndrome:
- Systolic blood pressure ≥ 130mmHg
- Diastolic blood pressure ≥ 85mmHg
- Fasting blood sugar level ≥ 110mg/dL
- Fasting triglycerides ≥ 150mg/dL
- Fasting HDL cholesterol < 40mg/dL
- Waist circumference ≥ 35" for women and ≥ 39" for men

Symptoms of unstable blood sugar:
- Fatigue and tiredness
- Difficulty sleeping

- Moodiness and irritability
- Difficulty focusing on tasks
- Lack of clarity

The reality for most people is that metabolic syndrome and type 2 diabetes can be controlled, improved, and even reversed with lifestyle changes, nutritional modification, weight loss, and especially exercise. A study conducted by Frank Hu, MD, of the Harvard School of Public Health and published in the *Annals of Internal Medicine* concluded that a brisk one hour walk each day could reduce type 2 diabetes risk by 34%. Studies have also proven that being physically active helps protect people with type 2 diabetes from heart disease; regardless of their age, body mass index (BMI), blood pressure, and total cholesterol. In other words, I tell people an overweight person who exercises regularly is much healthier (from a mortality perspective) than a skinny person who doesn't.

Exercise helps the body control blood sugar levels by increasing cellular sensitivity to insulin, allowing more glucose to be transported out of the blood and into our cells. In February 2002, the findings of the Diabetes Prevention Program study were presented in the *New England Journal of Medicine.* The study compared the results of lifestyle intervention including dietary changes and increased physical activity to the oral diabetes drug metformin and found that lifestyle intervention was far superior to the drug. Based on these findings, Clinical Lipid Specialist Ralph LaForge of Duke University set out to determine the blood-sugar-lowering effect of exercise via brisk walking and subsequently compare it to the effects of a popular diabetes drug. His research concluded that every intentional step (walking at close to full speed) has the same effect on blood sugar levels as .25 milligrams of metformin which is commonly prescribed for type 2 diabeties. This is powerful research and proves how beneficial exercise can be on our biochemistry.

According to the American Diabetes Association and the American College of Sports Medicine, exercise paired up with a low-glycemic diet, oral drugs, and insulin therapy (if necessary) are the cornerstones of diabetes treatment. Exercise fires up our metabolic machinery to burn more sugar. If you don't burn it, the body will store it as muscle glycogen, liver glycogen, and body fat. Do your body a favor by exercising and dramatically reduce the demands on your overworked pancreas.

In their Position Stand on Exercise and type 2 diabetes, the American College of Sports Medicine recommends starting with 10 to 15 minute exercise sessions and progressing to at least 30 minutes per day of low to moderate intensity activities. When weight loss is a primary goal then the duration needs to be increased to 60 minutes which is the minimum amount proven to help take weight off and keep it off. Both cardiovascular exercise (pain-tolerable but enjoyable movement-based activity) and resistance training need to be incorporated into the game plan.

Walking is the most common form of cardiovascular activity performed by diabetics and it can be done almost anywhere indoors or outdoors (see Chapter 5 for my progressive walking program). Resistance training with weights is critical because it will improve strength, enhance flexibility and joint range of motion, and most importantly for diabetics, it has been shown to improve glucose tolerance and insulin sensitivity. Your goal should be to lift weights two to three days a week working your entire body (all major muscle groups) with a well-designed program. If you are unfamiliar with structuring a weight-training program, seek professional assistance at your local wellness center, YMCA, or commercial health club. It will be well worth your time and expense (in some cases) to know you are doing the right exercises both safely and effectively.

> **Exercise Recommendations For Diabetics**
>
> **American Diabetes Association**
> *20-45 minutes at least 3 days per week*
>
> **American College of Sports Medicine**
> *30 minutes or more per day every day*

Osteoporosis

Osteoporosis and is a disease affecting more than 10 million Americans who have low bone mass and a structural deterioration of bone tissue. It is considered a silent disease because there are often no obvious symptoms until the day a bone breaks. Literally osteoporosis means "porous bone" and technically, it is classified as having a bone mineral density of 2.5 standard deviations or more below the young adult mean. Measurements are taken typically with a DEXA scan. Yes, the same DEXA I described for determining body composition. The precursor or warning sign of osteoporosis is called osteopenia which is having a bone mineral density from one to 2.5 standard deviations below the young adult mean. Over 34 million Americans are estimated to have osteopenia. The grim news…one out of every two women and one out of every four men will have an osteoporosis-related fracture at some point in their lifetime.

How does this happen? In most cases, this is a classic *use it or lose it* scenario. As we age and our activity levels decline, less and less new bone formation takes place and the outer surface of our bones, called the periosteum, essentially begins to erode. Minerals are leached from the bone into the bloodstream to meet the needs of our bodies. Studies have proven that without repeated stimulus, no new or very little bone formation takes place. Therefore repeated stimulus is the key and the earlier you start stimulating bone formation, the better. According to the "bone reserve" theory, during adolescence we lay down the foundation of bone development for the rest of our lives. In other words, the more solid bone you form in your teen years the less likely you will have problems related to bone density in the future. You have more of a reserve to draw from down the road of life. If you have growing children you should keep them active and moving so they build a solid skeleton to take them well into their golden years.

Like I discussed at length in Chapter 1, exercise stimulates bone formation by putting a mechanical load on the bones. Here is a quick and technically boring biomechanical recap. As long as the force of the load or the rate at which it is applied is sufficient to exceed what is called the minimal essential strain (MES), new bone modeling takes place causing calcium phosphate mineralization and a denser, harder bone surface to form. Resistance training (strength training) and weight-bearing activities are best for stimulating this process (osteogenic stimulus). Bones placed under enough strain by magnitude, rate, direction, and volume will bend slightly. This bone deformation signals specialized cells called osteoblasts to migrate to the areas of deformation. The osteoblasts secrete proteins and collagen molecules which eventually mineralize as calcium phosphate, adding structure and rigidity to the bones surface.

The most efficient and effective way to load bone and stimulate bone growth is through resistance training with weights. I'm not talking about picking up one pound dumbbells either. You have to push and pull weights that stress your bones, muscles, and connective tissues. You have to challenge your body to do more. Pick compound, multi-joint exercises that load the bones and joints longitudinally along their axis like variations of the squat, dead-lift, leg press, overhead press, and bench press to get the most benefits.

Movement-based activities that have been demonstrated to improve bone density are stair climbing, trail-hiking, dancing, and running. Sports and recreational activities that involve running and jumping like tennis, volleyball, racquetball, soccer, and basketball are also beneficial. They will not only serve your bones well, but they are also fun, competitive, social, and stress relieving too. The bottom line: you have to move your body and move some weights, no bones about it!

Osteoarthritis

Continuing with the saga of our bones and joints, osteoarthritis is a degenerative disease affecting over 21 million Americans. It is caused when the hard but slippery cartilage between the bones in our joints breaks down and leads to painful friction between bone surfaces. While medical research hasn't found a way to completely prevent it, studies have found that smoking, physical inactivity, obesity, and previous joint injuries can all make it worse. Previously, it was believed to be a "wear and tear" disease and people suffering joint pain were told not to exercise. Now we know it is a disease process that can be exacerbated by inactivity and therefore exercise is recommended and prescribed to reduce painful symptoms. In essence, the medical community has reversed its stance.

In fact, the Arthritis Foundation recommends exercise as one of the best treatments for osteoarthritis. Exercise increases flexibility and mobility of our joints and muscles and also improves circulation of nourishing blood to joint tissues. Even though exercising an arthritic joint can initially be painful and cause flare ups and inflammation, it should not discourage you from continuing. Icing painful joints after exercise can reduce inflammation and pain and some anti-inflammatory drugs may be necessary to manage painful symptoms. If you are suffering from osteoarthritis, discuss a proactive approach with your doctor that includes exercise. The long-term rewards will be worth the short-term pain, time, and effort.

In the future, scientists will have the ability to grow artificial cartilage to replace the damaged cartilage in arthritic joints. Advancements in artificial joint replacement materials and surgical techniques have also made it possible for people of almost any age to have severely diseased joints replaced. If you are waiting for either of these interventions, it still behooves you to exercise. People who exercise are better candidates for joint replacements and recover from the invasive procedures much quicker and with fewer complications.

Walking, swimming and cycling are some of the best forms of exercise for people with osteoarthritis and anyone for that matter, to improve overall health. The goal is to work up to at least 30 minutes of exercise five times per week. Resistance training with machines and free weights is also recommended to enhance the stability, strength, and range of motion of our joints to reduce the likelihood of problems and pain. Excess bodyweight can also improperly stress our joints and cause more wear and tear. Attaining and maintaining a healthy bodyweight should be everyone's goal for all the other reasons I've discussed, as well as for reducing joint problems like osteoarthritis too.

Back Pain

Although not technically a disease, back pain is one of the most pervasive ailments in our society today costing Americans well over $50 billion in medical expenses. Statistics show that 80 percent of adults in this country will experience debilitating back pain at some point in their lives. Besides the common cold, back pain is the most likely reason people visit their doctor and it puts more people out of work than any other single cause.

Treating back pain is big business and has given rise to "spinal health centers," chiropractic physicians, and orthopedic spine and back specialists. Back pain is caused by injury to or weakness of the muscles, connective tissues, vertebra, and discs of the spine which leads to pressure on one or more spinal nerves. Pressure on a spinal nerve causes intense pain to radiate out from the location of the pressure to surrounding tissues. It can make simple activities impossible without a lot of pain medication, weeks of rehabilitation, or in extreme cases, surgery.

The obvious question is why so much back pain? The answer is fairly simple. We are sitting on our butts more, have bigger bellies, have weaker muscular support of the low back, and are much more sedentary than our ancestors. When you mix this cocktail of conditions, the drink you get is back pain. Experts agree that the most likely cause is the loss of muscle mass and strength. When you have a large distended belly your center of mass shifts forward (anterior shift). This causes the muscles of the lower back to work harder to keep you upright. As these muscles become weaker from years of disuse, the spine and its complex arrangement of bones, discs, and nerves become like a house of cards. It is only a matter of time when the cards fall and something goes wrong. You could be pulling a roast out of the oven, pulling a toddler out of car seat, or simply reaching down to grab your car keys that fell on the floor and WHAAAM!!! You feel a swift pull or pop and the sudden pain in your low back takes you immediately to your knees. As you now lay in the fetal position from the excruciating pain, even breathing can be miserable.

If you are unfortunate enough to injure your back, the orthopedist, chiropractor, physical therapist, or athletic trainer who treats you will rehabilitate you by improving the strength of your lumbar muscles. Why wait to suffer an injury when back problems can be prevented with exercise in the first place. Remember *an ounce of prevention is worth more than a pound of cure.* The lower back is the foundation of our bodies connecting the head and upper torso with the hips and locomotive legs. This fact, coupled with the deep surrounding muscles which stabilize and move the spine has given rise to the term "core." Hundreds of books, instructional videos and exercise programs have been produced on core training and conditioning. Don't get too wrapped up in the hype and marketing though. Any comprehensive, whole body resistance-based training program will strengthen the muscles of the low back.

A properly working back is critical to a normal functional life because it is involved in so many activities of daily living — walking, standing, lifting things, reaching, and carrying. Do you want to hold your child in your arms or pick-up your grandson after he is born? You will definitely need a healthy back to do it and I encourage you to start and maintain a consistent exercise program if you aren't already doing so.

Incontinence

During sedentary aging, we lose muscle strength as our muscles atrophy from their lack of use and from the declining anabolic hormones in our body. With less muscle strength, we eventually can lose our ability to control our bladder. The pubococcygeus (PC) muscles, which form the pelvic floor, constrict the urethra and thereby prevent the flow of urine from the bladder and also play a vitally important role in sexual arousal and climax (whoo-hoo!). When these muscles are weak, you have less ability to dam the flow, so to speak. Anything which builds pressure in the bladder, like coughing, sneezing, laughing, or straining, can force urine out of the body against your will and low and behold, you have incontinence.

Believe it or nor, this is big business. Over 5 billion dollars are spent on adult diapers each year and expenditures will continue to grow as the baby boomers start to lose control of their flow. Kegel exercises were originally developed to strengthen the PC muscles in women experiencing incontinence after childbirth and have been adopted for incontinence treatment, in general. Regular exercise also helps strengthen these muscles and can simultaneously stimulate your pituitary gland to amp up your hormonal environment. Specifically, resistance training with weights causes your body to contract these muscles forcefully and over time, their strength and tonality will increase. With stronger pelvic muscles, your ability to dam the flow improves and the incontinence is prevented.

Over the years, I have trained many "vintage" clients in their 60's, 70's, and even 80's. When I initially start working with these clients, inevitably I have to get use to their frequent detours to the bathroom. What I have noticed unequivocally from this real world experience is that as their strength and stamina improve, the bathroom breaks decrease to one per session or stop altogether. If the body can hold back the flow while properly straining with weights, normal life should be no problem. Resistance training forces the PC muscles to work and get stronger. This is another classic example of *use it or lose it.*

So if you don't want the chore and expense of wearing adult diapers or don't want to face the potential embarrassment of wetting yourself when your best friend tells you a joke, then get to the gym and start lifting some weights as soon as possible. Sometimes strengthening the muscles you can't see can be just as important as strengthening the ones you can.

Alzheimer's Disease

Named after Dr. Alois Alzheimer who first documented brain abnormalities and degeneration in 1906, Alzheimer's disease affects approximately 4.5 million Americans and its associated medical costs exceed $100 billion. It is one of the most feared conditions of aging because it takes away memory, speech, and functional independence. It can leave people in a state of the living dead where they no longer remember their life experiences, their loved ones, or even their own name. This can take family caregivers on an emotional rollercoaster ride and leave them physically, mentally, and financially drained.

Alzheimer's disease is believed to be caused by degenerative changes to the brain including sticky vascular plaques, disjointed synapses, and rapidly decreasing neural connections. Starting in our thirties, the brain's weight, neural network, and blood flow all start to decrease unless you proactively do something about it by staying mentally engaged in society, consistently performing novel tasks, and especially exercising regularly.

Scientists have determined that the more we use our brains, especially during the first 12 to 14 years of life, the more brain reserve we build up. Like the bone reserve theory I discussed with osteoporosis, the brain reserve theory essentially concludes that people who amass more neural connections by using their noggin will have a reserve to draw from later in life. Research has found that having this brain reserve may thwart the ravaging symptoms of Alzheimer's disease or delay the progression of its symptoms. Autopsy studies have found that educated, functioning adults can have the physiological signs of the disease but were able to function normally and compensate with the extra brain reserve they attained early in life.

As we age, our brain cells (called neurons) start to decrease which can negatively affect our ability to remember names, faces, and where we left the car keys. The good news is that our brains are very plastic because they are constantly changing and neural connections can be forged throughout our lifetimes. We can maintain and even build our mental acuity and agility by reading, solving problems, doing crossword puzzles, and learning to play an instrument.

According to a growing body of evidence the best way to stave off degenerative disease of the brain is by exercise. Richard Snowdon,

Ph.D., author of *Aging with Grace*, has conducted a vast amount of research on brain aging and disease and concludes that: "If you have to choose between a crossword puzzle and exercising, get out the door and exercise your entire body." I say do them both simultaneously; get on a treadmill and solve a crossword puzzle while you walk.

Physical activity increases the nutrient and oxygen flow to the brain giving it more fuel to do its job. The brain by itself uses 25% of the oxygen we breathe in and controls every aspect of our thoughts, emotions, and body functions. Besides improving the fuel flow to the brain, exercise can also help control blood cholesterol levels. High cholesterol levels have been linked to brain decay in several studies.

Exercise, coupled with a low-fat, heart-healthy diet that includes lots of vegetables and omega-3 fatty acids, can be an effective way of reducing blood cholesterol levels and lower your risk of Alzheimer's disease. Research conducted by the University of California at San Francisco demonstrated that cholesterol-lowering statin drugs like Lipitor and Zocor may also help ward off Alzheimer's disease. But like I made the case in the heart disease section of this chapter, exercise is the best and most natural way of accomplishing this goal.

Finally, it is important to note that having a purpose, maintaining a positive mental outlook and being joyful have all been proven to not only extend life, but also to extend mental functioning and capacity late in life. If you keep yourself predominantly in a positive state of mind, you keep the body relaxed and flooded with stress-reducing hormones. Over time, this keeps everything running smooth and leads to less wear and tear on every internal system in our bodies, especially the brain. This can be done if you make the choice to do it and put forth the effort. Money doesn't buy happiness which has been proven over and over again. Surveys of lottery winners have determined that the extra money causes stress instead of reducing it. Having more quality time produces happiness. Stay active and learn to be a positive person. Learn to appreciate what you have instead of dwelling on what you don't have. As the title of actor, director Roberto Benigni's 1997 Oscar-winning movie suggests *La vita è bella...Life is Beautiful!* For more insight on adopting an uplifting approach to each day, I encourage you to read Norman Vincent Peale's timeless classic *The Power of Positive Thinking.*

Parkinson's Disease

Parkinson's disease is another devastating progressive disease caused when specialized cells of the brain stop producing dopamine. Dopamine is a neurotransmitter which carries signals between nerve cells in the brain and helps control motor function and mood. Without adequate dopamine, movement, speech, and swallowing become difficult. Tremors are the most common initial symptom of Parkinson's disease and other symptoms include slow movement, difficulty with balance, impaired fine motor control, slowed speech, and stiff muscles. Levodopa is the most commonly prescribed drug for treatment of Parkinson's disease. Science has yet to determine a cause of the disease, but a lot of research is being done to find a cure and to identify the best new treatments for people with the disease.

Since exercise naturally elevates dopamine levels in the brain, it has been identified as a possible means of preventing Parkinson's disease and has been increasingly advocated in treatment programs. A Harvard study found men who exercise have 40% less risk of developing Parkinson's than those who don't exercise. Since 40,000 Americans are diagnosed with this condition each year, this could potentially save 16,000 people annually from its ravaging effects on the body.

In treatment of Parkinson's disease, exercise has been shown to reduce symptoms, slow progression and improve quality of life. A meta-analysis of studies using exercise in the treatment of Parkinson's disease found exercise-induced improvements in gait, grip strength, coordination, fine motor control, flexibility, functional reach, balance, muscular strength, and mobility. These are most of the essential qualities of a functional life so it makes a lot of sense to include exercise in a successful treatment program.

If you (or someone you know) are suffering from this disease, see your doctor and have them prescribe exercise in your treatment program. Exercise, along with eating a healthy, balanced diet which includes lots of vibrant fruits and vegetables will go a long way to improving the outcomes of Parkinson's treatment. Exercise can also counter the depressive effects of progressive diseases like Parkinson's. I discuss exercise and depression at length in Chapter 3.

Preventive Maintenance

While I was visiting family out in the sticks of northern Alabama, it occurred to me that people are a lot like their cars and farm equipment when it comes to preventive maintenance. Now if you're not a Jeff Foxworthy fan or you've never been to that part of the country you may not understand the connection. Let me put it this way, when a lawn mower stops working or a car won't start, it stays right where it is. If a tractor breaks down, it has sealed its fate and it is now parked in its eternal mechanized cemetery, which in these parts is everyone's front yard. Judging from the shear amount of dead equipment and cars lying around, it is easy to determine there isn't much preventive maintenance going on there.

For the mechanically challenged (myself included), preventive maintenance is the simple things you do to maximize the functional lifespan of a machine. Things like: changing the engine oil, lubricating mechanical gears and rotating parts, tightening the nuts, bolts and screws, checking the electrical wiring, and putting on new tires before the old ones get bald. If you do these simple things on a periodic basis, you will prevent a catastrophic failure like an engine seizing up or an axle falling off. If you own a car, hopefully you are getting your oil changed every 3,000 miles or so. This is a classic example of preventive maintenance. Maybe you know of someone who has forgot to change their oil and ended up having to buy a new three thousand dollar engine because they forgot to get a fifteen dollar oil change.

I'm afraid people treat their bodies the same way and avoid scheduling some routine maintenance. Exercise is without a doubt the body's method of preventive maintenance. When done on a consistent basis, it will dramatically extend your functional lifespan, prevent painful ailments like back pain, and prevent a major catastrophic breakdown like a heart attack or stroke. Exercise keeps the moving parts moving and stimulates the body's internal lubricating process in our joints.

Like sharpening the blade of a lawn mower keeps it working properly, exercise keeps the mind sharp and helps you "cut" to the chase when you are collecting your thoughts. If you don't keep your lawnmower clean or leave it outside and exposed to the environment, it will inevitably rust as the iron oxidizes. Cancer is like rust on the inside and outside of our human machine and can be mostly prevented with exercise. Exercise also improves circulation to our locomotive feet which are like the wheels and tires on a car. Without tires, your car isn't going anywhere and without your feet working properly, you won't be going anywhere fast either. Three to four workouts a week for at least 30 minutes each are the physiological equivalent to the 3,000 mile oil change for your car. Unlike your car, however, you don't get to exchange your body for a new one if it breaks down. We only get one body to last a lifetime which makes preventive maintenance that much more critical. I hope I have made the point on the importance of preventive maintenance. Get yourself moving so you can keep yourself moving!

Injury Prevention

Scientific studies have proven the many benefits of exercise and I have attempted to cover many of them thus far, but perhaps one of the most overlooked benefits is injury prevention. I'm not just talking about athletes participating in sports either. This applies first and foremost to the resulting injuries from hidden obstacles, inevitable accidents, and unfortunate encounters of normal, every day life.

Exercise, particularly resistance-based strength training, improves balance and coordination making injury-producing falls less likely. More importantly, exercise builds stronger and more resilient muscles, tendons, ligaments, and bones which collectively keep our bodies moving and make them less likely to sprain, strain, tear, break, separate, or dislocate. Our joints act like mechanical hinges and rotating machinery. If a screw or bolt gets loose on a door hinge, it can cause a wobble or misalignment and the door won't open or close properly. When your joints get loose from weak muscles, ligaments, and tendons, like the door, things start moving around too much and the joint becomes less stable. The more things move around in and around our joints, the higher the likelihood of problems like injuries or wear and tear. Consider the HANS device that race car drivers wear to prevent their heads from whip-lashing or getting slammed around in the event of an accident. Our tendons, ligaments, cartilage, and intervertebral disks are the protective straps and padding which keep our joints from slamming around and allow the muscles to absorb most of the impact from trips, falls, and collisions. If you let them get weak from a lack of use, it's like racing without any protection and your likelihood of getting injured goes up dramatically.

Exercise also keeps the muscles more elastic which allows them to absorb more sudden force. Ever play with an old rubber band? It breaks easily doesn't it? Grab a new rubber band and you can stretch it over and over and it won't break. Strength training and dynamic flexibility training keeps our muscles limber and allows them to shorten and elongate without tearing. I am convinced that years of consistent weight training have allowed me to play contact sports, snow ski, jump out of planes close to 50 times, race motocross bikes, mountain bike through perilous terrain, compete in triathlons, play in state and collegiate-level racquetball tournaments, and participate in many recreational sports without any major injuries. After 40 plus years of being highly active, I have only one sprained ankle, one strained hamstring, and one broken pinkie to put in my exercise war chest. Either I am the luckiest person in the world or there is some definite truth to my exercise theory.

Strength training also keeps the modern athlete in one piece. If you have never suited up with a helmet and shoulder pads and played football, it will be hard for you to appreciate the forces the body can endure when you keep your muscles and connective tissues strong. It is estimated that the collisions in college and professional football are equivalent to a 35 miles-per-hour head-on collision in a car. Players suffer through this bodily violence repeatedly week in and week out during the season. All major university and National Football League football teams employ a staff of strength and conditioning specialists who are responsible for insuring team athletes achieve and maintain peak performance, but more importantly, keeping them on the field as much as possible. In March of 2009, I had the privilege of meeting and learning from the reigning NCAA National Champion Florida Gators football strength and conditioning staff at a clinic they conducted in Gainesville. Mike Mariotti, the leader of this phenomenal staff said: "Our first priority is always injury prevention because if the players aren't on the field, it doesn't matter how strong or fast they are." If you want to continue playing in the game of life well into your 80's and even 90's for the extremely diligent, engage your muscles in dynamic, strength-building exercises two to three days per week. You either pay now with time and effort or you will pay later with injuries and pain. It's your choice.

In this chapter and the previous one, I hope I made a foolproof case for incorporating exercise into your life. If you are a reasonable and prudent person, then you now understand most of the anti-aging and health benefits of exercise. But just in case you aren't convinced and need more evidence, in the next chapter I will discuss how exercise affects our mood, emotions, and how we feel. Kate learned all about the benefits of exercise first hand and her story follows these words.

"What a difference a year can make!"

In just one year following the exercise guidelines outlined in *The Magic Pill*, Kate lost over 50lbs of weight, lowered her body fat from 36% to a healthy 23%, lost 10 dress sizes, and dropped over 8 inches off her waist. More importantly, however, she dramatically lowered her risk factors for heart disease, stroke, cancer, and diabetes.

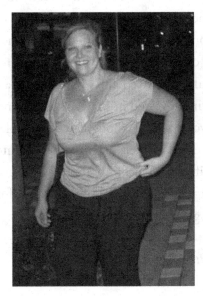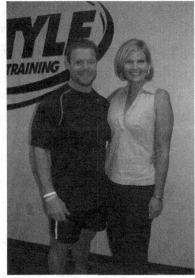

"During a summer visit home, my mom took a look at me and told me she was worried I was at risk for developing type 2 diabetes. I didn't believe her because I was only 28 years of age. But when I researched the risk factors, I realized I was inactive and had a Body Mass Index (BMI) greater than 27 (it was around 33 at the time). The thought of developing diabetes really scared me, so I decided to join a health club and get some help. Fortunately for me, the health club staff introduced me to Matt O'Brien and my life has not been the same since.

Working out with Matt became a great lesson in self-discipline and motivation. He systematically incorporated the principles of success he teaches to all his clients. The very same principles you will learn in this book. Getting up at 6AM every morning to head to the gym and even returning some nights for more cardio taught me not to make excuses and helped me get the results I was looking for. By changing my diet, constantly varying the exercises we did, and progressively increasing the intensity of my workouts, Matt helped me work through the inevitable plateaus and I continued to lose weight and gain muscle tone. Over time, I started enjoying the incredible feeling I had after the workouts and one day I even surprised myself when I looked in the mirror... Wow!!! Is that really me? My results weren't just cosmetic either. During my last physical, I had blood work done and my doctor's comment was 'You are definitely not going to die of heart disease.' My cholesterol levels, blood pressure, and resting heart rate were fantastically improved and I felt better than ever. I am so much better off for having invested in Matt's training and guidance. He pushed me to go beyond what I thought was possible, made working out fun for me, and helped me permanently incorporate fitness and sound nutrition into my lifestyle. Most importantly, I believe in myself again and have the self-confidence to do anything! Thanks for all of your help Matt! You've been a great inspiration."

- Kate Marcinek

CHAPTER THREE:

Better than Prozac

"Opportunities are like sunrises – if you wait too long, you miss them."
William Arthur Ward

Improve your Mood and Alleviate Anxiety

As the Bobby McFerrin song goes, "Don't worry, be happy!" Exercise helps lift your spirits and relieve the tension that life can dish out. It is estimated that over 17 million Americans are "depressed" and that estimate came out before the current economic crisis. Life can be like quicksand, slowly sucking us down into the restrictive muck of our daily routine and habits. We start sinking under the weight of responsibilities, parenthood, spousal demands, unanswered emails, unpaid bills and unless we recognize what's happening, eventually we are buried, suffocate, and die a premature, painful death.

Starting an exercise program is the lifeline you can grab onto and pull yourself out of the quicksand and establishing an exercise routine is the lifeboat that will keep you afloat. It gives you the freedom to move, express yourself, and experience the joy that is true life. Exercise helps you feel better, increases your sense of well-being, and boosts your self-esteem. Exercise, like therapeutic drugs, works best when you are consistent and the longer you are on an exercise program, the better the results — all without unwanted side effects.

At the time of this writing, there have been over 35 studies conducted which have proven that exercise reverses mild to moderate depression at least as well as medications and psychotherapy, and sometimes better. Technically, depression is defined as having feelings of sadness and/or a loss of interest in pleasurable activities for more than two weeks and can manifest itself with symptoms including: loss of appetite, insomnia, fatigue, feelings of guilt, poor concentration, reduced sex drive, and suicidal thoughts. Personally, I have suffered from depression in the past and it is no joy ride, let me tell you. Fortunately, I was able to pull myself out of the doldrums with my exercise lifeline and get myself back on track.

While researching and writing this book, I spent countless hours in the Starbucks around my hometown. People-watching is one of my favorite pastimes and I tend to be a fairly observant person. Thus, when my nose wasn't buried into a research text or my fingers weren't pounding on the keyboard of my laptop, I casually observed the cynical and selfish attitudes, behaviors, and comments of passersby and customers waiting for their coffee drinks. Though this is hardly scientific research and even accounting for the probability these individuals were caffeine-deprived and waiting for their fix, I deduced through this random sampling of Americana that a lot of people grumble, complain, and seem unhappy. This led me to wonder…are people seemingly miserable with life and all people, places, and things around them because of genuine unfortunate circumstances or are they really just unhappy with themselves?

Psychologists call this transference; when we take an internal negative emotion and transfer it to something external. Maybe you had a bad day at work because you forgot to do something and got yelled at by your boss. Then you come home and yell at your kids for not keeping their room picked up. You effectively transferred your internal feelings of failure to an external cause of anger. While this is a common, everyday occurrence leading to unnecessary bitterness, anger, and lots of sulking children locked in their bedrooms, exercise can provide an effective treatment to counteract a negative internal dialogue.

Exercise floods our brain with positive, mood-altering chemicals called endorphins. Endorphins are naturally occurring morphine-like chemicals that act just like morphine in regulating pain. The word endorphin is actually short for endogenous morphine, meaning morphine produced by the body. I'm sure you have probably heard about the "runner's high." The good news is you don't have to be a marathon runner to experience it. You are only one workout away from feeling better.

Any type of vigorous exercise can stimulate production of endorphins. Exercise has also been proven to increase production of the pleasure chemicals serotonin and dopamine much like antidepressant medications do. Together with endorphins, they significantly improve pain-regulation, feelings of well-being and can noticeably improve your outlook on life. People who exercise regularly are less prone to depression and are able to better cope with daily stress.

Besides feeling better, this exercised-induced "pleasure cocktail" of endorphins, dopamine, and serotonin could be the healthy cure for obesity. Research conducted by the US Department of Energy's Brookhaven National Laboratory and published in *The Lancet* in 2001 identified a definitive link between dopamine receptors and obesity. Scientists in the study found obese people have fewer receptors for dopamine in their brain and may eat more food volume and eat more often to stimulate the dopamine "pleasure circuits" much like a drug addict trying to get their fix. In the case of obesity, food is the drug and overeating is the fix. Since drugs that alter dopamine levels are often highly addictive, they concluded that exercise was a more viable alternative to stimulating pleasure and satisfaction via this dopamine pathway. If more people would learn to produce dopamine and other feel good chemicals with exercise, we would not only be happier and more productive, but also a lot thinner too!

Some people suffer from seasonal affective disorder which is appropriately abbreviated as SAD. SAD is a form of depression that typically occurs during the dark winter months or when you are buried in a basement office with no windows like I was early in my career in hospital administration. People who don't get to see the light of day often sleep a lot, crave sweet foods (causing weight gain), and become socially withdrawn. According to the Mayo Clinic staff and the American Medical Association, exercise and light therapy can be prescribed as a treatment for SAD and other forms of depression. While medical science hasn't officially called exercise a cure for depression, they admit it will remarkably improve its symptoms.

Here's the deal with me. If I don't exercise, I am not the same person. In fact, I recently went five days without working out because I rationalized that this book should take precedence and I needed to devote every free second I had to writing it. What I found out was I couldn't write at all, I lost the efficiency of my thought process, and I became extremely frustrated with myself. I started beating myself up a little bit (not literally) because I felt I wasted my time. Then it dawned on me that I hadn't exercised and it began to make sense. In fact, as I am writing these very words right now, I just finished a good workout and low and behold, the words are back. Maybe it's not Pulitzer Prize winning material, but at least it's the accurate expression of my thoughts and I'm thankful for what is flowing through my fingertips onto these pages. The point is this: time spent exercising makes us feel better and will make us *more* productive, not less (as we can easily convince ourselves sometimes). The time you spend exercising will easily be recouped when you accomplish tasks more efficiently and have more stamina to work longer, if necessary.

I know if I didn't exercise almost every day, I would be a lot less happy and my wife would probably want to kick me where the sun doesn't shine. Many of my clients tell me exercise is therapeutic for them and helps them cope with stress. They come in with tension and anguish written all over their face and leave with a calming smile. Everyone feels better when they exercise. That much I can absolutely guarantee. Stress is an inevitable consequence of life. Unfortunately, this not only affects us, but also those closest to us. When we are upset, we often take out our anger on the ones we love. Between my junior and senior year of college I had surgery to fix a deviated septum and was under doctor's orders not to exercise while I was recovering. By the fifth day, I was extremely edgy and snapped at my girlfriend at the time and treated her extremely unfairly. She did absolutely nothing to deserve it and I had every reason to thank her for taking care of me, but I didn't. Instead, I took out my frustrations on her and only later did I make the connection with my bad mood and the lack of mood-altering exercise I was getting. Once the doctor cleared me for "light activity" I went out and hit about 500 golf balls at the driving range and felt much better.

Does this sound familiar to you? Sometimes we blame our bad moods on our situation in life, but more often than not, it is just a physiological plea for exercise. Most of the time we can't control our current circumstances, but we can control how we respond and react to them. You too can learn to treat exercise like a giant "happy pill." Whenever you get moody, down, upset, or irritable, hit the gym, bike trail, sidewalk, or basketball court as soon as possible and inevitably, you *will* feel better and life's problems will seem to magically disappear. If for no other reason than this, exercise is worth it. Your friends and loved ones will thank you, trust me!

Corinne
Age: 46
School Teacher

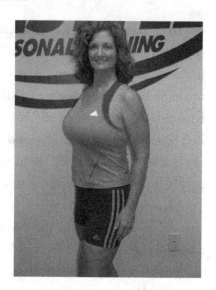

THE FACTS:
In 41 days…

- Lost 14.4 pounds
- Lowered her body fat by 5.5%
- Achieved a healthy BMI of 25.4
- Lost over 2 inches off both her waist and her hips

"Incorporating exercise into my life has helped me in so many ways. My self-esteem is way up and I'm an all around happier person. I've lost weight, gained strength and confidence, and improved my overall health. In fact I would even say exercise is my psychiatrist in terms of helping me deal with stress. Matt is much more than my trainer, he's a friend I can count on. I thank him from the bottom of my heart for all he has done for me."

Relax and Reduce Anxiety

Exercise can help your muscles and mind relax and dramatically reduce the anxious feelings which overwhelm us from time to time. We are born with an innate "fight or flight" response. If you subscribe to *Evolution Magazine*, you would know this bodily process was originally intended to protect us from getting devoured by saber-tooth tigers and other fierce creatures with a taste for human flesh. You either held your ground for the fight of your life or you took flight like an African gazelle running from a hungry cheetah on the plains of the Serengeti. The fight or flight adrenaline boost also revved us up for the hunt so that we could track, capture, kill, and eat the meat of wooly mammoths.

Ultimately, this physiological mechanism insures our long-term survival as a species.

Biochemically speaking, the fight or flight response is triggered by a cascade of hormones released into the bloodstream by the adrenal glands which includes epinephrine, norepinephrine, cortisol, and aldosterone. Cortisol, epinephrine and norepinephrine (adrenaline) work together to raise blood pressure and blood sugar, elevate our heart rate to circulate more blood to working muscles, dilate our pupils making vision sharper (to see the lion lurking in the bushes), increase respiration to get more oxygen into the blood, constrict our blood vessels to restrict blood loss (if we are cut or mauled), open up the nasal passageways (so we can smell the prey miles away), and raise the hair on our bodies (so we can look like a werewolf – ok, maybe not).

Back when we were on the hunt or running away from animals with big teeth, this response gave us the extra boost in energy, stamina, speed, and strength we needed to survive. Like gas on a fire, we burned off the negative effects of this survival mechanism. But today the only thing we run towards when stressed is the vending machine in the break room. Our bodies don't get to burn off the extra fuel produced, which causes toxic effects on our bodies. Too much cortisol, for instance, can lead to weight gain, irregular menstrual periods in women, loss of muscle, trouble sleeping and emotional problems such as depression.

We all still have the fight or flight response and most people experience it on a daily basis. Have you ever found out you had a huge report due the next day that you completely forgot about? How about your boss telling you: "See me in my office in five minutes and it isn't going to be pretty!" What about when you are running late to a meeting and you get on the freeway only to discover traffic is backed up and everyone behind you is honking (as if it's your fault)? Maybe you come home and your spouse berates you for forgetting to put the milk back in the fridge that morning? Or my mom's personal favorite...when I was a kid and would ask her for a check to pay for a field trip that day right as she was just about to leave for work. And my personal favorite...when you are rushing home to make dinner for your spouse and you stop into the grocery store to get just one thing, run to the "Express Check-out" register and wait ten minutes for someone to slowly dig through their purse to write a $4.19 check to cover the cost of the tabloid magazine they are buying to fill all of the free time they must have to read it!

I'm sure you can think of countless other examples which make your blood boil, temperature rise, heart jump, stomach drop, and face turn red. All of these are modern examples of the fight or flight response and collectively, they cause what most people call "stress" in our lives. The chronic effects of stress, anxiety, and angst left unchecked, are high blood pressure, irritability, foul temperament, overeating, fat storage, and eventually, elevated risk for heart disease, stroke, and type 2 diabetes.

Anxiety is an emotion we all have experienced before a job interview or getting in front of a group of people to speak. It can cause fear and worry, our hearts to pound out of our chest, sweating, and nervous behavior like nail biting or tapping our feet. Some anxiety can increase performance, but too much can become a major problem. In extreme cases, too much anxiety can cause a psychiatric condition called generalized anxiety disorder or GAD for short. People who suffer from GAD typically have feelings of chronic distress, worry, and fear and physical symptoms like muscular tension, headache, dizziness, hot flashes, and breathlessness. If you have a brief episode of these feelings, it's called a panic attack.

If you don't learn how to mitigate stress, anxiety and all their modern-day cousins, you are taking years off your life. The great news is exercise is the cure for the toxicity and anxiety of our stressful lives. Just thirty minutes of exercise a day has a relaxation and anti-anxiety effect by lowering our stress-producing hormones. One study found that thirty minutes of exercise just three times a week significantly decreased circulating amounts of the stress hormones adrenaline and cortisol. Less stress hormones equals less stress — makes sense, doesn't it?

Think of yourself as a steam engine. The stress-producing circumstances of each day are like the hot coals under the boiler.

The more stress you have, the more coals you have heating the water. Eventually, the water starts to boil which builds up steam pressure in the boiler. If you continue to add coals, the pressure in the boiler continues to rise and eventually, unless it is released, it will rupture. A small crack in the boiler might be the ill-timed bark at your co-worker, yelling at your spouse and children, or road rage on the freeway. With enough repeated stress on the boiler, it can explode violently leaving a complete meltdown in your life. This can be prevented with routine exercise.

Exercise is your release valve for the building pressure in the boiler. The more stress and responsibility you have in your life, the more critical it is to get some form of exercise. It will help you regulate the pressure by altering your stress response and it also provides a distraction from the stressors causing the pressure. It would also be beneficial to learn and practice stress management techniques like meditation and proactive coping mechanisms like sublimation. With a mature approach, these can prevent pressure build-up like taking coals off the fire (reducing the heat) or dousing the coals with water to stop the heat entirely.

I have seen exercise produce modern miracles in the stressful lives of my clients. I have trained several high-level executives in the restaurant, television, and financial industries and seen them go from overweight, sleep-deprived, stressed out maniacs to calm, rested, thoughtful leaders who grew their business wisely and without ill-consequence to their health. One of my clients is a senior executive for one of the largest restaurant chains in America and he was suffering from classic "type A" personality stress when he came to see me. His high blood pressure, high cholesterol and lack of sound sleep were starting to take their toll on his health and his steam engine was probably ready to blow. By applying his high-intensity personality to working out instead of worrying whether the next new entrée would be a success or not, he was able to reduce his stress-induced pressure. This helped him sleep better, lowered his cholesterol and blood pressure, and kept his executive team from beating him on the head with a dead fish because he was much happier and stopped snapping at them. Make sure you release your own steam with repeated exercise and the stressors in your life will seem much more manageable.

Reduce Muscle Tension

Exercise can also reduce the tension and metabolic waste products in your muscles much like a Swedish or deep tissue massage would. When you do repeated movement exercises like riding a stationary bike or walking briskly in your neighborhood, you are contracting and relaxing the large muscles of your legs and hips hundreds, if not thousands, of times. Each contract-relax cycle draws more nutrient-rich blood into the working muscles and circulates out the toxic waste products of cellular metabolism. With enough repetitions of the contract-relax cycle, muscles will use up available energy, fatigue, and be much more relaxed, less tense, and less sore. When you lift weights during resistance training, you facilitate an even deeper contraction of the muscle tissue which can help reset the tension levels in the muscle. Combining both cardio and resistance-based exercise into your weekly routine is an effective way to keep your muscles less tense and more relaxed.

A lot of the muscle pain and tension we suffer from can be quickly relieved with a single bout of exercise. Physical therapists and athletic trainers often use electrical stimulation on their patients and athletes to force specific muscles to contract and relax. With enough cycles of electrical stimulation, even the most stubborn muscle pain will go away. I learned this my freshman year in college when I pulled a muscle in my back playing football. The pain made it hard to breathe and virtually impossible to play, but 15 minutes of electrically induced contract-relax cycles relieved the pain enough for me to get on the field. Unfortunately it didn't give me any bionic powers or morph me into a super-athlete though. Exercise can serve the same purpose for you that the electrodes did on my back. You will feel much more relaxed, have less pain, sleep better, and the tensions of life will melt away.

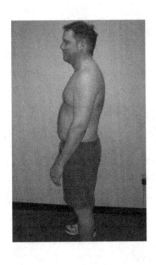

Jarrett
Age: 38
Engineer

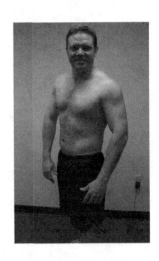

I lost over 13 pounds, lowered my bodyfat by 5%, and lost 4 inches from my waist. Most importantly, I greatly improved my cardiovascular health and lowered my blood pressure.

"Working with Matt has helped me refocus on my health and life balance. I have greatly improved my cardiovascular health and reduced my blood pressure to a healthy level. I learned that with focus, dedication, and support, amazing results are achievable.

Exercise also helps me release the pressure of a stress-filled day. I have a hectic schedule and have to travel frequently. Making time for exercise to maintain life balance is essential to your health. The successes you gain in energy, mood, and physical fitness are so worth the small sacrifices you have to make when you make fitness a priority. This is a chance to change the present and the rest of your life! I am amazed at the fun I have had and how the results have been so much more than just physical."

- Jarrett Potts

PART TWO:

EDUCATION
The Knowledge

CHAPTER FOUR:

Invest in Yourself

"The first wealth is health"
Ralph Waldo Emerson

The Costs of Exercise

If I was to offer you two options: Option 1 - giving you a single penny on day one and doubling what you have each day for 30 days (2 cents on day two, 4 cents on day three, etc.) or Option 2 - giving you one million dollars in cold hard cash at the end of the month, which option would you take? It may surprise you to know that if you took the doubling penny option, you would end up getting 536 million, 870 thousand, and 912 pennies or $5,368,709.12. That's five million three hundred sixty-eight thousand, seven hundred and nine dollars and twelve cents if you were writing it in your check book! Besides dealing with all the pennies, that is a much better deal than the million dollars. One of my college professors taught me this example to illustrate the power of compounding. While earning 100% interest compounded daily is hardly a realistic possibility, it does make the point that compounding can be powerful.

Exercise is like compounding interest. The earlier you start and the more consistent you add little investments of your time week in and week out, the greater the dividend payments will be to your functional health down the road in your 60's, 70's and 80's. Like your financial advisor would tell you to start investing now in whatever amount you can afford, I, being your health advisor, am telling you to invest in your health with a little exercise on most days of the week. The earlier you start, the greater the benefits to your health and the more you will decrease your risk of getting those diseases we talked about in Chapter 2. Let's invest some time discussing the financial side of exercise.

Get a Gym Membership (*Cost of Gym membership*)

When I used to sell gym memberships many moons ago, it never ceased to amaze me when someone told me they couldn't afford the $30 to $40 dollars a month it cost to have access to a million dollars worth of equipment and the life and health-changing opportunity it provided. Where else in life can you lease a million dollars worth of equipment for one or two dollars a day? Either you pay it now, or you will pay it later.

Like all things in life, I know there are exceptions, but let's be real for a second. If you can afford to go out to dinner at least once a week, then you can afford a gym membership. Recently, my wife and I went through Dave Ramsey's Financial Peace University (I highly recommend it for the budget-minded person in all of us). One of the course assignments we had to do was adding up how much money we spent on restaurant meals. Many people discovered they were spending 300 to 400 dollars a month (or more) eating out and one guy I talked to was spending over 800 dollars each month. If you're spending anywhere close to this, that's a lot of money that could better serve your health and your budget.

Frankly, it saddens me to see people get into the vicious cycle of going to restaurants one, two, three or even more nights a week, unknowingly eat too many calories, gain weight, feel bloated and miserable and then repeat the process week in and week out. As the weeks and years start passing by and the pounds start piling on, despair and discomfort from the excess weight becomes a recurring issue. Yet many people continue to seek happiness from the very thing causing their despair in the first place, eating. When they finally get the courage to do something about it or are fed up with buying bigger clothes every three months, they come into the gym and make the choice that they can't afford a $40 dollar-a-month gym membership. So for all posterity, for the health of the world, and for the future success of health clubs across the country, let's break this down for a minute.

Most health clubs operate on a membership system. When you join, they are going to require an enrollment or initiation fee, a card fee, and some initial prorated membership dues and then you will pay recurring monthly dues to maintain your membership. Membership dues are based on the level of service, geographic location, and single location or multiple location options. There are exceptions to this, but this is how most companies work. Generally, the card fee and dues are set in stone, but the enrollment fee can vary from day to day and you can save yourself a few bucks by asking someone in membership to call you during the next special, which usually coincides with the end of the month. If the end of the month is a long way off, I wouldn't wait. Isn't your health worth the 10 or 15 extra dollars you might save by waiting? By the time you exercise for those three weeks, you won't miss the money, your health will start to improve, and you will feel a whole lot better about yourself.

Here's how a typical health club membership breaks down:

Gym Membership:

Initiation Fee:	$29 - $79
Card fee:	$10 - $20
Monthly Dues:	<u>$15 – $50</u>

Total to Start: **$64 - $149**

Recurring Dues: *$15 - $50 per month (plus tax)*

Now compare this to the average per person cost of eating at a restaurant:

Dinner at Restaurant:

Cost of Entree:	$15 - $28
Appetizer:	$7 - $11
Beverages:	$0 - $15
Dessert:	$0 - $9
15% tip:	<u>$4 - $10</u>

Total (per person):   **$26 - $73**

If you are only eating out once a week and there are just over four weeks in a month, then each month you're spending somewhere between 104 and 292 of your hard-earned dollars on food you could easily and more economically prepare yourself. I have nothing against restaurants and I enjoy being pampered, waited on, and not having to deal with the dishes as much as anyone, but I'm making a point here. Even if you take the average, you're looking at spending $198 a month. If you skip just one meal a month, it is highly likely that you will have no problem affording a typical gym membership. For all practical purposes, the cost of one restaurant meal equates to an entire month at the gym.

I know many people who earn a living as a school teacher, church pastor, shift worker, carpenter, construction laborer, administrative assistant, or line cook. Right or wrong, these are not high salary professions, yet they all find room in their budget for a gym membership. Let me give you a specific example to illustrate the point of prioritization. Jessica is a social worker in her mid-twenties who doesn't bring home a lot of bacon. Somehow she affords to pay not only for a gym membership, but also hired me for personal training too. One day I was curious (and explained to her I was writing this chapter), so I asked her: "How do you afford to pay for personal training given your financial circumstances?" I was half expecting her to say her parents paid for it or she had an inheritance, but she replied simply: "I decided exercise and my health were a high priority in my life. So I cut back on eating out and drinking to have the money in my budget."

Well said Jessica and if she can do it I know you can too. And don't make the "I have kids" argument because most decent health clubs include free childcare (or costing at most $10 or $15 a month) with their membership. It is all about how you want to prioritize your life and I hope I have made a convincing case so far in this book that *exercise is a must have in your life.* If you want more information on hiring a personal trainer or how much it costs, I discuss it in Chapter 10.

> *"Those who think they have not time for bodily exercise will sooner or later have to find time for illness"*
> Edward Stanley

The Costs if You Don't Exercise

Now consider the cost of *not* exercising. Let's assume for a minute that you don't make the smart choice and follow my exercise advice. Like most Americans, you can expect to gain an average of two to seven pounds of body fat each year starting in your 20's. Remember the scale doesn't tell you the whole truth. It may say you only gained seven pounds last year when in reality you gained 10 pounds of fat and lost three pounds of muscle. For each decade of life that translates into 20 to 70 extra pounds of needless fat you will carry on your body. By the time you are in your 60's, you could be hauling around 100 pounds of dead weight that is burdening your heart, joints, liver, arteries, and self-esteem. Essentially, you are now a walking heart attack time bomb with high cholesterol, high blood pressure, and osteoarthritis and you will be taking a minimum of five prescription drugs (most likely 10 to 15) to prolong life and treat your pain, diabetes, high blood pressure, high cholesterol and your inevitable depression.

Assuming you have health insurance and take formulary or generic drugs, your co-payments for these prescriptions will be a minimum of $100 a month for the best plans, but more likely closer to $250. In fact, one study estimates: *for every 10 pounds of excess weight, Americans spend an additional $500 annually for healthcare.* This equates to an additional $208 per month if you are 50 pounds overweight (50lbs divided by 10 = 5 multiplied by $500 = $2500 per year divided by 12 months = $208). If that doesn't irk you, I have heard of some absurd amounts being paid for prescription drugs by extremely obese individuals. One of the contestants on NBC's *The Biggest Loser* said he was paying over $15,000 per year for all the drugs he was taking because of his weight and the diabetes that came with it.

Now let's assume you also decide to protect your family's financial future and carry some type of life insurance. The extra weight is going to cost you big time in additional premiums, if you can even qualify. Your rate classification will be impacted by your mortality risk factors and cost you $100 to $200 more per month than if you had a healthy weight and normal blood pressure. Consider the following example: $500,000 term life policy for a 55 year old, male, non-smoker who is within weight guidelines and normal blood pressure would cost about $150 per month. The same policy for someone 100 pounds overweight with high blood pressure would cost around $450 per month, if they were lucky enough to get coverage.

So let's add up these additional monthly costs and see where we are so far.

Prescription co-pays:	$150
Healthcare costs:	$208
Extra Insurance Costs:	$300
Total Extra costs per month:	**$658**

For $658, you could afford a health club membership, a personal trainer for two sessions a week and even a massage each month. Most importantly, you would feel much better about yourself, be more productive, have better functional health, not be popping prescription medicines every day, and statistically, live longer. Like I said, *you either pay a little now or you will pay a lot later.*

We haven't even considered the impact to your productivity, average salary, and financial earning power. Studies show healthy, vibrant people are more likely to get hired or promoted, have more earning power, miss less work, and make more money, on average, than their overweight counterparts. People who exercise regularly are more productive and less likely to call in sick. One study of U.S. postal workers in Washington D.C. found that the active mail carriers who walked their routes had a 300% less risk for heart disease then the sedentary clerks and route walkers also missed less days of work due to illness.

Consistent exercise will also buy you extra time. I can't even begin to quantify how much an extra day of life is worth. Most people would consider an extra day to spend with a loved one priceless. How about an extra year? How about five extra years? The point is that if you exercise three to four days per week on most weeks per year, for most years in a lifetime, you could successfully add seven to eleven years to your life. If one extra day is priceless, how much would eleven years be worth?

Does the tail wag the dog or are you going to decide to wag your tail and do something about it? Don't wait a day longer, it is never too late to start exercising and the benefits can be felt almost immediately. Just a 10% weight reduction can significantly reduce your risks of heart disease, cancer, and stroke and you will notice the physiological changes within weeks. You will feel better, have more energy, and start to believe in yourself and what you can accomplish!

Michelle
Age: 35
Housewife and Mom

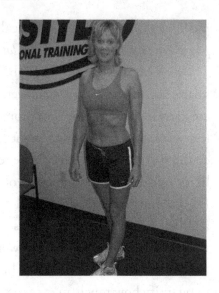

THE FACTS:
In 42 days…

- She lost over 8 pounds of body fat
- Increased her muscle mass by 2.66 pounds
- Lowered her body fat by 5.6%
- Dramatically improved strength and muscle tone

"Following Matt's guidance has made me stronger, healthier, happier, and a more self-confident person. My life has improved so much. I have become stronger physically, mentally, and emotionally. I have gone from a skinny, frail and insecure woman to a toned, strong, and confident one who likes what she sees in the mirror… especially the legs! Taking control of one area of my life, my health that is, has led to improvement in all other areas of my life too."

The Barriers to Entry

If you decided to start a new company, most business experts would tell you to have a great business plan. And if you put together any business plan worthy of venture capital financing, you better make sure you consider the barriers to entry into the marketplace, as well as your expected competitions' too. Likewise, when you consider making the commitment to exercise, you should be aware of the potential barriers, challenges, and obstacles you will face along the way. The capitalists want a decent return on their investment and so do you.

Without a doubt, the number one barrier to entry for most people (especially at a large commercial gym) is fear. Fear of the unknown.

Fear of being judged or being glared at. Fear of not belonging or being outside your comfort zone. Fear of not knowing what to do. You have to learn to acknowledge these fears and supplant them with the much larger fear of dying an early, painful death if you don't get in there and exercise.

That being said, I know it can be tough. I've been working out for over 25 years at gyms all over the world and even I get the nervous jitters anytime I walk into a new facility. These are natural feelings and it is completely normal to be nervous, apprehensive, and even afraid. Take comfort in the fact these feelings will all pass with time, familiarity, and the pleasure you will receive from your workouts. Once you establish your routine, your fear will be replaced with comfort, joy, and positive emotions and you will even start to miss it when you don't come — believe it or not.

Another barrier or challenge you may face is time. Time management is critical to success in any venture, business or otherwise. If you don't plan your time, time will slip away leaving you with less of it to accomplish the tasks at hand. Surveys of successful business executives and start-up entrepreneurs found that most of them budget their time each week. Likewise, I recommend you sit down with a weekly time management calendar like a Franklin Planner and plan out your week. Allocate time for work, grocery shopping, meal preparation, household chores, your children's play time and youth programs (if you have kids), personal hygiene, sleep (7 to 8 hours), special projects, leisure, and of course, exercise. Don't forget to include travel time to and from and time for a shower after you exercise. I guarantee you that time spent planning your week will be returned to you in spades. A small investment of 10 to 15 minutes to plan each week will make you much more efficient and you will get much more done. Every professional football team starts each game with a game plan. Start each week with your own game plan and things will go much more smoothly.

Making time for exercise will likely require an adjustment if it isn't already part of your current routine. Some people find that exercising first thing in the morning, before work and other obligations, is best for them. It starts the day on a positive, energizing note and it is the least likely time something else can interfere (like work commitments, having to pick up a sick child from school, being worn out from a stressful day). For other people, exercising after work or during an extended lunch break may be best. If you truly are not a "morning person" then I would recommend budgeting your exercise time for immediately after work. I have seen the "night owls" try exercising early in the morning and inevitably they hit the snooze button too many times and end up missing their workouts or cutting them short. Learn to capitalize on your afternoon energy and pack a gym bag to take with you each day. Go straight to the gym after work so you avoid the time and energy-sapping temptations that lurk in our homes. If you must go home, don't stop even for a second to sit down, turn on the TV, or log on to your computer. Go in, change, have a snack and out the door you go. If you are exercising at home, follow the same rules with the exception that you start your exercise routine instead of heading to the gym.

I could come up with other challenges you will face but the bottom line is this: Don't let small obstacles or distractions become huge barriers between you and your health. Budget your time, conquer your fears, and prioritize your life to incorporate the most important use of your time; exercise! In the next chapter you will learn the exercise fundamentals so you can make the most of the time you devote to the exercise *Magic Pill*.

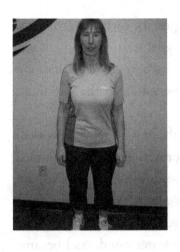

Jill
Age: 48
Housewife

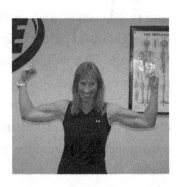

In 10 weeks, I lost 16 lbs of bodyfat, lowered my bodyfat by 8.5%, and dropped 14 inches off my body. Most importantly, I lowered my cholesterol level and risk factors for heart disease.

"I am very proud of the body I now possess. My personal trainer Matt O'Brien and I have worked tremendously hard, transforming my once undefined, overweight shape into a powerful, sculpted form. As a result I have emerged from my intensive training stronger in body and mind. I am back in the 'driver's seat' of my life.

At the age of 48, I have accomplished what I wish I had done ten years ago. I had allowed my physical fitness to slip away until I got to the point where I thought it was hopeless. I approached Matt, and discussed with him my need to be back in good shape. Matt spent a great deal of time chatting to me, in order to establish my past exercise and eating habits. He also spent time getting to know my personality, character, my motivation to succeed and my level of commitment. It was extremely reassuring to have that level of attention, since time taken to consider me as an individual allowed me to trust Matt; he always had my best interests at heart.

His knowledge and passion for fitness and good nutrition, and his personable manner, gave me great faith in his ability to put me on the right path to health and fitness. He helped me focus by giving me structured exercise and nutrition plans. My goal strangely enough was not weight loss; I purely wanted to be in the very best physical condition for my age. The weight reduction that happened along the way was a pleasant byproduct.

My blood pressure dropped significantly, my bodyfat decreased, my lean muscle increased and my mood improved greatly as I pounded out my pent up emotions induced by the stresses of life. I now have muscle and tone and my body shape has altered and is now more athletic in appearance. My energy levels have increased drastically and I now achieve much more in a day, with a clearer mind. As I became fitter and happier, those around me also benefited from my improved outlook on life.

I know for certain that I would not have arrived at this fantastic place in my life without Matt as my personal trainer. Matt's ability to convey his vast knowledge and passion for fitness and nutrition, his genuine unwavering interest in my progress, and his continual encouragement, made me feel my success is every bit as important to him as it is to me.

Thank you Matt for giving me my health, fitness and life back."

- Jill Gear

CHAPTER FIVE:

Exert Yourself

"There are only two options regarding commitment; you're either in or you're out. There's no such thing as life in-between."

Pat Riley

Commit Yourself to Exercise

Personally I believe this is the most important chapter in the book. This is where the rubber meets the road, so to speak, and you will learn how to obtain all the numerous benefits we discussed previously. Exercise is the most efficient and effective method of keeping you young, preventing disease, keeping you sane, and propelling you to more success in life. You are going to learn the current exercise guidelines and key concepts like heart rate monitoring, rating of perceived exertion, the F.I.T.T. principle, cardio and weight training, and exercise principles like specificity, progression, and variation. This chapter is Fitness 101 and will give you most of the fundamental knowledge of exercise you will need.

Because of the diluted amount of information and self-proclaimed expertise that exists today, it is very easy to be confused about what and how to do anything, particularly when it pertains to diet and exercise. It is unfortunate that some people can manipulate scientific information and sensationalize results to prey upon people's hopes and fears in order to sell the "latest and greatest" program, book, or DVD. My goal is to help you minimize the exercise clutter that's out there and learn the basic and timeless principles of exercise which you can use for the rest of your life. For the purpose and duration of this book, I use the term exercise interchangeably with physical activity. I would define exercise as any sustained and purposeful activity which elevates your heart rate, uses the large muscles of the body, expends energy, and causes you to break a sweat.

People often ask me: "What is the best way to exercise?" and they look at me like there is a one sentence answer. This question is like asking a litigation attorney: "How can I win an injury case against a major drug company?" or asking an auto mechanic: "How do I overhaul an engine?" There are no "one size fits all" solutions when it comes to exercise and what might be right for one person might be completely wrong for someone else. I have spent the better part of 20 years studying exercise science and I'm still learning each day.

Learning to exercise is a lot like learning a foreign language — it is best to learn with a teacher and it takes years to speak fluently. The best proven way to learn a language is through immersion; where you live, eat, read, walk, and talk in the native country whose language you're trying to learn. This is the method our government uses to train agents and emissaries to become language specialists. One of my good friends spent 18 months in Argentina "immersed" in this type of learning and became extremely proficient in the official language of Spanish and even a little of Argentina's other indigenous languages like Quechua and Guarani. For most of us however, packing up our stuff and moving to Beijing to learn Mandarin Chinese is an unrealistic possibility. Most people would therefore enlist the help of a school, teacher, or a language learning system to assist them in the process.

Similarly, immersing yourself by living in a gym or health club 24/7 wouldn't be realistic either. You're not going to learn all there is to know about fitness overnight and I highly recommend you hire a personal trainer to serve as your initial coach, teacher, and mentor. Don't get me wrong, there are many self-starters out there that can use the resources provided in this book and other books, magazines, web sites, and instructional DVDs to get phenomenal results on their own. But reality for most people is that a helpful hand will expedite their results. You be the judge and do what works best for you. In any case, I recommend you join a health club which has established training protocols, group fitness classes, and instructional programs to help you learn the fitness language.

It never ceases to amaze me when I get asked: "Hey, you got a minute? How should I get in shape?" To which I reply with a lot of patience: "That's gonna take more than a minute, you have a lifetime?" The point is this: it takes time and constant exposure to technique and program knowledge to become proficient. Would you attempt to complete a complicated 1040 income tax return without the help of a good accountant? If you aren't familiar with exercise science, strength training, and cardio programming, do yourself a favor and at a minimum, find a decent personal trainer or fitness specialist to help get you started. Keep them on your personal staff of professionals like your attorney, accountant, doctor, and therapist to periodically adjust your program, monitor your progress, and ensure some form of accountability for your training and results. (For more information, details and suggestions about hiring a personal trainer see Chapter 11.)

And for you "been there, done that" know-it-alls out there, I have a few words of advice for you...You haven't and you didn't! Exercise science and training programs are constantly evolving, improving, and yielding better, faster, and more scientifically-based results. Don't ever think you are on top of it. I live it, breath it, try to stay current on all of the exercise and nutritional research, attend countless seminars and workshops each year, and even so, I am not too proud or naïve to think I'm too good for someone else's opinion or assistance. I invest thousands of dollars each year learning from other people in my field. A new approach can be beneficial to anyone. If for no other reason, doing things in a new way will be novel to the body and provoke some type of adaptation. Even changing something as simple as your repetition speed can lead to improved results. So check your ego at the door and get a fresh opinion. Not only will people think you're more intelligent for being smart enough to hire an expert, but your body will most likely break out of the perpetual rut it's been stuck in the past few years.

Getting Started

To get you started, I want to give you some basic information, kind of like learning how to say: "Yes, No, Where's the Bathroom, and May I have a beer please in German (*Ein bier bitte*). I have included a basic walking program you can use almost anywhere and my menu-based system for designing a resistance-based exercise program which will help you learn how to construct your own workouts. These are tools to help simplify the process of exercise program design as long as you're working out, which hopefully will be for the rest of your life. With this knowledge, you should be able to go to any health club (or your own home gym if you are that fortunate) and get started with an effective program.

There are fundamentally two types of exercise or "exertion" you need to know and understand: aerobic and anaerobic. You are probably familiar with the more popular terms "cardio" and "lifting weights." In the next section, we will take a quick look at muscle physiology and anatomy. You will learn the difference between the aerobic and anaerobic exercise and why both are equally essential to your ultimate health.

Energy Systems and Muscle Fiber Types

There are three energy systems (called metabolic pathways) the body uses to move the body and its constituent parts. The *phosphagen system* uses adenosine triphosphate (ATP) and gives us about 25 seconds of 100% all out effort (like sprinting at maximum speed). The *lactic acid system* uses anaerobic (without oxygen) glycolysis to convert stored glycogen in the muscles and liver to give us about two to three minutes of high intensity work (like lifting heavy weights or pushing a fully loaded wheel barrel). The *oxygen system* uses aerobic (with oxygen) metabolism to provide lasting energy for movements and activities lasting longer than two to three minutes. The capacity of this system is only limited by the availability of oxygen and fuel. This system is extremely efficient and can use glycogen (sugar stored in the liver and muscle), blood glucose, stored fat, and even protein to produce energy for movement.

The type of activity you are doing will determine which metabolic pathway is being used, but the reality is that all three energy systems are being used in some capacity all the time. Workouts can be designed to emphasize different pathways like high-intensity interval training (HIIT) which can emphasize the phosphagen system, high-intensity weight training which emphasizes the lactic acid system, or long-duration, low-intensity cardio training which emphasizes the oxygen system.

The skeletal muscles which move our bodies by pulling on bones through their tendonis attachments are composed of different fiber types. Type 1 fibers are the red, slow-twitch and predominately aerobic type fibers that provide contractile effort for long duration activity at low intensity levels, like walking or slow jogging. Most people have about 45% of their total muscle mass in type 1 fibers. Type 2 fibers are the white, fast-twitch predominantly anaerobic type fibers that contract at high intensity workloads for a relatively short duration. There are several sub-types of type 2 fibers that are differentiated for varying roles. Type 2a fibers, about 10% of our total muscle mass, are "transition fibers" that bridge the gap between traditional long distance and short, intense exercise. A good example would be an 800 to 1500 meter race or the classic "miler" would have well developed type 2a fibers. Type 2b are the classic fast-twitch strength fibers that an Olympic weight lifter or power lifter would have a large proportion of. On average, 45% of our muscle mass is type 2b. Type 2c fibers are undifferentiated fibers that can essentially go "both ways" depending on which demands are placed on the body. If you spend the majority of your exercise time lifting weights, these fibers will take on the attributes of the fast-twitch fibers giving you more strength. If you are a runner, swimmer, or any other distance athlete, the 2c fibers will adapt to perform slow-twitch functions giving you more endurance.

Over the years, my training has evolved as I learned new information, incorporated new exercise methods, and tested out different philosophies. I've put all of this practical experience into developing an incredibly time-efficient workout system. I originally designed this method of training for my own use, but found it incredibly effective for my clients too. Training this way will emphasize all muscle fiber types and simultaneously stress all three energy systems, effectively giving you the most bang for your workout buck. We all have tremendous demands on our time in our rush-rush society and I am no exception. Later in the chapter I will share this workout philosophy with you. I call it the "Menu Workout" system. But before we get to it, let's take a look at how this exercise thing all started. What you learn may surprise you.

The History of Exercise

While modern science, the media, and the authors of the countless books on diet and exercise want us to believe they know something new, unique, and different, the truthful reality is the core principles of exercise and nutrition were discovered and understood hundreds and even thousands of years ago. Don't believe me? Read the following insight from Hippocrates recorded over two thousand years ago!

> *"All parts of the body which have a function, if used in moderation and exercised in labors to which each is accustomed, become thereby healthy and well developed, and age slowly; but if unused and left idle, they become liable to disease, defective in growth, and age quickly."*
> Hippocrates (circa 400 BC)

Want a more recent example but still ancient by scientific standards? Consider Artie McGovern who was the original "trainer to the stars" back in the 1920's and 1930's. I never would have known he existed if my wonderful mother hadn't given me his book *The Secret of Keeping Fit* (originally published in 1935 by Simon and Schuster), which she picked up at an antique store about five years ago. Artie lived and worked in New York City and his clients included Jack Dempsey, Marshall Field (yeah, the one the stores are named after), Morton Downey (the original not the junior), William Sloan, Arthur Murray, John Phillip Sousa, and most notably, Babe Ruth, who he helped lose 30 to 40 pounds and get in playing shape prior to each baseball season. Given the Babe's penchant for excess, I'm sure this was no small feat. The Father of Fitness estimates Babe Ruth gained and lost close to 7,000 pounds over the last 10 years of his baseball career.

When I read his book, I was downright flabbergasted to learn that most of what we do today as elite trainers has been around for a long, long time. Here I am a leading-edge, well-educated, certified strength and conditioning specialist thinking he knows some new, state of the art, proprietary training techniques, only to discover that mister McGovern beat me to the punch over 80 years ago. Needless to say, I enjoyed a quick piece of humble pie and became fascinated with the possibility of learning something from one of the original master trainers.

What did I learn? I discovered that other than some verbal semantics like "reducing," which we call "weight loss" and "dieting" today, the two underlying principles of fitness and weight control haven't changed. Move more and eat less. More specifically, he proclaimed that the four success factors for getting lean are: diet, exercise, relaxation, and sleep. We would like to think that our infatuation with being fit and trim is a modern-day phenomenon, but his clients and the public, in general, were obsessed with "reducing" back in the roaring twenties and the "Great Depression" thirties too. Artie even went on to describe all the (and I quote) "diet faddists and diet crazes" people were exposed to during his career. He stated way back in 1935: "Nearly every fad diet is concocted for the purpose of selling some book, some institution, some patent food, or some person. The more sensational or radical the diet, then usually the better the sale." To think we are living in the enlightened age is somewhat whimsical and funny now.

No summation of the history of exercise would be complete without mentioning the great Jack LaLanne. If Artie McGovern is the father of fitness, then Jack is the eternal "Godfather of Fitness." Born in San Francisco, California in 1914, Jack pioneered the modern day health club when he opened his first health spa in 1936. He had a fitness television show which ran for over 34 years and also invented most of the original exercise equipment used in commercial gyms today. Most people know of Jack from his amazing feats of strength and endurance which he performed to champion the benefits of exercise. Jack LaLanne has dedicated his life to encouraging people to exercise as a way of improving their life. There are literally thousands upon thousands of exercise facilities today serving millions of Americans in their quest for a better, healthier life and their roots are all traceable back to his life's work.

We all now have access to great exercise equipment and training programs. The point of telling you this is simple. Don't feel you will miss out if you're not at a self-designated "elite exercise facility" training with a celebrity "trainer to the stars." I've trained with some of them and they aren't any different from the rest of us and they don't have access to any magical machines or information. We all have access to the same research and training information; now more than ever. You can have just as much success at a small-town YMCA that you can have at any facility in New York or Los Angeles when you learn and apply the fundamental principles of success I will share with you in this book.

Before You Start Exercising

Before you get started, I again want to reiterate the importance of consulting with your personal physician prior to beginning this or any other exercise program. If you smoke, are extremely overweight, experience chest pain or dizziness, have bone or joint problems, or have any chronic conditions such as heart disease, diabetes, high blood pressure, arthritis, or shortness of breath, you must consider this advice mandatory. Most of you probably fall into the gray area where you're not sure about your health risk factors, which is why most commercial health clubs and wellness centers use a *Physical Assessment Readiness Questionnaire* (PAR-Q) to determine if you need to see your doctor prior to starting an exercise program. If you have access to the internet, just type PAR-Q into your search engine and you can find the questions for yourself. Regardless of your condition, work with your doctor to get you into a suitable exercise program as soon as possible.

Exercise Guidelines

In August 2007, the American College of Sports Medicine (ACSM) and the American Heart Association (AHA) published their revised physical activity guidelines, which state: "all healthy adults ages 18 to 65 years need moderate-intensity aerobic physical activity for at least 30 minutes on five days each week or vigorous-intensity aerobic physical activity for at least 20 minutes on three days each week. In addition, activities that maintain or increase muscular strength and endurance should be performed for at least two days each week. It is recommended that 8 to 10 exercises using the major muscle groups be performed on two non-consecutive days. To maximize strength development, a resistance (weight) should be used for 8 to 12 repetitions of each exercise resulting in willful fatigue."

ACSM and AHA Exercise Guidelines:

All healthy adults ages 18 to 65 should perform:

- *moderate intensity cardiovascular activity for 30 minutes on 5 days of each week*

   OR

- *vigorous intensity cardiovascular activity for 20 minutes on 3 days of each week*

   AND

- *8-10 strength training exercises for 8-12 repetitions each on 2 days of each week*

The ACSM is the largest sports medicine and exercise science organization in the world. According to its website, this organization has over 20,000 worldwide members dedicated to advancing and integrating scientific research to provide education and practical applications of exercise science and sports medicine (www.ACSM.org). The AHA (www.americanheart.org) was founded in 1924 and is the nation's largest and oldest voluntary health organization dedicated to reducing disability and death from diseases of the heart and stroke. Their website points out that heart disease and stroke are the number one and three killers of Americans claiming over 870,000 lives each year.

If you are over the age of 65 or are 50 to 64 with chronic conditions like arthritis, then the ACSM also recommends adding balance training and having a physical activity plan to the exercise guidelines. It is important to note that the new guidelines specify "the recommended amount of aerobic activity is *in addition to* routine activities of daily living." They also point out that "more is better" when it comes to exercise stating "activity performed above the recommended minimum amount provides even greater health benefits." This, of course, has its limits and assumes people aren't going out to run a marathon every day. Remember the "moderation principle," which I will be discussing in detail in Chapter 10: "Everything in moderation, including moderation."

What is moderate intensity exercise you are probably wondering? There are many ways to gauge intensity and the easiest answer to this question is: exercise hard enough to break a sweat but where you can still hold a conversation. This is called the "talk test." When performing vigorous intensity exercise, you would only be able to talk in broken sentences of three to five words at a time and you would feel your heart pounding and your lungs burning. An example of moderate intensity exercise would be brisk walking at about 3.8 to 4.2 miles per hour for 30 to 40 minutes. Vigorous intensity exercise for most adults would be jogging at about 5.8 to 6.2 miles per hour for 20 to 30 minutes or climbing 15 flights of stairs two or three times.

In the fall of 2008, the U.S. Department of Health and Human Services issued the 2008 Physical Activity Guidelines for Americans which were developed from the comprehensive expertise and exhaustive research of the Physical Activity Guidelines Advisory Committee.

Besides concluding that regular physical activity improves overall health and reduces the risk of many adverse health outcomes, the official report included both aerobic (endurance) and muscle-strengthening (resistance) physical activity in its recommendations. These guidelines recommend that all adults get at least 2½ hours (150 minutes) of moderate-intensity physical activity such as brisk walking or 1¼ hours (75 minutes) of a vigorous-intensity activity such as running or playing a sport like soccer each week. In addition, the guidelines also recommend adults should do muscle-strengthening activities like weight training on two or more days each week.

The exercise guidelines were also extended (with some modifications) to older adults, pregnant women, adults with disabilities, adults with chronic medical conditions, children, and adolescents. Now *no one is off the proverbial exercise hook*, because according to the Guidelines Committee, the "benefits of physical activity far outweigh the possibility of adverse outcomes." Sorry Charlie, no more excuses now. It's time to take the exercise plunge if you haven't already. For additional information visit their web site at www.health.gov/paguidelines/.

Despite the numerous proven benefits of exercise and all types of physical activity, the statistics for Americans are really grim.

- 25% of adults get none
- 50% of adults don't get enough
- 33% of children in grades 9 to 12 don't exercise

So the choice is yours. Each week of your life, do five days of moderate activity for at least 30 minutes or three days of vigorous activity for at least 20 minutes. Another option, and in my opinion preferable, is to mix it up by doing one or two days of vigorous activity and three to five days of moderate activity each week. Or you can do what I do, which is to combine vigorous and moderate activity into one workout, maximizing the benefits of exercise in the minimum amount of time. I don't care which method you choose, but the bottom line is you have to do something each week. Think of it as the mandatory, life-saving, life-extending prescription that it is. Like the Nike slogan tells us, "Just Do It!"

You may not be able to do 30 minutes of continuous exercise right now and that's okay. Rome was not built in a day and like all the roads that lead to Rome, we will get you there too; one step at a time. The good news is that studies found that three separate 10 minute bouts of exercise can be equally effective as 30 continuous minutes and using the concept of progression, you will gradually build the duration of exercise up each day until you are there.

Likewise, some of you may be so busy that you can't carve out 30 consecutive minutes. If this is your personal truth then you have my sympathies; I've been there before and don't intend to ever go back. Even so, you can proceed with the understanding that you will make it a goal to get 150 cumulative minutes of exercise each week. By employing some simple strategies like parking your car further from the office or entrance to the grocery store, walking while your kids are at soccer practice, taking the dog for a longer walk, taking the stairs instead of the elevator, getting up 15 to 20 minutes earlier in the morning, walking on a treadmill while you watch your favorite shows, and walking your kids to the bus stop, you can find the time to do something great for yourself. Plan for exercise and exercise your plan!

Exercise Guidelines and Children

Since we are in the midst of a childhood obesity and diabetes epidemic, I want to make the special case for children to get a substantial amount of exercise. If we don't break the chain with this generation and put the health and fitness train back on the tracks, then ultimately our country will perish. The prosperity of America in years to come depends on the future ingenuity, productivity, and teamwork of our children.

The Physical Activity Guidelines direct children and adolescents to exercise for 60 minutes every day with vigorous, muscle-strengthening, and bone-strengthening physical activities included on at least 3 days of the week.

It wouldn't be fair to hold a child accountable to these exercise guidelines. It is absolutely the responsibility of their parents to mandate, enforce, regulate (or whatever else you prefer to call it) activity every day. It is also the responsibility of the parent to lead by example, which means you have to get your exercise in too. Kids are very perceptive and if you plan to hypocritically prescribe exercise to your children while you sit down on your own overweight, out of shape butt, they will call you out big time or worse, keep it to themselves. As I learned studying military history, all great leaders lead by example. As a parent, you are your children's heroic leader. You have to demonstrate that your health is important to you by keeping yourself in shape and making the time to fit exercise into your own life. What's good for the goose is good for the gander, especially when it comes to exercise.

Yes, this may require some effort or even some additional expense on your part if you are currently a parent or planning to be one. But just like you wouldn't dare allow your child to miss a medical vaccination or an educational opportunity, you can't allow them to miss out on the benefits of exercise either. I'm not a lawyer, but I would say it is child neglect if you don't get your kid involved in some form of exercise. And don't be fooled that exercise is the child's decision. Given a choice, most kids would rather play video games, watch TV and eat candy than play soccer or ride their bike. Remember who the boss is! I hear parents say: "Little Johnnie just doesn't want to exercise" far too often. It isn't up to them. Their minds aren't developed enough to know the consequences of their decisions and their primitive brains will evolve with a low self-esteem and little self-worth by allowing them to get their way all the time.

I'll share with you the trick my parents used to get me and my brothers to exercise when we were growing up. They would give us the option: "Either you go out and play or I will give you some more chores to do. It is your choice." Of course given those two alternatives, we always chose to play. They also kept us involved in organized sports virtually year-round to keep us active — football in the fall, soccer in the winter, baseball in the spring, and swimming in the summer. Each season had its sport and the associated friendships and life lessons we learned. I'll get off my soapbox now, but I sincerely hope I have driven home the point to get children involved even if they themselves don't want to. Like I thanked my parents when I grew up, they will thank you too.

Getting Maximum Results

If you want to fit into your clothes, use the F.I.T. principle. If you want to fit into smaller clothes, use the very F.I.T. principle. There are 4 key concepts to getting maximum results from exercise and unfortunately most people miss

Very F.I.T. Principles for Success		
Very	=	Variation
F	=	Frequency
I	=	Intensity
T	=	Time and Type

the boat. Now you too are going to be one of the 'enlightened' few and by incorporating all of them into your own fitness program, you WILL accomplish your fitness goals in the shortest time possible. I have come up with the moniker "very F.I.T." to help you remember them.

Variation

The first principle is probably the least practiced and the least understood: *variation*. It is by far the most important to ensure you continue to get results from exercise. You probably know someone who is very routine. They wake up at the same time, eat the same breakfast, go to the same job, and do the same workout everyday. As you will learn, having a nutritional routine is a great thing, but you want your fitness routine to be anything but!

Let's take a look at a character we'll call Sam. Sam is a 47 year-old mid-level manager, happily married father of two, and for the past two and a half years, he has worked out Monday through Friday at 6am rain or shine. Sam starts every workout with a 30 minute jog on the treadmill at six miles per hour and then does exactly two sets of the same 12 weight machines for 12 repetitions each set. When he is feeling particularly strong, he may up the weight he uses on each machine by five pounds, but more often than not, he uses the same amount of weight from week to week. He finishes each workout with a five minute stretch on an exercise mat then hits the showers ready to tackle his hectic day at the office.

From a first impression, most people would say that Sam has an exceptional workout routine and he is extremely disciplined. Personally, I would congratulate Sam on his work ethic and practicing the 'F' and 'T' of the FIT principle. But here's the rest of the story. Despite his efforts, Sam is unhappy because he is 20 pounds overweight and has an ever-present "spare tire" around his midsection. Often he gets frustrated because he is putting in over 5 hours a week of intense exercise and eats healthy, but his weight hasn't changed in the past year and his pants are still tight. He continues to exercise because he feels great, has more energy at work, and his doctor says his blood-work "looks outstanding." What is Sam doing wrong?

Sam needs to kneel in tribute to the Variation Goddess and start mixing things up in the gym. Even though it is a little cliché now, I'm going to quote Einstein's definition of insanity one more time to drive home the point.

"Insanity is doing the same things over and over and expecting different results."

Variation is about changing or "varying" everything about your workouts so your body continues to adapt. Think of exercise as the stimulus for change in the body. If you constantly provide the same stimulus, your body quickly adapts to it and will get more and more efficient at accomplishing the task at hand. Now this is ok if you are training for a specific event or sport, where you want to economize your efforts to get better performance. But when you are an everyday Joe or Jane trying to lose weight or get in shape, efficiency is a bad thing. You want your body to be the least efficient possible so it burns the most amount of calories in the least amount of time. It's like a car that gets less gas mileage in the city when it is constantly changing direction and speed, compared to the relative efficiency of cruising at 60 mph on the highway. To lower your gas mileage in the gym or in any workout, you need to constantly change what you do.

The body adapts very quickly to any new exercise stimulus or protocol. The last thing you want is to fall victim to the same daily or weekly exercise "routine" month in, month out. If you don't change the stimulus at least periodically, the body's neuromuscular and endocrine systems will "flat-line" in terms of progression and performance enhancement. In order to continue improving and getting the results you seek, you have to manipulate the exercise variables in your workouts and training.

There are many ways to change your exercise program and it isn't as complicated as it may otherwise seem. You can vary the modes of exercise (cycling, treadmill, free weights, machines), the volume of exercise (total sets and repetitions or the distances traveled), the order of exercises performed, the speed of performing each repetition (slow or fast), the surface an exercise is performed on (stable or instable, flat or inclined, hard or soft), the rest intervals between sets (20 seconds to 2 minutes), the workload (light or heavy), the rate of loading (power and plyometrics), and the list goes on and on.

If you are training for endurance events like 10K runs, marathons, or triathlons (when you crave pain), then you can also add variation to your workouts by changing the terrain you train on (hills, sand, roads, and trails), the distances you train (daily and weekly), adding resistance (bigger tires, less efficient bikes, baggy clothing), adding some speed work on a track, integrating sprints or hills periodically to your distance runs (Fartlek training), and interval work (alternated with base training).

Variation is probably the single most important benefit my clients get having me as their trainer. No two workouts are alike and their bodies are constantly adapting to different modes of exercise. You don't have to have a degree in exercise science to apply these principles. Just like you might take a different route to work to save time or get a change of scenery, you can change the "roadmap" of your workouts too. The more you vary them, the better your results will be.

Frequency

The next principle is simple enough: *frequency*. If you aren't pounding the pavement, turning the pedals on your bike, getting to the gym, or "sweating to the oldies" at least 3 to 5 days a week, then you have to make this happen Pronto! If you don't approach this as if your life depended on it (and it probably does), you are unlikely to give it the priority it deserves in your life. If I could do it for you, I honestly would because I love exercise and care about people big time. Unfortunately, it doesn't work this way. Besides me not making money exercising for others, you won't be making any headway either if you don't make the time each week to exercise.

Whenever I meet with a potential client for the first time, I tell them (as I point to the entrance to the health club) "the absolute hardest thing about working out is coming through that front door." I tell them their job is to "get here and I will take it from that point on." So practically speaking, they have one concern on their mind: just get to the gym. The carrot that I give them, which is absolutely true, is "you will always feel better when you leave." I can't tell you how many times my clients have told me they were thinking about not coming saying to themselves: "I was tired." "I had a long day." "My kids were driving me nuts!" But they always thank me for getting them through the door, because they leave feeling energized, alive, and filled with a sense of accomplishment. Always begin with the goal in mind. Your goal in this case is to exercise for 3 to 5 days a week, regardless!

Intensity

More than anything else, I attribute my own success in athletics, personal training, and my own fitness to this principle of success: *intensity*. Or should I say INTENSITY!!! Intensity is what separates the men and women from the boys and girls, the athletes from the weekend warriors, and the great leaders from the average managers. Without the proper intensity, you will waste a lot of time in the gym and in your life. A recent study found that 67% of women exercisers lifting weights were not exercising at an intensity level that would actually produce results. And before you guys say "I told you so" there was another study which confirmed that men weren't much better (60%). Learning to exercise with the proper intensity is probably the single most important thing you can do to ensure you get a lifetime of successful results from exercise.

Do you remember studying for a final exam in high school or college? You may have been thinking at the time, "How am I going to cram a semester's worth of knowledge into my brain in 10 hours of studying." You did it with intensity! The pressure of an impending exam and fear of subsequent failure creates a mental and physical environment in the body which allows you to do more in less time. By releasing a cascade of hormones, the body prepares itself for academic battle. The mind is more alert and focused, information retention and memory recall improve, and you're able to pass the exam with flying colors.

Like you "crammed" for this exam, you can use similar techniques to cram in more exercise too! I really want you to understand this concept, so I am going to teach you several methods to gauge intensity. Most importantly, I want to help you develop the athlete's and warrior's attitude so you can attack your workouts with the same vigor as a Harvard freshman attacks her exams during finals week.

So how do you determine intensity when it comes to exercise? If you were an exercise physiologist working in a university lab, you would probably measure exercise intensity with ventilatory threshold, lactate threshold, VO_2 max, or METS (metabolic equivalents). Let's be frank for a minute here. Most people probably think METS is a baseball team from New York and VO_2 max is a new energy drink. Since you probably aren't working on a research study and don't have access to a computerized spirometer or maybe you don't want to compute the complicated formulas for determining some of these measurements, I prefer to use two fairly simple methods for gauging intensity levels during exercise: perceived exertion and target heart rate.

Rating of Perceived Exertion (RPE): In 1970, Gunnar Borg developed a 6 (no exertion) to 20 (maximal exertion) scale to allow exercisers to subjectively rate their feelings while exercising. I prefer a simpler and more intuitive method of gauging exercise intensity using a scale of 1 to 10, where 1 is your everyday, walk to your car intensity and 10 is a flat out sprint up ten flights of stairs, where eventually, you will have to stop because your heart is pounding out of your chest. You can apply the 1 to 10 scale to corresponding maximum heart rate percentages, where 5 would be 50% of your maximum heart rate and 7 would be 70%, and so on.

Translating it another way, a 3 would be considered a sedentary intensity, a 6 would be considered moderate intensity and 8 to 9 would be considered vigorous intensity. Or you could use the pain scale I use with my clients where 1 is "I'm still asleep"; 3 is "I could do this all day"; 5 is "You've got my attention"; 7 is "Oh my God, this hurts"; 9 is "You're killing me!" and 10 is "I'm dead..." I've only seen 10 hit three times in my training career and fortunately for me and my clients, they all survived...although it did require some ice, a towel, 15 minutes of sitting in a chair praying for air, and a lot of extra TLC (tender loving care).

Working at a true 10 intensity level is a very uncomfortable place to be and not realistic for most people. Personally, I've only hit 10 once in the past few years. In 2007 I was running a 41 floor "stair climb challenge" for the American Lung Association. I was racing (for fastest time) one of the Ironman triathletes I train. She beat me by 15 seconds and it truly felt like my heart was beating out of my chest. My heart rate monitor informed me I had a heart rate of 195 beats per minute! It took me 15 minutes sitting head down in a chair to get the burn out of my lungs and 15 days to recover from the bruise to my ego.

Don't worry, I am not recommending you exercise at this intensity under the ruse: "No pain, no gain." There is a feasible limit and 10 is way beyond what is required to get results. Whether it's cranking out two more muscle-searing reps of squats at a pain intensity of 7 or running incline intervals on a treadmill at 85% of your maximum heart rate, an intensity of 6 to 8.5 will get you great results. Pain is a little too subjective, so if you want a more objective accountability tool for gauging exercise intensity, use your heart rate to guide you. Let's learn how to calculate your own maximum heart rate and how you can apply it to your workouts.

Maximum Heart Rate: Although experts agree there is no universal method to accurately predict maximum heart rate because of significant variances based on age and gender, for the practical purpose of determining exercise intensities for cardiovascular exercise we will use the long accepted empirical formula: 220 minus your calendar age equals your estimated maximum heart rate. For example, I'm 40 years old (at the time I'm writing this) and would calculate my estimated HR_{max} using this method:

Formula: **220 – Age**   **$= HR_{max}$**

Mine: *220 – 40*   *= 180 (beats per minute)*

Yours: *220 – ＿＿＿ = ＿＿＿ (beats per minute)*
　　　　　　　　Age　　　HRmax

Now you may be saying: "Hey, wait a minute. You just told me you had yours up to 195 climbing those stairs last year. Oh, and you lost the race to a woman." Thanks for reminding me, but this illustrates the anti-aging effect that persistent training can have on the heart. Like Dr Michael Roizen, coauthor of *You: The Owner's Manual*, author of *The RealAge® Makeover*, and creator of the RealAge® concept points out, we can have a younger heart. Using his RealAge® concept, I can take my actual maximum heart rate of 195 and subtract it from 220 to get the physiological age of my heart. I'm curious…what is it? *(220 – 195 = 25)* Lucky for me, I have the heart of a 25-year-old. But like the Roman philosopher Seneca said over two thousand years ago "luck is what happens when preparation meets opportunity." I have had a lot of preparation (as well as some favorable genetics) and so will you. With your max heart rate determined, you can now determine exercise intensity as a percentage or "target" of this maximum heart rate. This is called your target heart rate and I can't emphasize enough how using target heart rates in your training will more or less guarantee you results. There is no better way to gauge your exercise intensity levels.

Target Heart Rate: Target or training heart rate is the range or zone of heart rate desired during exercise. Using the 1 to 10 scale discussed previously, you will want to start out exercising in the 6 to 8.5 range which corresponds to 60% to 85% of your estimated maximum heart rate. Exercise physiologists call this the "zero to peak method" and it is determined by multiplying the max heart rate you calculated previously with the lower and higher percentages of your exercise range. Continuing with me as your faithful example, I would calculate my target heart rate range of 60% to 85% like this:

HR$_{max}$ x 0.6 (60%)   = **Lower training range**

Mine: 180 x 0.6 = 108

Yours: _____ x 0.6 = _____
      (HRmax)   (Lower Range)

HR$_{max}$ x 0.85 (85%)   = **Upper training range**

Mine: 180 x 0.85 = 153

Yours: _____ x 0.85 = _____
      (HRmax)   (Upper Range)

Ok, you now have the estimated target heart rate range for your training and you should write those numbers down or memorize them. This is the zone you want to keep your heart rate in when you first get started and I highly recommend a Polar, heart rate monitor (or comparable brands) to help you monitor your heart rate while you exercise. Trying to take your radial or carotid pulse while exercising is a

> ### Heart Rate Monitors
>
> Heart rate monitors are a great tool to have in your exercise tool box and cost anywhere from $60 to $120. Most brands will allow you to program in your target heart rate zone or the device will calculate it for you. Like having a screaming personal trainer by your side, they can be set to alert you if you fall outside your training zone, keeping you motivated and accountable. More current models also include calorie counters to show you how many calories you burn during your workouts.

lot like going on a scavenger hunt and the detection devices included on some types of exercise equipment often fail to give a reading, which can be extremely frustrating when you're exhausted on the treadmill. So before you break the screen on an exercise bike because it won't tell you what you're heart is doing, pick up a decent heart rate monitor from your local sporting goods store or through a reputable online retailer. Just make sure it has a constant heart rate display so you always know what your heart is doing.

After you have been exercising for awhile or if you are already in pretty decent shape, the quality of your heart muscle and its ability to pump blood, called stroke volume, will improve. Since a trained heart can respond differently to exercise than a sedentary one, you will see the importance of the next, and more accurate (but more involved) method of determining your target or training heart rate called the "heart rate reserve or Karvonen method." The Karvonen method factors in resting heart rate (HR_{rest}) to calculate the target heart rate (THR):

$$THR = ([HR_{max} - HR_{rest}] \times \%Intensity) + HR_{rest}$$

Using myself as an example with a HR_{max} of 180 and a HR_{rest} of 53:

At 60% intensity: ([180 – 53] × 0.60) + 53 = 129 bpm

At 85% intensity: ([180 – 53] × 0.85) + 53 = 161 bpm

This gives me a much different target range of 129 – 161 beats per minute when compared to the 108 – 153 bpm I calculated previously using the easier peak method. As you can see, I now have a more tightly defined and higher average training zone using this method. To calculate your own target heart rate zone using this method, you will need to find out what your resting heart rate is.

Determining your Resting Heart Rate

This is calculated first thing in the morning, before you get out of bed and best accomplished by wearing a heart rate monitor all night and looking at the displayed heart rate when you wake normally, without an alarm that shakes you out of bed with 130 decibels of screaming noise (this will jolt your heart unnaturally, if you haven't already guessed). If you don't have a heart rate monitor (you mean you didn't rush out and get one yet?) or don't want to wait until you do, you can determine your resting heart rate by taking your pulse for 60 seconds first thing in the morning when you wake peacefully. Locate your radial pulse by turning your right or left palm up and placing the index and middle fingers of the opposite hand on the wrist joint towards the thumb side. If you have trouble finding it, try to locate your carotid pulse by placing your index and middle finger on the top of your neck just under the jawline beneath your ear and slightly in the direction of the chin. Find which location works best and practice so you are familiar with it before you attempt to do it when you are groggy and half asleep in the morning. Make sure you have a watch with a second hand by your bed so you can determine 60 seconds accurately.

Once you have your resting heart rate HR$_{rest}$ you will also need the max heart rate you previously determined by subtracting your age from 220. Plug these numbers into the following formulas and calculate the answers.

Calculate your training zones:

60% target HR = ([_____ - _____] x 0.6) + _____
     (HRmax)   (HRrest)   (HRrest)

85% target HR = ([_____ - _____] x 0.85) + _____
     (HRmax)   (HRrest)   (HRrest)

Now you are armed and dangerous with information you can use to get more intense and more effective workouts. Whenever you do cardiovascular exercise or circuit-type weight training, strive to keep your heart rate in this range. This will ensure you are working at a high enough intensity to guarantee you results. Exercising at this intensity will likely cause your resting heart rate to go down over time so recalculate your ranges every three to four months. You will also use this heart rate range in both the cardiovascular and strength training programs I provide at the end of this chapter. So the time spent calculating it was well spent. Speaking of time, we now press on to the last of the fitness principles of success, time and type.

Time and Type

The final two principles of success are simple to understand yet require a little planning and discipline: *time* and *type*. How long should we exercise for and what types of exercise should we be doing? Like we discussed at length in the *Exercise Guidelines* section of this chapter, the American College of Sports Medicine and the American Heart Association both recommend you should exercise for at least 30 minutes on most days of the week to ensure good overall health. The Physical

Activity Guidelines for Americans recommend that adults get at least 2½ hours of moderate-intensity physical activity such as brisk walking or 1¼ hours of a vigorous-intensity activity such as running or playing a sport like soccer each week. This covers the "time" requirements and answers the "how long do I need to exercise?" question. What kind of exercise should you do? All credible guidelines recommend *both* cardiovascular exercise (walking, running, biking) and muscle strengthening activities like weight training which covers the "type" of exercise. But what does this really mean?

Let's put things into "real world" perspective and agree that almost everyone can carve out 200 minutes over the course of a week to dedicate to exercise. Research has proven it is the cumulative exercise volume performed each week that is most important, regardless of how you break it down specifically. NOTE: For you talkers out there, each minute means you're running on the treadmill, not running your mouth. Likewise, when you are training with weights, resting for ten minutes between sets so you can socialize or catch up on the latest gossip or sports scores doesn't count toward your exercise time either. Carve out the time and exercise with a purpose.

- ■ Breakdown of 200 minutes of cumulative weekly exercise:
  - 7 days a week for 30 minutes
  - 6 days per week for 34 minutes
  - 5 days per week for 40 minutes
  - 4 days per week for 50 minutes
  - 3 days per week for 65 minutes

The first step is to identify how you will split up the time so you can determine your weekly plan. If you can only get to the gym three days a week, then you will need to plan on exercising for 65 minutes when you go. You will divide each workout into a weight training portion and a cardio portion – i.e. warm-up for 5 minutes, do weight training for 30 minutes and then do cardio for 30 minutes for a grand total of 65 minutes.

If you plan to go to the gym five days a week, then you know you must exercise for at least 40 minutes each visit. Since you are exercising more frequently in this scenario, you may want to split up your workouts into dedicated cardio workouts three times per week and dedicated strength training two times per week, in an alternating fashion – i.e. Monday, Wednesday, and Friday do cardio training for 40 minutes and Tuesday and Thursday (or Saturday instead) do weight training for 40 minutes. If you are participating in a vigorous sport like basketball, hockey, or soccer once or twice a week, this could replace two of your cardio workouts. Just keep in mind that it's best to separate your weight training workouts by at least 48 hours to allow your working muscles to fully recover.

If you are really pressed for time and want an efficient exercise protocol, combine your weight training with integrated conditioning like jumping rope, stair climbing, or treadmill intervals and you knock out two birds with one stone. I use integrated conditioning with many of my clients to maximize caloric expenditure and increase their average heart rate over the course of the workout. Essentially, you alternate two or three strength training exercises with 60 to 90 seconds of vigorous cardio-type activity. In 30 minutes of exercise, you can effectively do both cardio and weight training in this manner. This is one of the essential components of my exercise philosophy I discuss later in the chapter.

Putting it All Together – Exercise Programming

There are so many different ways to exercise and thousands of books have been published outlining individual programs you can do. My intent with this book was not to give you a specific program to follow, per se, but to get you to start and continue to exercise. The specific program you follow isn't as critical as doing it with proper form, doing it with adequate intensity, and doing it consistently. If you want to practice the variation principle, get yourself two or three exercise programs to follow and alternate them weekly or monthly. I will be publishing my own exercise program manual in the very near future, but I do want to give you something to work with to get you started.

For the remainder of this chapter, I give you both a cardio and strength training program you can use. First I will outline a 52 week walking program you can follow to take you from the couch to the finish line of good health. It incorporates all the "Very F.I.T." success principles to maximize your results. I will also share with you my *Menu Workout* system and philosophy to help you successfully plan your weight training workouts. These two programs can be the meat and potatoes of your exercise program for awhile, but eventually you will want to expand your horizons with other programs and activities.

Walking Program

There are so many benefits to walking that I could write a whole book about it (and maybe I will someday). But suffice it to say that regular walking can be done almost anywhere and it will do wonders for your health and well-being. Recent research has determined that regular (brisk) walking can lower the risk of heart attack, stroke, and type 2 diabetes, as well as lower elevated cholesterol and triglyceride levels, improve peripheral circulation, improve insulin sensitivity, and decrease blood pressure. One research study even equated walking to the therapeutic effects of a popular diabetes drug and you get all the positive results without the cost or negative side effects. You don't have to walk a marathon to get the benefits either. As little as a mile a day can do the trick, but for most people, set your sights on three miles a day as your ultimate goal.

I have developed a one year walking program that will take you from "ground zero" (essentially someone who as never exercised) to an extremely high level of cardiovascular fitness. The only tools you will need are a good pedometer (to count your total steps and steps per minute), a heart rate monitor to gauge your intensity level, and either some open road or a treadmill — preferably both. Having both exercise options will give you much needed variety and a treadmill will eliminate the "it's raining so I can't walk today" excuse. It doesn't matter which intensity gauge you use, but you will definitely need the pedometer to count your steps instead of logging miles.

Many studies have proven the benefits of using a pedometer in walking programs. The general consensus of the studies I reviewed is this: when compared to people not using a pedometer, those who did use one increased their exercise compliance, increased their motivation, and walked significantly further distances. A study conducted by San Diego State and Arizona State Universities and funded by the Centers for Disease Control and Prevention determined a step count of 100 steps per minute to be the minimum required to reach a moderate intensity level. Having a pedometer provides an accountability tool so you can gauge your progress, log your steps, and build on what you have done on previous days. There are many good ones on the market and they are available at most sporting goods stores or via online stores. Expect to pay about 15 to 25 dollars.

The following walking program uses total steps to govern the time or duration. To monitor your intensity levels you will use steps per minute (a setting on most pedometers) and percentage of maximum heart rate (as we learned to calculate earlier in this chapter). If you can't get to the assigned steps per minute value in the chart without exceeding the assigned percentage of maximum heart rate value, then use your heart rate to govern intensity until your fitness improves. If you only have a pedometer to use, then periodically check your heart rate with your radial or carotid pulse during each workout to ensure you are in your training zone. You will also be incorporating interval training with work-recovery cycles to add variation, raise your metabolism and improve overall fitness. See the applicable end notes for specific instructions.

Weeks	Frequency	HR Intensity	Time	Ratio	Steps	SPM	SEE NOTES
	per week	%HRmax	minutes	work to rest	total (est.)	steps per min	
Build Aerobic Base							
1 - 2	2	60	15	N/A	1,200	80	
3 - 4	3	65	15	N/A	1,275	85	
5 - 6	3	65	20	N/A	1,700	85	
7 - 8	3	70	20	N/A	1,800	90	
9 - 10	3	75	25	N/A	2,375	95	
11 - 12	4	80	30	N/A	3,000	100	
13	**WEEK OFF (Strength Training Only)**						
Interval Training							
14 - 15	2	85 - 55	28	2 : 2	3,000	110 - 90	1
16 - 17	3	90 - 60	30	1 : 1	3,000	115 - 85	2
Endurance Training							
18 - 19	3	65	40	N/A	4,000	100	
20 - 21	3	65	45	N/A	4,500	100	
Interval Training							
22 - 23	3	85 - 65	30	2 : 1	3,210	110 - 100	3
24 - 25	3	90 - 55	30	1 : 2	2,950	125 - 85	4
26	**WEEK OFF (Strength Training Only)**						
Endurance Training							
27 - 28	4	80	50	N/A	5,500	110	
29 - 30	3	65	60	N/A	6,000	100	
Alternate Training							
31 - 34	3 - 4						
Workout 1	Endurance	65	60	N/A	6,000	100	
Workout 2	Interval	90 - 55	42	1 : 2	3,950	125 - 85	5
Workout 3	Endurance	65	60	N/A	6,000	100	
Workout 4	Interval	85 - 55	40	2 : 2	4,000	110 - 90	6

Combination Training							
35 - 38	3						
Workout 1	*Combination*	65 - 90	48	10 : 2 x 4	5,000	100 - 115	**7**
Workout 2	Endurance	65	60	N/A	6,000	100	
Workout 3	*Combination*	65 - 90	60	a:5:2x4 / b:2:2 x 8	6,500	100 - 120	**8**
39	**WEEK OFF (Strength Training Only)**						
40 -46	*Repeat Alternate Training Protocol*						**9**
47 - 52	*Repeat Combination Training Protocol*						**10**

NOTES

1. Walk vigorously for 2 minutes then walk easily for 2 minutes (Repeat 7 times)

2. *Walk at max speed for 1 minute then walk easily for 1 minute (Repeat 15 times)*

3. Walk vigorously for 2 minutes then walk easily for 1 minute (Repeat 10 times)

4. *Walk max speed (or jog) for 1 minute then walk moderately for 2 minutes (Repeat 10 times)*

5. Walk max speed (or jog) for 1 minute then walk moderately for 2 minutes (Repeat 14 times)

6. *Walk vigorously for 2 minutes then walk easily for 2 minutes (Repeat 10 times)*

7. Walk at moderate pace for 10 minutes then vigorously for 2 minutes (Repeat 4 times)

8. *a: Walk at moderate pace for 5 minutes then jog for 2 minutes (Repeat 4 times)*

   b: Walk at easy pace for 2 minutes then jog for 2 minutes (Repeat 8 times)

9. Extend Workouts 1 and 3 (Endurance workouts) to 75 minutes

10. *Extend Workout 1 to 60 minutes by repeating 10 : 2 ratio 5 times*

The MENU Workout Plan

There has been a lot said, written, and postulated about how to properly workout with weights (resistance training) and I think this has only served to confuse people about what to do when they get to the gym. Consider this brief synopsis of exercise jargon: cardio, endurance, functional, core, agility, flexibility, balance, power, plyometrics, periodization, specificity, split routines, combination training, cross-fit training, cross-training, and circuit training. Sound like French to you? Unless you're an exercise physiologist it should. A lot of people like to spew out the lingo in an attempt to convince others they know what they are talking about. Beware of exercise linguists because if they really cared about you, they would talk to you in terms you can understand.

That being said, which type of exercise program should you follow? For most people, you should be doing some combination of all of these exercise protocols in a systematic, progressive, and enjoyable way. Confused or overwhelmed? Intimidated? Don't know where to begin? Rest assured because you are not alone. This is why hiring a good personal trainer is such a good investment. He or she will eliminate the guess work for you and take you through a properly designed, appropriately intense, progressive workout program ensuring you get positive results without getting injured. (For more about hiring a personal trainer, see Chapter 11.)

For the rest of you who choose not to hire a trainer to get you started, I wanted to develop an easy to follow system of program design to enable you to intelligently construct your own workouts to get maximum benefits and timely results. Wow, that was a mouthful! In other words, I want to give you a simple system to get you results from your workouts. Without further adieu, let's look at the menu.

Unless you were born in a cave and then raised in a jungle, I think it is a sure bet to assume you have eaten at a restaurant at some point in your life. If you're like most Americans, it is probably two to three times a week. Now I'm not talking about going to a typical fast food burger joint where your only decisions are whether or not to get fries with your burger, getting a combo meal or just the sandwich, upgrading to the value-size or super-duper-size, or similar non-formative decisions. I'm talking about a sit-down restaurant where you have about five pages of menu to peruse and decide what you are going to eat to satisfy the seemingly insatiable appetite you think you have. I will also assume that unless you are eating at The Cheesecake Factory, and you are having trouble picking from their 18 or so pages of menu temptations and still leave yourself enough room for a delicious and unique flavor of dessert, that you are able to, under normal circumstances, navigate the menu and make decisions about what you and your restaurant guests are going to eat and drink.

My exercise philosophy for working out with weights and machines is like ordering from a restaurant. You have an appetizer (warm-up), a salad or soup (joint-specific functional exercises and agility), a main course (compound, multi-joint exercises), side orders (isolation, single-joint exercises or integrated conditioning), and a dessert (core training and flexibility exercises). Sound simple enough? Just like you wouldn't order the same thing over and over if you ate at a restaurant three to four times a week, you will want to mix up what you order off my workout menu too. Eventually, you will also want to start going to different restaurants with completely different menus (training variation) or try a particular type of food like French, Italian, or Chinese (specificity training).

By following this program design method, you can feel confident you are performing properly orchestrated, resistance-based workouts. So expand your palate and workout repertoire. Design your workouts by creating different meals from the menu. Before you go to the gym, plan out what you are going to do and (ideally) write it down. Having your workout planned out ahead of time gives you a roadmap to follow and will dramatically improve the quality, intensity, efficiency, and accountability of your workouts. Pick out an appetizer for your warm-up, maybe include a salad of plyometrics, then select a main course of whole body exercises with a couple of sides, and finish with a flexibility cool-down for dessert.

The following is a simplified version of my *Menu Workout*™ plan that you can use to get started. You will still need to become familiar with each exercise and I recommend you seek a professional to teach you proper form, technique, and joint mechanics. If you have internet access you can put the name of the exercise into a search engine and many video links will come up so you can see how it is performed. Since

I don't have control over what people post online, I can't guarantee that the form will be correct. Hopefully it will be close enough to give you an idea of what to do.

Some of the exercises I included in this menu may not be suitable for all individuals. I have provided it primarily to teach you how to structure a workout, not necessarily as a "one size fits all" workout plan, because there isn't such a thing. For the sake of instruction, I have highlighted certain exercises on the menu as an example workout I would have my clients do during an exercise session. The highlighted workout is included at the end of the chapter and you will see that I can get my clients through all of it in less than an hour. Plan your workouts, move with a purpose, and you will accomplish amazing things!

THE MENU WORKOUT™

STARTERS

WARM-UP *raise core temperature*	SETS	REPS	TIME	REST
Walking on a treadmill	1	N/A	7-10 min	N/A
Riding a stationary bike	1	N/A	7-10 min	N/A
Using an elliptical trainer	1	N/A	7-10 min	N/A
Jumping Jacks	3	25	7-10 min	30 sec
Light stretching	1	N/A	7-10 min	N/A
Jumping Rope	3	60	7-10 min	30 sec

SOUPS

AGILITY *neuromuscular coordination*	SETS	REPS	TIME	REST
Agility Ladder Drills	3	N/A	5 min	30-45 sec
Cone Zig-Zags	3	N/A	5 min	30-45 sec
Shuttle Runs	3	N/A	5 min	30-45 sec

SALADS

PLYOMETRICS *dynamic muscular activation*	SETS	REPS	TIME	REST
Line Hops	1 - 3	10 - 20	5 min	1 min
Squat Jumps	1 - 3	5 - 15	5 min	1 min
Cone Jumps	1 - 3	10 - 20	5 min	1 min
Depth Drops	1 - 3	5 - 15	5 min	1 min
Box Jumps	1 - 3	5 - 15	5 min	1 min

MEDICINE BALL *dynamic muscular activation*	SETS	REPS	TIME	REST
Overhead Bounce *"kill the ant"*	1 - 3	10 - 20	3 min	1 min
Overhead Jump Toss *"shootin' hoops"*	1 - 3	10 - 20	3 min	1 min
Lateral Throws *"swinging a bat"*	1 - 3	10 - 20	3 min	1 min
Diagonal Bounce *"wood chops"*	1 - 3	10 - 20	3 min	1 min

SIDES

SIDES ONLY SERVED WITH MAIN COURSE ENTRÉES

ISOLATION EXERCISES		STABILIZATION EXERCISES	
Leg Extensions	Quadriceps	Isoprone Abs	"Planks"
Leg Curls	Hamstrings	Single-leg Squats	Legs and Hips
Calf Raise	Gastrocnemius / Soleus	Lateral Lunges	Legs and Hips
Shrugs	Trapezius	Scaption	Shoulders
Side Lateral Raise	Deltoids	SB* Curl-ups	Abs / Core
Chest Fly	Pectoralis Major / Minor	SB* Chest Press	Chest / Triceps / Core
Bicep Curls	Biceps aka "The Guns"	SB* Squats	Legs / Core
Tricep Extensions	Triceps	BOSU™ Squats	Legs / Core
Wrist Curls	Forearms	BOSU™ Push-ups	Chest / Triceps / Core
* - Stability Ball (Swiss Ball)		BOSU™ Deadlifts	Legs / Core

MAIN COURSE ENTRÉES

WHOLE BODY *for the hearty appetite*	SETS	REPS	TIME	REST
Squats	3	8 - 12	5-8 min	60 - 90 sec
Deadlifts	3	8 - 12	5-8 min	60 - 90 sec
Front Squats to Push Presses	3	8 - 12	5-8 min	60 - 90 sec
Hang Cleans or Single-arm Dumbbell Cleans	3	8 - 12	5-8 min	60 - 90 sec
Barbell Stiff Leg Deadlifts to Bentover Rows	3	8 - 12	5-8 min	60 - 90 sec
Kettlebell or Dumbbell Swings	3	8 - 12	5-8 min	60 - 90 sec
Standing Barbell or Dumbbell Push Presses	3	8 - 12	5-8 min	60 - 90 sec

LEGS	SETS	REPS	TIME	REST
Squats *Bodyweight, Machine, Hack, Smith, Barbell*	3	8 - 12	5-8 min	45 - 60 sec
Leg Press *Machine, Lying, Horizontal*	3	8 - 12	5-8 min	45 - 60 sec
Bench Step-ups *Bodyweight, Dumbbell, Barbell*	3	8 - 12	5-8 min	45 - 60 sec
Lunges *Bodyweight, Dumbbell, Barbell*	3	8 - 12	5-8 min	45 - 60 sec
Front Squats *Dumbbell, Barbell*	3	8 - 12	5-8 min	45 - 60 sec
Deadlifts *Straight-leg, Romanian, Single-leg*	3	8 - 12	5-8 min	45 - 60 sec

BACK and BICEPS	SETS	REPS	TIME	REST
Pull-ups *Palms Away*	3	max	3-5 min	45 - 60 sec
Chin-ups *Palms Toward*	3	max	3-5 min	45 - 60 sec
Machine or Cable Pull-downs *Wide or Reverse Grip*	3	8 - 12	5-8 min	45 - 60 sec
Bentover Barbell Rows *Overhand or Reverse Grip*	3	8 - 12	5-8 min	45 - 60 sec
Dumbbell Rows	3	8 - 12	5-8 min	45 - 60 sec
Machine or Cable Rows	3	8 - 12	5-8 min	45 - 60 sec

CHEST, SHOULDERS, and TRICEPS	SETS	REPS	TIME	REST
Barbell Bench Presses *Flat, Incline, Decline*	3	8 - 12	5-8 min	45 - 60 sec
Dumbell Bench Presses *Flat, Incline, Decline*	3	8 - 12	5-8 min	45 - 60 sec
Push-ups *On Knees, Standard, Feet Elevated, Weighted*	1 - 3	max	3-5 min	45 - 60 sec
Dips *Assisted, Bodyweight, Weighted*	1 - 3	max	3-5 min	45 - 60 sec
Overhead Press *Dumbbell, Barbell - Seated or Standing*	3	8 - 12	5-8 min	45 - 60 sec
Upright Rows *Cable, Dumbbell, Barbell*	3	8 - 12	5-8 min	45 - 60 sec

DESSERTS

AFTER YOU CLEAN YOUR PLATE

CORE AND ABS	FLEXIBILITY AND REHAB		
	Static Stretching		*Self Myofacial Release*
Crunches *Floor, Machine, Stability Ball*	Calves	Cobra	Calf
Curl-ups / Sit-ups	Quads	Scorpion	Hamstring
Reverse crunch / Pike Leg Raises	Hamstrings	Neck	Quad
Hanging Knee or Leg Raises	Hip Flexors	Traps	Glutes
Decline Board Curl-ups	Glutes	Deltoids	Hip Flexor
Cable Woodchop *(high to low)*	Lower back	Bicep	IT Band
Cable Woodchop *(low to high)*	Lats	Tricep	Lower Back
Cable Lateral Rotation	Chest	Forearms	Romboids
Machine Crunch	Spinal Rotation		Lats
Cable Crunch	Lying Leg crossover		Traps
Russian Twists			

Foam Rolling (spanning right section)

157

Trainer's Notes

Warm-up: Performing a good five to seven minute warm-up is important before you begin more vigorous exercise. Essentially it is a progressive physiological preparation for your heart, lungs, working muscles, joints, ligaments, and tendons. It decreases the likelihood of cardiovascular complications and musculoskeletal injuries. An effective warm-up will include the large muscle groups, elevate the heart rate, increase body temperature, and lubricate the joints with synovial fluid (oil for the joints). If you are exercising first thing in the morning, you may need a longer warm-up (10 to 15 minutes) to get the body ready for intense exercise.

Dynamic muscular activation: After a thorough warm-up, your muscles are ready for agility and plyometrics type exercises which can put a significant amount of stress on the muscles and joints. Agility exercises facilitate neuromuscular coordination which can improve the way your brain recruits muscles when you move. Plyometric exercises involve rapid eccentric contractions (lengthening) followed by rapid concentric contractions (shortening) which challenges the nervous system to recruit fast-twitch muscle fibers to perform these powerful, explosive movements. This is why you should do them at the beginning of the workout when your body is fresh. I'm not saying it is impossible to do them at the end of the workout, just inadvisable. You will be more likely to injure connective tissue (tendons and ligaments) if you attempt these type exercises when your muscles are fatigued.

Stability training: When it comes to working out, stabilization exercises are like McDonald's french fries...everyone loves them. I often see trainers trying to impress their clients by doing countless exercises on stability balls, BOSU trainers, core boards, and Airex balance pads and some of the things people can do should be considered for the next Cirque du Soleil show. The reality however, is this: unless you are a hockey player, ice skater, professional skate boarder, or are competing for a position in the Flying Wallendas, you don't need to devote much time to stabilization training.

The problem with spending the majority of any workout on an unstable surface is its effect on force production and muscular threshold recruitment. Exercise physiologists have proven conclusively that force production decreases significantly when you are on an unstable surface. Many trainers point to the fact that training on an unstable surface improves dynamic muscular activation which I would agree with. In other words, more of your muscles are firing to keep you balanced. This shouldn't be confused with force production though, which is the amount of force your muscles produce during contraction. If you compare the increase in muscular activation you get on an unstable surface with its corresponding decrease on force production, you are left with less total muscle fiber contractions compared to doing the same exercise on a stable surface with more weight (better force production). Stable surfaces are also more functional in that they more closely resemble what people actually encounter in the real world. Don't get me wrong, I still believe stabilization training is important, especially as people get older. Just try to limit the time you spend on these exercises to about 30% of your workout. This is why I have included them as a "side order" in my *Menu Workout* philosophy.

Main course exercises and side orders: Design the bulk of your workouts (60 – 70% of allotted time) to accomplish compound, multi-joint, main course exercises like the suggestions I've included and intersperse them with two or three "side order" type isolation and stabilization exercises. Advanced weightlifters who are exercising four or more days of the week can divide their training into a "split routine" by focusing on specific muscle groups during each workout (i.e. legs on Monday, back and biceps on Tuesday, and chest, shoulders, triceps on Wednesday then take a day off and start the sequence over).

The most efficient way of training is by using a "push-pull" system of training alternating push (away from the body) type exercises with pull (toward the body) type exercises or by alternating upper body exercises with lower body exercises. This allows you to perform the maximum amount of workload volume in the minimum amount of time and simultaneously keep your average heart rate higher. While your push or upper body muscles are working, the pull or lower body muscles are recovering and vice versa. If you want to take it a step further, mix in a side order type exercise after the push-pull exercises to make a circuit. By mixing up the menu, the possibilities are endless!

Flexibility and core training: In the summer of 2007, I attended the National Conference of the National Strength and Conditioning Association in Atlanta and one of the most controversial and well-attended lectures was titled: "Flexibility: Friend or Foe?" During the presentation, intelligent arguments both for and against stretching were made and to date there is no definitive research proving that stretching reduces your chance of getting injured. What is agreed upon is that stretching after your workouts can speed your recovery and decrease muscle soreness. So I would say if you have five to ten extra minutes at the end of your workouts, stretch until your heart's content or learn how to release tension in your muscles with foam rolling.

Similarly, core and abdominal training should be reserved for the end of the workout so these stabilizing muscles of the spine and torso are fresh during the intense main course exercises you should be focusing your workouts on. Many people don't realize how much work their abdominal muscles get when you are doing a heavy set of squats, a reverse grip pull-down, or even the classic push-up. If you perform your main course exercises with appropriate intensity, your core and abs will get sufficient work. Treat crunches and similar exercises like dessert and do them at the end of your workout.

Integrated conditioning: For maximum efficiency from your available workout time (especially if you can only workout two or three days a week), you will have to include some conditioning type training with your weight training. This technique is also extremely beneficial for anyone with the primary goal of losing weight or for individuals who compete in sports which require strength and conditioning like mixed martial arts or wrestling. To employ integrated conditioning into your *Menu Workout*, simply perform two or three strength exercises then immediately do 30 to 90 seconds of a cardio type activity. Jumping rope, jumping jacks, box step-ups, riding a stationary bike, running some stairs, or doing a treadmill jog are ideal for this purpose. Instead of resting on your butt between sets (like so many people I see at the gym), you will be working your butt off — literally and figuratively.

Let me give you a typical example I like to do with my clients. I will have them perform an intense set of bench press or push-ups (push exercises), followed immediately by heavy pull-downs or pull-ups (pull exercises), then have them run up and down five flights of stairs (integrated conditioning). We may repeat this sequence two to three times depending on how much time we have and what their level of conditioning is.

Want another example? If I'm in a particular foul mood or just want to torture someone, I will have them do a set of Smith machine squats (push), followed by a set of barbell bent-over rows (pull), followed by a set of barbell push-press (push), and complete the journey of the "pain train" with a set of jump pull-ups (pull). Then just like your favorite pitchman would say during an infomercial: "But wait! There's more. If you order right now, you will get a set of jump squats absolutely free! " All kidding aside, this is an intense sequence that will challenge even the best athletes, yet I can coach my clients through it after consistent effort on their part.

Cardio and weight training on the same day: If you plan on doing your weight training and a separate cardiovascular-type workout on the same day, I would recommend you do the weights first then do your cardio. If you ask 10 trainers what they would recommend in this scenario, you would probably get five who would say do cardio first and the other five would say do weights first. The logic I use in my recommendation is based on fuel preference and the overall effect on metabolism. Since weight training will have the most overall impact to your metabolism and uses blood sugar and muscle glycogen as its preferred fuel, it makes sense to me to prioritize it in a combination workout.

By performing your weight training first, you will deplete glycogen stores so that when you follow it with cardio training, you will ignite your fat-burning furnace sooner than you would if you do the cardio first (relatively speaking). If you do cardio first, you will use up some muscle glycogen and lower your blood sugar levels, which will affect your ability to lift weights with true intensity. Exercise studies support me in this belief and over the course of 12 weeks, you will be stronger, leaner, and have a higher metabolism by lifting weights before your cardio. Many of my clients have learned this the hard way when they do cardio before our training sessions thinking they were going above and beyond. Inevitably though, they run out of gas before we finish because they depleted their fuel stores on the treadmill. That being said, if you feel like doing your cardio exercise first gets you going and puts you more in the exercise groove before you lift weights, then by all means, do what works for you. I am just thankful you are doing both and I would congratulate you on that.

Cross-Training: When it comes to your total training plan, make sure to incorporate activities you enjoy to prevent boredom, monotony, and burnout. If you love being on the water, you can incorporate kayaking, surfing, waterskiing or windsurfing into your exercise plan. If you like competition, join a recreational league for whatever sport or sports you enjoy. Just make sure you schedule them consistently because kayaking the bayou once every 45 days does not constitute an exercise plan. If you don't make it to the trails for some mountain biking or to the water for some wakeboarding, then get your butt to the gym for a workout.

Gym Etiquette: If you are using a commercial exercise facility for your workouts, it is important to realize that you are sharing the space, time, and equipment with others. Just like you wouldn't want someone to invade your home with foul language, dirty shoes, or a careless attitude, you shouldn't be inconsiderate either when you go to the gym. They say ignorance is bliss and unfortunately I've seen lots of ignorant people over the years. Consider yourselves enlightened after you read and follow these twelve basic rules of gym etiquette.

1. **Sweaters:** Wipe down equipment after you're done using it. No one wants to sit in your puddle of sweat.

2. **Gym clutter:** Put the free weights and weight plates back into their appropriate place when you're done using them (even if the person before you didn't because two wrongs don't make a right).

3. **Daydreamers:** Don't "daydream" on equipment for more than 2 minutes. Focus on what you're doing while you're there and lift with a purpose.

4. **Walkers:** Don't waste time lifting a one pound dumbbell when 8 lbs is what you should be lifting (I call this "walking in the gym").

5. **Talkers:** Don't hold a detailed conversation with someone who is trying to exercise. A quick hello is ok, but save the socializing for when you are both finished.

6. **Screamers:** Screaming like a circus monkey is unnecessary and distracting to others. Motivation comes from within.

7. **Potty mouths:** Profanity and discussing inappropriate topics within earshot of others is inappropriate and violates the rules and regulations of most health clubs. Avoid it.

8. **Cell phone addicts:** Long-winded conversations and constant chirps from text messaging drives most people nuts. If you must have your phone with you, turn the ringer off and take your conversations outside.

9. **Equipment hogs:** If you are circuit training or doing 10 sets of squats on the only squat rack in the gym, you must allow

people to work in. In other words, you can't hold 10 pieces of equipment or one unique piece for your exclusive use. Share and you may get a new friend or spotter in the process.

10. **Litter bugs:** Don't leave your trash, empty bottles, or used paper towels for someone else to clean up. A little respect goes a long way.

11. **Cling-ons:** If you are walking on an incline treadmill at 15 degrees but holding on for dear life, back the angle down a bit and let go. Grabbing on and leaning back negates the relative angle and the additional calories you are trying to burn.

12. **Streakers, Stinkers and Sneakers:** Wearing improper attire, splashing on too much perfume or cologne, wearing clothes that haven't been washed, or wearing open-toed shoes or sandals can be distracting to others or dangerous to yourself (save the bikini top sports bras and flip-flops for the beach).

Example workout: The following example workout illustrates how I take items from the Menu and put it into a meal. This particular workout would take approximately 70 minutes (57 minutes of work with 13 minutes of rest). You can construct an infinite amount of workouts in this way, as long as you stick to the tips I described previously. I always divide the workout into three phases: phase one - *Starters*; phase two - *Main Courses and Sides*; and phase three - *Desserts*. Pay particular attention to the time spent on each area of the Menu. The warm-up coupled with agility, plyometrics, and medicine ball work takes 16 minutes or 23% of the total workout time. The main courses and sides take 45 minutes or 64% of the total workout time. And the dessert which includes core work and flexibility takes 9 minutes or just under 13% of the total time. Based on the allotted time, you can see where the "meat and potatoes" of this workout can be found. If you have less time per workout, simply stick to the percentages so that most of your available time is spent doing the exercises in the main course section of the *Menu Workout*.

EXAMPLE WORKOUT

STARTERS

WARM-UP *raise core temperature*	SETS	REPS	TIME	REST
Walking on a treadmill	1	N/A	7 min	N/A
AGILITY *neuromuscular coordination*				
Shuttle Runs	2	N/A	3 min	45 sec
PLYOMETRICS *dynamic muscular activation*				
Cone Jumps	2	20	2 min	1 min
MEDICINE BALL *dynamic muscular activation*				
Overhead Bounce *"kill the ant"*	1	20	1 min	N/A
Lateral Throws *"swinging a bat"*	1	10	1 min	N/A
Totals:	**9**	**50**	**14 min**	**2 min**

MAIN COURSE ENTRÉES and SIDES

Triple Set *complete each in succession*	SETS	REPS	TIME	REST
Front Squat to Push Press	3	8 - 12		60 - 90 sec
Pull-ups	3	max	15 min	*after each*
BOSU™ Squats	3	20		*triple set*
Triple Set *complete each in succession*		120		
Leg Press	2	8 - 12		60 - 90 sec
Deadlifts *Romanian*	2	8 - 12	10 min	*after each*
Calf Raise *Seated*	2	12 - 15		*triple set*
Super Set *complete back to back*		70		
Barbell Bench Press *Incline*	2	8 - 12	5 min	45 - 60 sec
Dumbbell Rows	2	8 - 12		
Super Set *complete back to back*		40		
Upright Rows *Cable, Dumbbell, Barbell*	2	8 - 12	5 min	45 - 60 sec
Push-ups *Feet Elevated*	2	max		45 - 60 sec
Totals:	**25**	**300**	**35 min**	**10 min**

DESSERTS

CORE AND ABS	SETS	REPS	TIME	REST
Crunches *Stability Ball*	2	20	90 sec	30 sec
Hanging Knee Raises	2	10	90 sec	30 sec
FLEXIBILITY AND REHAB				
Static Stretching				
Lower back	1	1	30 sec	N/A
Hamstrings	1	1	30 sec	N/A
Self Myofacial Release				
Glutes	1	1	90 sec	N/A
Lower Back	1	1	30 sec	N/A
Romboids	1	1	30 sec	N/A
Lats	1	1	30 sec	N/A
Traps	1	1	30 sec	N/A
Totals:	**25**	**300**	**8 min**	**1 min**

CHAPTER SIX:

Motivate Yourself

> *"When you work you fulfill a part of earth's furthest dream,*
> *Assigned to you when the dream was born,*
> *And in keeping yourself with labor*
> *You are in truth loving life,*
> *And to love life through labor is to be*
> *intimate with life's inmost secret."*
>
> Kahlil Gibran, *The Prophet,* circa 1923

Are You Lost in Love or in Love to be Lost?

Just last weekend I traveled to Charlotte, North Carolina to visit a really great friend of mine and we definitely had a blast. While I was enroute I had to change planes in Atlanta and had a little time to kill. Since Hartsfield is such a busy airport, I decided to make some observations about the people I saw walking by and put the dismal statistics on overweight and obese Americans to the test. Since the numbers lead us to believe that two out of every three people are overweight in our country, I expected to see herds of cattle-size humans meandering by on their way to the feeding trough of fast food restaurants in the food court. Fortunately, this was not what I saw in the thousands of people I observed that day. Maybe we're not as bad off as the media, actuaries, and research scientists have made us out to be; or maybe overweight people don't fly; or maybe we have learned to better disguise our weight; or maybe all the heavy people were hitching rides in those golf cart sky cabs with the annoying horns barking at you from behind. Whatever the case was, my little experiment didn't corroborate the scientific data… but then again, my observations were hardly scientific.

Once I arrived back in Tampa, I did finally see what I was looking for but it led me to an unexpected conclusion. On the tram ride back to the main terminal, I saw a couple in their late 50's or early 60's who were talking to each other in that easy and familiar husband and wife kind of way. The wife was thin and unassumingly attractive, put together well, and had an air of calm about her. The husband lumbered painfully in his khaki slacks and the green short-sleeve golf shirt he had stretched over about 150 excess pounds of good living. His face was red, his breathing was labored, and he seemed anxious and uncomfortable. During my half hour drive home, my thoughts kept drifting back to this man and his wife. I knew that if he didn't change the course he was on, he was on his way to an early grave, no doubt about it. I thought to myself: *Is she prepared to lose this man? What's going to happen when his apparent lack of self-control takes its inevitable toll? Is he even aware that he is trading many future years with his wife for the temporary pleasures of today?*

Despite having a wonderful weekend, I was suddenly upset. I was visualizing a future of pain, suffering and loss. Granted, I can't see into the future, but the prognosis for this man's condition is pretty grim. Either he immediately make some serious lifestyle changes or the consequences of his excess weight will make them for him; except instead of being positive, quality and quantity of life improving changes, they would be changes which involved hospital stays, emergency surgery, cardiac rehabilitation, nutritional intervention, and moving around with dependency on a wheelchair and a caring, but suffering, spouse.

So I ask you now: Do you have a spouse or someone you care about who is on their own self-made path to destruction? Are you on your own ruinous path towards health complications or burdensome dependency on someone else? Are you prepared to live without the person you spend your life with? Are they prepared to live without you? *Are you in love to be lost or are you lost in love and want to do something about it?* If you aren't selfish enough to exercise for yourself, please be selfless enough to do it for the ones you love.

My experience in dealing with these situations over the past 12 plus years has taught me that you can lead a horse to water but you can't make them drink. Like putting on excess weight is an individual decision, taking it off must be an individual decision too. That doesn't mean you can't help them. Drug addicts and alcoholics often need a family intervention to get them to take the necessary steps to institute change in their lives. Likewise, it may take your love, patience and understanding, along with a strong loving nudge in the right direction to get someone you care about to change. I think the best approach is to put yourself in the frame of mind of what your life would be like without this person. Could you manage? I know we all have our fleeting moments when we think we'd be better off without our spouses, family, friends, or significant others, but this is hardly realistic. Think about all the things you would miss about them -- their smile, their laugh, their trusting love, their sweet caresses, their quiet presence by your side, their fireside conversations, their reliable companionship, and all the qualities that make them so unique. Then take the time to write them down in a love letter. You can start the first paragraph with the sentence: "This is what I love about you..." Then start the second paragraph with the sentence: "This is what I'm going to miss about you..." Let them know how many people are touched by their life and how they would be affected if something happened. Let them know you truly care and you want to offer your help and support. And especially, lead by example. Make sure you are taking care of yourself too. I have written this chapter to help facilitate the motivation to start and continue exercising. Whether it's for you the reader, a friend, or someone you love or care about, I hope it helps.

A Labor of Love

The next step to success may prove to be the most difficult for you, but you absolutely, positively must take action and for most people that means getting rid of the excuses that have held you back in the past. In

Napoleon Hill's revolutionary book *Think and Grow Rich* he outlines 30 reasons why people fail. He calls two of these reasons, procrastination and indecision, "twin brothers" because they are so similar in their impact to our lives. Don't put off the decision to start exercising for any reason, because the earlier you start the more lasting and substantial the benefits will be. In fact, ignoring the logical voice in your head telling you to exercise could be detrimental to your immediate health. Some people are just a day or two away from a catastrophic, life-changing health event which can be prevented or delayed with exercise. Remember, the benefits of exercise are immediate and for some people, life saving.

I have heard all the excuses for not exercising (trust me) and I have even fallen victim to these evil demons myself from time to time... *"I'm too busy. I don't have the time. I have kids. I have better things to do. I can't afford it. I don't have the energy. It's too cold out. It's too warm out. I don't know what to do. I can't do it alone. My spouse won't do it. It's too late for me to start. I am too sore. My feet hurt. My back hurts. I have a headache. My favorite TV show is on."* And I could go on and on, but we must learn to change our internal dialogue to a more empowering one. One of my goals in this book is to show you how.

I am on a personal crusade to get America moving!

I will warn you right now that your biggest potential obstacle to success (in any endeavor and especially exercise) will be your own personal motivation. It is absolutely essential for you to keep your motivation high. Let me repeat that... *It is absolutely essential for you to keep your motivation high!* Motivation has the power to move us to take action, but unfortunately, it also has the power to keep us stuck in the lifeless, energy-sapping vortex of the couch too! Galileo originally explained the concept of inertia and Sir Isaac Newton made it his first Law of Motion which is simply stated: An object in motion stays in motion while an object at rest stays at rest (unless an external force acts upon the object).

Applying this concept to your life, it is easier to keep moving in a positive direction once you are moving and it may take some external force, a.k.a. effort, on your part to get the exercise ball rolling in the first place. Inertia is why I tell my clients and friends to go straight from work to the gym without stopping home, because of just that — stopping. Inertia is also why I do body composition measurements every two weeks when a client of mine begins an exercise program. I want them to see the positive changes of exercise happening to their bodies so that they will be motivated to keep the changes going.

Something motivated you to invest in this book, as well as carve out the time required to read it. You must constantly remind yourself of whatever it is that got you to take action in the first place. Later in Chapters 13 and 14 I will cover goals and goal setting in more detail, but you can never underestimate the power goals can have in your life. Every great accomplishment ever accomplished began as an idea. Right now you probably have an idea of what you want to accomplish with exercise (or other areas of your life too) and I implore you to write it down. Pretty please with a cherry on top! Don't over think it. Just complete this sentence... *I want to* _____ *by exercising* _____ *times per week.*

Do this simple task then read what you wrote down at least twice a day (once in the morning and once before you go to bed) and you will be absolutely amazed with the results you will achieve. By writing down a goal and then reading it every day you cement your desires into your subconscious mind. When this happens, the power is unmistakable. It will guide every decision you make (and we make thousands of decisions every day) in the direction of your goal. Without even realizing it, you will be heading in the right direction. Write down your goals and read them again and again!

As far as exercise is concerned, starting a fitness program (initiative) and sticking with it (persistence) will be your first challenge. If you are exercising at home, your hurdle will be getting out the front door for a power walk or onto the treadmill in your spare bedroom. If you are using a health club, follow the advice I give to people at the gym, I tell my clients the hardest part of each workout we do together is walking through the front door. If they promise me and more importantly, themselves, to get through the door, I promise them they will feel a lot better when they walk out the door. And inevitably, they always do. I tell them to focus on the intense feelings of accomplishment and self-worth they have when they leave, so they can recall these same feelings the next time they are having trouble getting the motivation to get to the gym. Hopefully with this technique, along with your powerful goals, you will be compelled to *make the time!*

Everybody can carve out 30 minutes a day to do something crucial for their long-term health and well-being. You have to approach this with the attitude "I can't afford not to!" because you really can't. Excuses are like a virus. They are hard to cure, aren't well understood, can spread person to person, and wreak havoc on our bodies. Prevention is the best medicine, so *make the time!*

Do as I say and do as I do – I practice what I preach

Looking back on 2006-2007, there was a twelve month period in which I was intensely busy. I worked 50 to 60 hours a week, bought one house, sold another house, got married, moved myself and my wife, painted 2,000 square feet of condo walls, studied for and passed my Certified Strength and Conditioning Specialist (CSCS) certification exam, took 9 clients through a 6 week "Biggest Winner" contest, traveled in and out of the country, and researched and wrote a good part of this book. Even with all of these time-devouring commitments, I still carved out three to four hours a week to exercise and move my body. Now please don't get me wrong. I am not telling you this because I want people to think I'm Superman or that I deserve a medal or anything else for that matter. I tell you this simply to illustrate what is possible when you set goals, prioritize your time, and make a commitment to yourself.

Most of my clients and many of the people I know live very busy lives filled with work deadlines, taking care of children, and commuting around town. Yet they carve out time in their schedules for exercise. Some come to the gym and/or exercise outdoors five days a week, some four days, some three days, and some come just twice. By planning and prioritizing their time, they are able to make the time for exercise. This relatively small investment of time and effort helps them live better, healthier, and happier lives. And so can you by following the *1% Principle*.

The 1% Principle

There are ten thousand and eighty minutes in each week of our lives. Dedicating 120 minutes (two total hours) to exercise each week represents just over one percent of your available time and how you choose to use it can add years to your life. This is the *1% Principle*. This small relative amount of time can have a HUGE positive impact on the other 99 percent. By following this principle each week you will: look and feel better, improve the quality of your relationships, improve your self-esteem, improve your attitude, increase your energy, enhance your productivity at work, improve the quality of your sleep, heighten all five of your senses, increase your self-confidence, improve the quality of sex you have and increase the likelihood you will have it, improve your functional health, and most importantly, extend the quality and quantity of your life. No other thing in life can make this claim. Not money, fame, sex, drugs, rock and roll, or even time itself can make this claim. Prioritize your life. Do you think you can find the 1% in your life? I certainly hope so.

Over the course of a week this translates to: 20 minutes on six days, 24 minutes on five days, or 30 minutes on four days. If can only workout on three days of the week, then do at least 40 minutes to get in your 120 minutes of exercise. If you can't even find this time (and you would have to be very persuasive to convince me why), then make your weekends your "health days" by exercising for 60 minutes each day. If you are a glutton for punishment you can do century rides on your bike or train for a 10K run. If you are inclined to like a little less pain, you can go on a two-hour hike, learn to kayak, or play tennis with a competitive friend, or find something else you enjoy. In the grand picture of life I don't care what type of exercise you do, just that you make it a consistent priority throughout your lifetime. Obviously if you have more time, say 2% or even 3%, than devoting more time to exercise will give you more results and benefits. But Rome wasn't built in a day and if you are new to exercise, make one percent your goal and build from there.

How much is your time worth?
If someone was to offer you $10,000 cash money to go sit in a room for 30 minutes, three times a week, I guarantee that you and most Americans could find the time to do it, regardless of any current circumstances. *Exercise should be no different!* We are in an obesity crisis and epidemic in this country and you can choose to be part of the solution or you can choose to be part of the problem. Which direction do you want to go in? Which side of the fence are you on? Being indecisive is not an option because the worst kind of decision is no decision. This may not pertain to you individually, but you probably know someone who could stand to lose some weight for their own health. Obesity is one of the primary risk factors for heart disease and with over 450,000 American adults under the age of 85 dying of heart attacks each year, it's time we do something about it.

Maybe you don't think this affects you and you may be thinking "Why bother?" Let me give you a piece of informational beef jerky to chew on. When our health insurance premiums continue to climb to offset the skyrocketing health care costs of treating problems associated with obesity, you may start to pay attention. The American Insurance Industry estimates that for every 20 pounds of weight people gain, they will spend an additional $500 per year on medical bills. When they can't afford to pay, guess who does? We do. The capable subsidize the health of the incapable. It's a vicious cycle. Medicare and Medicaid are both government programs we pay for with our tax dollars and if our current health trends continue, taxes will have to be increased to cover the additional costs.

You could also end up caring for a loved one or a good friend who is incapable of caring for themselves due to the ravages of an obesity-related disease. Obesity increases risk factors for stroke, heart attacks, cancer, and diabetes, as well as many other diseases. In the year 2000, Americans spent in excess of 119 billion dollars on obesity-related medical costs. By the year 2012, it is estimated to reach 1 trillion dollars! We can't sit around and allow this to happen. Let's get moving America! Just like when someone quits smoking reduces their risk of getting cancer, exercise reduces the risk of obesity and all its associated illnesses. For most people, obesity is something you can prevent or control.

> **"Today's generation of children is the first in history to have a shorter life expectancy than their parents."**
> Rear Admiral Steven K Galson, U.S. Surgeon General (2008)

You or someone you know may dramatically shorten the quantity of years lived and/or the quality of life we are so privileged to have. You may have children who join the thousands of others now suffering from type 2 diabetes, which use to predominantly affect only adults. Based on current estimates, one out of every three children born in the year 2000 will have diabetes sometime during their life. It's time to do something about it… *make the time!*

According to a 2005 published report by Dr William Haskell of Stanford University, 25% of American adults age 18 to 65 get absolutely no leisure time activity and less than 50% of all U.S. adults meet the current guidelines for exercise. My hunch is that it is less than this. Doesn't it seem odd to you that we live in the age of technology in which all these time-saving devices are supposed to help us? Yet somehow we seem to have no time. In my opinion, technology has just made us busier and consumes any opportunity for leisure with more competing demands for our time and attention.

Laptop computers, cell phones, pocket PC's, portable DVD players, text messaging, Blackberries, PDA's, Bluetooth technology, iPods, barcode scanning, touchscreens, drive-thru windows, and "Call ahead" ordering at restaurants are all supposed to help simplify our lives. But how could they? It seems to me that life is now extremely complicated and we have even more expectations placed upon us because of these "convenience" devices. Just 10 years ago, you were allowed to fax documents when you got to your next stop on a business trip. Now you have to email them immediately from wherever you are with your Windows Mobile enabled phone or your laptop using a WiFi network. Taking a flight on a commercial airplane may be the last sanctuary from the information age left. But even that's changing as some airlines are installing technology to get you connected to the internet from 36,000 feet in the air. Yikes! Somebody help us!!!

Well that somebody has to be you. You have to get a handle on your life and all of its demands on your time. I am extremely thankful for the education I received at the U.S. Air Force Academy. Despite taking what seemed like every subject known to man, I can honestly say the best education I received while I was there was in "time management." We had so many demands on our time besides the requisite coursework: military studies, squadron duties, athletic requirements, marching, mandatory meal times, formal military inspections, parades, key personnel visits and speeches, reveille and retreat ceremonies, homework, leadership training and many other responsibilities "as assigned." If you didn't learn to manage your time, you would fail — bottom line. Failure was not an option for me so I learned to prioritize my available time based on what was most important. When push comes to shove, I know you can learn to do it too.

"You can't build a reputation on what you are going to do."
Henry Ford

One simple technique is to incorporate the use of the self-starter "Do it Now" into your life. Whenever you feel procrastination creeping into your thoughts, immediately say to yourself "Do it now!" then go do whatever it is you are telling yourself to do. By using this self-starter consistently, you will rapidly become a doer instead of a dreamer. This technique will reprogram your self-conscious mind to take action and ultimately, you will get more things done. For example, when you come home from a long day at work and all you feel like doing is sitting on the couch, putting your legs up, and relaxing but you hear this little voice in the back of your mind saying "I need to get in my exercise." That's when you say to yourself out loud "Do it now!" and you have to go do it. When I come home at 9pm after a 12 hour day training clients the last thing I feel like doing is working some more, but I say "Do it now!" and force myself to make my food and protein shakes for the following day, pack my gym bag and set it by the door, and prepare something healthy to eat for dinner. If I am not prepared for the next day, then I am planning to fail.

Take a look at the following excuses people have for not exercising and their accompanying action statements. Action statements are empowering, counter-therapy to the disempowering, de-energizing effects of excuses. If these toxic excuses commonly pop into your head or out of your mouth, use the action statement next to it as an antidote. These don't cover all the excuses but you can get the hang of the technique and apply it to any excuse you can come up with.

Excuses...	Action statements...
I'm too busy	I will be more efficient
I don't have time	I will make the time
I can't fit it into my schedule	I will reprioritize my schedule
I work too many hours	Exercise will help me be more productive
I have kids	I will enroll my kids into activities
I don't know how	I will hire a personal trainer
I'm afraid, intimidated, fearful, etc.	I will get over my fears once I get started

We can always find reasons not to do something; the challenge is to find a way *to do* it. Learning to prioritize and incorporate exercise, fitness, wellness, and sound nutrition into your life consistently and permanently, like a good education and a positive attitude, will serve you over and over. A truly small investment of time and effort, will lead to a more fulfilling, enjoyable, productive, functional, emotionally balanced, and longer life. Learn to make the time for exercise because you absolutely cannot afford to go without it.

Do it anyway!

Just the other day I overheard someone telling their workout buddy: "I can't do cardio because it is too boring." This is the most common excuse I hear when it comes to cardiovascular exercise and you know what I say to this excuse? *"So what! Do it anyway!"* Sitting in a hospital for four months recovering from a quadruple bypass is probably pretty boring too. Or maybe being prematurely admitted into a nursing home because you can no longer take care of yourself might be pretty boring. Or maybe losing your feet and ability to walk due to poor circulation from type 2 diabetes might cramp your style a bit too. I can't think of anything worse than losing your functional freedom to do the things you want to do. I realize that sometimes these situations are not avoidable, but the reality for most of us is that they are.

One of the best gems of advice I can give you is to never tell yourself "I can't do something." I have a great friend and old Air Force

4 Reasons for Exercise Dropout

1. Inconvenience (time or location)
2. Lack of variety
3. Lack of enjoyment
4. Exercising alone

buddy named Jeff who always used to tell his airmen: "Can't never could, so don't be can't." Can't is a self-defeating word and it programs your subconscious to follow through. *Beliefs create reality,* so if you believe you can't do something, then reality will confirm your own self-limiting expectations. Come on, believe in yourself a little bit. Because the flip side is also true. Like W. Clement Stone and Napoleon Hill stated in their book *Success Through a Positive Mental Attitude:* "Whatever people can conceive and believe, they can achieve."

I like to tell my clients: *The body can do it if the mind will allow it.* If you choose not to do something, make it a choice. Instead of saying: "I can't play cricket" say "I choose not to play cricket because I don't look good in white." Or instead of saying: "I can't hit a golf ball 300 yards" you could say: "I choose not to hit a golf ball 300 yards because I don't want to invest two hours a day practicing and refining my swing power." There's a big psychological difference. Other than defying the physical laws of the universe, there are few things we truly can't do. As it applies to cardio training, do whatever you have to do. Watch TV, read a book, load up your mp3 player with audio books or music you truly enjoy, join an exercise group or club, or take fitness classes.

If you are the responsible nurturing type, buy a dog of a breed that requires a lot of exercise. Not only will you both benefit from the obligatory exercise, but you will satiate your maternal or paternal instincts and gain an unconditional friend to boot. This gives you an all important purpose in life and studies show that pet owners live longer. If you can't handle all the responsibilities of dog ownership but still enjoy their company, many communities have instituted dog walking programs. Call your local animal shelter or Humane Society and ask if they have a volunteer dog walking program or position. They will most likely welcome you with open arms and open paws.

If you are a mother with a small child, buy one of those deluxe big wheel strollers and map out a couple of neighborhood routes to alternately walk each day. One of my clients heeded this advice and when she reported back to me, I learned there are now strollers outfitted with integrated speakers, an iPod docking station, cup holders and even cruise control. Ok, I'm kidding about the cruise control, but I hope you get the point. She now gets beneficial exercise, some quality time with her husband (if he goes with), and some fresh air for both her and her daughter.

If you think you can't afford something like this, don't rule it out. Check out web services that specialize in recycling usable goods like Yahoo's FreeCycle and FlipSwap. Also look at craigslist, Play It Again Sports, the Salvation Army, local thrift stores or query your friends and family. They may have a stroller they're not using or know someone who is ready to get rid of one. Remember the six degrees of separation? Put the word out and you may be surprised how rapidly you find what you are looking for.

If you have a favorite TV show or enjoy watching sports like I do, arrange your life so you can knock out two birds with one stone. On a past Sunday during football season, I wanted to watch my favorite football team play. So I drove a little out of my way to one of our health clubs which has individual flat panel TVs on all the cardio equipment. Unfortunately my team lost, but the time flew by and I ended up doing more exercise than I was originally planning. When you take your mind off what your body is doing, cardio time goes by much faster. There are many great gyms out there and with the increasingly competitive environment for your membership dollars, you should be able to find a club with some kind of mental distraction for your cardio time.

If you prefer to exercise at home, get one or two good cardio machines and a small flat screen TV. In as little as 100 square feet, you can have your own cardio gym and watch your favorite show while you work your heart and burn fat at the same time. Record motivational or educational TV shows you enjoy and save them for your exercise time. You will soon begin to associate cardio with these pleasurable activities and will look forward to it. Exercise your body and mind simultaneously. What a winning combination.

If you are passionate about reading, use your exercise time to read. One of my clients has read hundreds of books while burning calories on our treadmills, elliptical trainers, and exercise bikes. Her enthusiasm for reading is now permanently linked with cardiovascular exercise. I'll give you a quick tip from my own personal experience. Get yourself a large binder clip to hold the pages open while you crank those pedals. It will keep your hands free and save you a little frustration with the pages turning by themselves. If you are a technofile, you might want to invest in a Nook, iPad, or Amazon's Kindle. These display devices allow you to flip through the pages of a book without flipping pages. You can also enlarge the type for better visibility, if necessary. Just think, you could be burning through the pages of my next book while burning calories too.

My "Health Stimulus Package"

Like George W. Bush signed into law the Economic Stimulus Package in 2008 to infuse some much needed dollars into the economy, I am proposing my Health Stimulus Package to get Americans moving to create health, wealth, and abundance in our great nation. Maybe you currently are unable to afford all the healthy "perimeter foods" at the grocery store because their cost has increased over 20% (my grocery bill is around $110 a week for just two people), but you can't *not* afford to invest 30 to 60 minutes of your time exercising three to five days a week. If you're forced by budgetary considerations to eat more of the cheaper processed foods in the center of the store, at least you can offset most of their negative health and waistline consequences with consistent trips to the gym.

I consider myself very fortunate today because I can afford organic produce, hormone and antibiotic-free milk, eggs and low-fat dairy products, as well as fresh fruits, vegetables, lean meats, fish, and double fiber bread. But I'm all too familiar with the impact a dwindling bank account or lack of a paycheck can have on your trips to the grocery store. I know there are many people out there who are currently suffering under the stress of the current global economy. I encourage you to persevere and keep hope alive in your life. Precious metals are purified with high heat and we are often made better after times of stress too. I have experienced the highs of success and the lows of failure and both have shaped me into the person I am today. Experiences, both good and bad, give us perspective. Embrace each season of your life as a time to learn and grow, even if you have nothing to eat but peanut butter and jelly sandwiches…

Peanut Butter and Jelly Sandwiches

There was a time in my not-so-distance past when I was at my lowest of lows financially, my fridge and pantry were almost completely bare and I was surviving on hope, prayers and a lot of ramen noodle soup, peanut butter and jelly sandwiches, and 4-for-a-dollar boxes of mac-n-cheese. The dreaded day came when my gas tank and bank account were both empty, I wasn't sure when I would make another small sales commission, and even the peanut butter I was scraping by on ran out.

My saving grace during this time in my life was my sister Michelle who came by one day to swap cars for a supposed "errand" requiring my larger vehicle. I remember being embarrassed when I told her I didn't have much gas left but she just shrugged it off. When I got into my car after work that night, my previously empty gas tank was full and I came home to a refrigerator full of food and a completely stocked pantry with a big jar of my favorite peanut butter sitting front and center on the middle shelf. I literally collapsed on the floor and started crying. Sometimes you don't know how much you miss something until it's gone and then you get it back. Even simple things like bread and peanut butter can be taken for granted.

That day marked an important turning point in my life when I decided to give up building other people's dreams to pursue my own passion in fitness training and I've never looked back. It was on that night that I sat down and originally conceived the idea for this book and wrote down a goal for myself to complete it. With about four years of persistent effort and the powerful guiding light of my goal, this book is now in your hands. The moral of the story is good things can come from the dire circumstances in our lives.

I am so grateful for all of life's experiences which collectively shape who we are and what we can accomplish. Don't ever give up on yourself even when the going gets tough. You can never underestimate the value of your family and friends. They will be there with you to celebrate the victories and lend a helping hand when things aren't going your way. I still have a peanut butter and jelly sandwich once a week to remind me to enjoy the simple things in life and never take them for granted.

The point of telling you that story is that I understand there are times, circumstances, and situations in our life which dictate what and when we get to eat. Not everyone can afford the luxury of stocking their grocery carts with the unprocessed, whole foods I and countless others recommend. But everyone, I'm convinced, can afford to exercise like I have done throughout my life. Exercise can offset most of the caloric, glycemic, and hormonal impact of eating high *calorie per dollar* foods like rice, pasta, chips, potatoes, pizza, donuts, cookies, and dessert cakes. My daily workouts kept me physically and mentally fit when I had nothing else going for me, and like my sister, they were and still are my saving grace. If you can relate to this story or know of someone caught in a similar predicament, the best thing you can do for yourself or for them, is to start exercising. As an investment of your time, energy, and effort, exercise will pay a lifetime of dividends to your health. If what I've communicated makes a difference in your life, I sincerely hope you will pay it forward to someone else.

Since I wet your appetite with some food talk, I can't think of a better time to segue to the skeleton in many people's closet...nutrition. Even though exercise is the most important component of your health, the impact of the foods we eat (good and bad) can't be overlooked. What we should eat, how much we should eat, and when we should eat are all addressed in the following chapter. You will most importantly learn my *Ten Commandments of Nutrition* which will serve to guide you in every future decision concerning food. The truth will set you free!

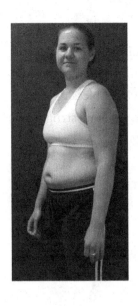

Kimberly

Age: 25
Project Manager

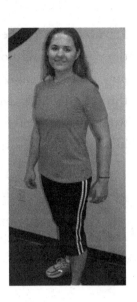

What started as a New Year's resolution changed my life!

In six months, I lowered my bodyfat by 12% and lost over 34 pounds of bodyfat, lost 7 inches off my waist, and lost 5 inches off my hips… and gained my life back!

"The last six months have changed my life. As my New Year's resolution, I set out to lose the 30 plus pounds I gained since high school. What I didn't realize though was the shell I crawled into because I was ashamed about my weight. Because it came on slowly but steadily each year, I didn't feel like anything was wrong. That was until I saw an old picture and the reality of the extra weight and 6 more dress sizes set in.

At first I was sad and felt powerless, but then I decided to do something about it and that's when I met Matt. He sat down with me and we talked about what got me into this situation and how we were going to get out of it. He is a great listener and together we came up with a plan to get me to my goal.

My strength has improved, I lost close to 35 pounds, and I have my health back. My cholesterol and blood pressure are back down and

I'm no longer in the obese category. At 25 yrs old, I shouldn't have those worries and now I don't. I used to dread going to the store but now I actually enjoy shopping and have more confidence to do other things. Thanks to Matt for all his help. He truly is a blessing and I would recommend his training and information to anyone struggling like I was."

- Kim Knitt

CHAPTER SEVEN:

Nourish Yourself

"One's philosophy is not best expressed in words;
it is expressed in the choices one makes.
In the long run, we shape our lives and we shape ourselves.
The process never ends until we die.
And, the choices we make are ultimately our own responsibility."

Eleanor Roosevelt
1884-1962, American First Lady

Do you *Eat to Live or Live to Eat?*

Personally, I am definitely a *Live to Eat* personality type, but I practice an *Eat to Live* philosophy by exercising good nutritional judgment most of the time. Which are you? Do you constantly think about food or do you sometimes forget to eat? If you have trouble making food decisions or feel like you could go without eating, you are an *Eat to Live* type. If you could gnaw off your own arm when you haven't eaten for two hours, you are a *Live to Eat* type. My wife likes to joke that she is already thinking about dinner when she is eating her breakfast. She is a strong *Live to Eat* type and when she gets cranky, I know I better get her something to eat *on the double before there is trouble* (before she chews on me).

A Tufts University study of volunteers over the age of 56 who performed weight training exercises for 30 minutes, three times per week, were able to eat 300 more calories per day without gaining weight! This is great news for us *Live to Eat* types and one of the countless reasons I exercise personally. In this and the next chapter, I will discuss nutrition for nourishment and weight loss in great detail. But suffice it to say that if you like to eat like I do, than exercise can be your constant companion to prevent some of the negative consequences of eating too much. That being said, how you eat and what you eat can be just as important to your waistline and overall happiness as exercise is. So let's spend some quality time discussing nutrition.

The Nutritional Road Map to Dietary Success

Waiting to eat until you feel hungry is like waiting to breathe until you feel your lungs burn from a lack of oxygen. I assume you don't go around holding your breath and then suddenly take in a big gulp of air. Likewise, don't "hold your meals" or take big gulps of food either. This is the logic with eating small, frequent meals. Like respiration allows your lungs to constantly supply the cells of your body with oxygen via the bloodstream, frequently eating nutritious, portion-controlled meals allows the digestive system to supply the body's cells with vital nutrients via the bloodstream, as well. These nutrients are essential for tissue repair, hormone function, growth, and energy production. Without them constantly available, the body doesn't perform efficiently or heal properly and we start to feel bad.

In this chapter, I want to present you with a general nutritional philosophy on what and how we should eat and drink. After 20 years of personal experimentation with different eating plans, diets, nutritional protocols, or whatever else you want to call them, as well as extrapolating useful information from countless books and scientific articles on nutrition, I have come up with the fundamental "meat and potatoes" of sound nutrition. I also reviewed the documented dietary habits of long-lived cultures like the Okinawans, Sardinians, and the Nicoyans. I took all that I've learned and boiled it down, reducing it to a simple sauce to complete this informational meal. If you read, understand, and incorporate the nutritional principles discussed in this chapter into your life, you will feel and look better, sleep better, have more energy, and ultimately decrease your risk of most disease. This will synergistically compliment any exercise plan you follow and lead to even better health outcomes. Bon appétit!

Are you running on empty?

Hunger is caused by a complex hormonal feedback system which is triggered when our nutrient fuel tank starts to get low. Going without food for long periods of time (more than four hours) is like drowning without oxygen getting into your lungs. Your body begins to starve and as a survival mechanism, puts out very powerful warning signals to force you to eat. These signals cause sugar, salt, and fat cravings, ultimately leading to uncontrolled, subconscious, and excessive eating. Using an automotive analogy, you probably don't like to risk driving around when the fuel gauge reads "E" for empty, especially when you're facing a long stretch of road with no chance to fill up. (That is unless you are a college student who redirected their gas money into the beer money account and are waiting for the next parental subsidy payment to arrive.) Driving around with a "Full" tank of gas isn't necessarily the best scenario either. With a full tank, your car must move a lot more extra weight (around 6 pounds per gallon) and therefore gets lower gas mileage. So an ideal scenario would be to keep your fuel tank between a quarter and half full. This maximizes gas mileage, allows your car to accelerate faster, and makes it perform better but also ensures you will have enough fuel to get to the next fuel station three to four hours down the road.

Putting food into our human fuel tank follows the same logic. When you eat a huge meal, your body gets less gas mileage and we feel sluggish. The circulatory system has to redirect, or shunt, a lot of blood to the digestive system, leaving less available for the rest of the body. We essentially force the body to prioritize a significant amount of available resources to handle the biochemical burdens of digestion. This is why we feel lethargic after eating a Thanksgiving type feast (although you've probably been led to believe it's the tryptophan in the turkey). When you overburden the body in this way, it rewards you with the overwhelming desire to take a nap. Our regulatory systems say: "Hey bud, it's time to shut you down for awhile so we can go to work on the 2,000 calories you just ate."

The digestive track can process and assimilate only a limited number of nutrients at any given time. Overeating also forces the pancreas to release an excessive amount of the hormone insulin. Think of overeating as wringing out your pancreas like a sponge, squeezing every last drop of available insulin into the bloodstream. That is a lot of unnecessary wear and tear and if you do this habitually over a number of years, you will most likely develop insulin resistance. This is the first biochemical warning sign of type 2 diabetes and something we must try to avoid. The extra calories from large meals are eventually stored as fat and repeating this process over and over leads to weight gain and eventually, to obesity.

If you are already a diagnosed type 2 diabetic or think you may be prediabetic (called "metabolic syndrome" or "syndrome X"), then consult your physician and seek the guidance of a registered dietician. The complications of this disease can be devastating and include weight gain, loss of eyesight, increased risk of heart disease, and serious circulatory problems. Eating a nutritious, low-glycemic diet coupled with sufficient amounts of exercise can make a significant difference. A little prevention goes a long way.

Eating too much food (in terms of calories) is the most prevalent problem with the American or "Western" diet because, quite frankly, we are moving much less these days thanks to automation, computerization, and industrialization. The dichotomy between energy consumed versus energy expended continues to diverge. Despite increasing our sedentary behaviors, we are consuming more calories than we used to. Since the late 1960's, restaurant portions have increased by about 30% and we have reprogrammed our palates as well as expanded our plates to accommodate more food. Put these two facts together and we our moving less and eating more. This is the recipe responsible for our type 2 diabetes and obesity epidemics.

So in addition to controlling the amount of food and drink (by volume) we are eating and drinking, it is important to be cognizant of the caloric density of the foods and drinks we consume. The industrialization of the food supply has allowed farmers and food manufacturers to increase production enough to exceed the caloric demands of the ever-increasing world population. Grocery stores are filled to the brim with cheap, highly-processed, high-calorie foods. If you compared the amount of calories you could fit into a standard size grocery cart from a grocery store in the 1940's with what you could today in a modern supercenter, the difference would be profound. Obviously this is better than the alternative, but the negative consequence of food processing is that we now have extremely calorie-dense "convenience foods" that Mother Nature never intended our bodies to eat. By refining foods to improve shelf-life, transportability, and processing options, our food suppliers have solved one problem but created another. When whole foods are refined, a lot of the fiber, nutrient, and water content are removed. This has left consumers with a limitless supply of high-calorie, low-nutrient foods that can be eaten virtually anywhere at anytime. Unfortunately, most of the highly nutritious and hunger-satisfying fiber and volume of the food has been removed giving us our present day problem…we can eat high-calorie meals in just a few bites.

If you think back to when our great Nation was founded back in the 1700's and tried to put together a 2,000 calorie meal with the foods available then, you better have a table ready to hold all that you would have to eat. I'm visualizing three ears of fire-roasted corn, two yams baked in the family hearth, a small loaf of bread made from stone-ground wheat and churned butter, and a large bowl of cured meat stewed with some mixed garden vegetables. This is a huge meal that would have easily fed a hungry family of four.

Today, we can put 2,000 calories on one plate in the form of cheese fries; or in a bag in the form of corn chips; or in a box in the form of chocolate brownies; or in a carton in the form of ice cream; or in a microwaveable bowl in the form of a "family-size" chicken pot-pie. We have so many calorie-dense, low-volume, low-fiber, low-nutrient food choices today that typically we end up eating lots of calories even though we aren't eating that much in terms of quantity or volume. Simply switching back to the way we used to eat (unprocessed, nutrient-dense, high-volume, high-fiber foods) would resolve the obesity epidemic, decrease our waistlines, and some would argue (including myself) reverse and prevent most of the disease in our country. This is the essence of my food philosophy and something you can learn to adopt into your own life.

The Glycemic Index

Researchers, nutritionists, and dieticians wanted a system to classify the impact a food or macronutrient has on blood sugar levels. Thus the glycemic index (GI) of food was born. It classifies foods by their rate of conversion to blood sugar on a 100 or 150 point scale depending on which index you use. The higher the glycemic number of a food, the faster it converts to blood sugar in the body. More recently it has been determined that high glycemic foods and meals also raise triglyceride levels in the blood which we discussed at length in Chapter 3. Studies conducted by the Harvard School of Public Health and many other prestigious universities have linked the risk of type 2 diabetes and cardiovascular disease with the overall GI of the diet consumed. High GI diets have a higher risk and vice versa. Generally, the lower the glycemic index of a particular food, the better.

For some GI charts, glucose is used as the basis of comparison for other foods and assigned a value of 100. On other GI charts, white bread is assigned a value of 100 and foods are compared to its relative impact on blood sugar levels. Glycemic index charts based on white bread being 100 will give you a much higher GI value for the same food on a GI chart based on glucose. A baked potato, for instance, can therefore have a GI of 111 or 146 depending on which index you are using. To avoid confusion, make sure you are using the same scale when comparing different foods.

It is important to familiarize yourself with the GI of the foods you are eating now and maybe consider replacing some of them with lower GI options. For example: Baked Russett potatoes have a GI of 111 but boiled red-skin potatoes which are chilled can be as low as 56. Jasmine rice is 109 on the glycemic index but Basmati rice is around 57. Most green, fibrous vegetables are around 25 on the glycemic index. Can this be a useful tool in planning how you eat? Absolutely. Is it fool proof? Not exactly.

The problem is that we rarely eat foods individually. Or in other words, we most often eat foods in combination. You would have to calculate the calories of each food and factor the corresponding glycemic rating of each food to determine the glycemic load of the entire meal. Also, some foods like watermelon have a high-GI, but because they have a relatively low amount of carbohydrates by volume, have a low glycemic load. And on the flip side, many types of pasta have a low glycemic index, but have a lot of carbohydrates per serving and will have a relatively high glycemic load. It is therefore better to understand the glycemic index as a fundamental guide to help you make smarter food choices. Many index listings of food are available online (use your internet search engine and type in glycemic index of foods) and in print and I encourage you to formulate eating habits based on low-GI foods. You will be able to eat more food volume and avoid most, if not all, of the moods swings and cravings associated with high-GI foods.

For most people, picking lower glycemic foods will help keep insulin levels lower, stabilize blood sugar levels, and reduce low blood sugar crashes and their associated hunger pangs which scream "Feed me now! Feed me now!" However, two instances when a high-glycemic food or drink may be advantageous are immediately after resistance-based weight-training workouts and during long-duration (over two hours) endurance training or competition (like marathons and triathlons). In the case of post-workout nutrient timing, a high-GI drink combined with protein facilitates a desired insulin surge from the pancreas and helps the body replenish the muscle and liver glycogen stores depleted from anaerobic-type weight training. Insulin is the hormone required to transport nutrients into muscle cells. The presence of insulin in our bloodstream immediately post-workout creates an anabolic environment which speeds the natural muscle building and repair process and also helps shuttle more energy into the cell in the form of glucose. In long-duration events of over 90 minutes, high-GI drinks, gels, and energy bars can provide relatively instant energy for your working muscles. Unless you are doing these types of activity, however, it is generally advisable to stay with low-GI foods.

Our Carbohydrate Addiction

We are a nation of carbohydrate addicts and I would be willing to bet that you are one too. Don't believe me? Try to go for one week without eating potatoes, pasta, rice, or anything with sugar or flour in it (cakes, crackers, bread, pretzels, bagels, muffins, dinner rolls, cookies, ice cream, soda, juice). Heck, I bet it would be tough to go for three days without enjoying the high we get from sugar, bread, or starchy carbohydrates. Tell you what, try going for just one day without eating a single carbohydrate. For most people it would be an impossible task. Carbs are so much a part of everything we eat and drink. Crackers, bread, fruit, corn, cereal, chips, pretzels, soda, juice, milk, and beer all have carbohydrates. Think you could go just a day without any of the items on this short-list of foods?

In case you are wondering, it is possible. Two arctic explorers, Vilhjalmur Stefansson and Karsten Andersen, did it for a year in a landmark study from 1929 to 1930. After one of their scientific expeditions, they reported the fatty meat diets of the northern Eskimos and their apparent good health; but experts disagreed this was possible. To prove their research was accurate, they volunteered to be kept at Belleview Hospital in New York for one entire year while eating nothing but fatty meat (simulating the diets of the Eskimos). Even though they ate a substantial 2,500 calories, they both lost weight (about 6 pounds). Doctors monitored their health throughout the experiment and determined their blood chemistry and blood pressure remained normal and they developed no vitamin deficiencies. Both men appeared and felt in excellent health. Does this mean you should trade-in your cauliflower for caribou meat and eat nothing but animal flesh the rest of your life? Of course not. Do I subscribe to this self-imposed meatfest personally? No I don't, because of my moderation mantra and the fact that I like chocolate cake, but I do think it's better than the diets most people live off of now.

While it is commonly misbelieved we are a nation on a "low carb" kick, truth be told, the average American gets 67 percent of their calories from high-calorie, highly-processed, low-nutrient carbohydrates. Surprise, surprise. We may think we are eating low-carb, but like Brain Wansink illustrates in his book *Mindless Eating*, we often eat unconsciously. When I ask someone trying to lose weight what they ate yesterday, they selectively remember only the chicken breast and side of broccoli they had for lunch, but somehow fail to remember the mocha latte and bag of pretzels they had with it.

We also are a nation of constant snackers, most of which are carbohydrates. If you have ever attended any "off-site" business meeting, you will probably remember the tray of bagels, muffins, and donuts set out on your arrival into the conference room to tide you over between breakfast and lunch. Then after lunch, out comes the delicious tray of cookies to quell our hunger until dinner. Before dinner is served, out comes the basket of rolls or the hot loaf of bread just to get us through the chasm of starvation until our food arrives. See any nutritional patterns here? Just eliminate the between-meal carbohydrate snacks or what I will coin "tweeners" and you would eliminate about 200 to 300 grams (800 to 1,200 calories worth) of excess high-glycemic carbohydrates.

Nutritionists and registered dieticians love to promote the benefits of eating carbohydrates and I agree with them to some extent. I have been to countless seminars on nutrition conducted by leading sports nutritionists and a popular argument they make is: "Have you seen marathon runners? Marathon runners aren't fat and they eat lots of carbs. So carbs don't make us fat." I always cringe when I here this because most Americans already eat like a marathon runner but can't even say marathon when it comes to exercise. We are in an obesity epidemic and people don't need any encouragement to eat anymore of anything, much less carbohydrates. While a marathon runner can get away with eating three and four thousand plus calories a day, most American's version of a marathon is when they forget something in their car and have to make two trips to the driveway. We either have to dramatically increase activity levels (which most people aren't willing or don't have the time to do) or take out the caloric "fluff" in our diets.

Please don't think I'm impervious to the temptations of these foods because I'm not. (In fact, I'm munching on some cheese crackers while I write this sentence in an attempt to get my blood sugar up so my brain will help me compose the next sentence.) Whenever I see a tray of brownies in the break room, I turn and run away because I know I don't have the willpower to avoid them if they are staring me in the face. When I was in the corporate world and faced the conference table challenges of bagels, cookies, and muffins, I'll admit it was hard to avoid them completely. The trick that helps me fight off the cookie monster is eating a decent-sized green apple. I find the apple (at about 80 calories and 5 grams of fiber) leaves me feeling full and curbs the temptation to eat something with a lot more calories.

Being smart about what and how we eat is a necessary evil. But learning to consistently eat low-glycemic vegetables paired with some lean protein can change the way you think about food. Now is it realistic to think you will eye a piece of broccoli like an ice cream addict eyes a Ben and Jerry's ice cream truck? Probably not, but your cravings for foods will definitely change. I have a client named Jill who told me the changes in the foods she craved were remarkable after she followed a whole-food, low-carbohydrate (by calorie) eating plan. Remember you are in charge of your body, not the other way around. Generally, the more you eat something, the more you will begin to crave it. Just choose wisely.

What to Eat?

So much has been written, said, hypothesized, speculated, researched, and reported about how to construct the ratio of carbohydrates, protein, and fat in our diets that I could write ten books on the subject. Ten years ago when I was doing research for my own nutrition plan, I read the then popular diet and nutrition books and looked at the prevailing research of the time and concluded that a Dr Barry Sears Zone Diet 40-30-30 ratio of 40% carbohydrates, 30% protein, and 30% fat is a fairly sound approach to a lifetime nutrition plan. First it complies with my moderation mantra by not completely eliminating or severely restricting any specific macronutrients. Second, it allows a balanced approach to eating. Third, it allows for a lot of variety to keep from getting bored with food choices. Recent research has vindicated this approach and specifically, put the ratio at 44% carbohydrates, 26% protein, and 33% fat for optimum sustainability and performance enhancement. This is the ratio recommended to elite athletes by the world's top sports nutritionists and it will work for you too. When in Rome, do as the Romans do!

For most people, this ratio will reduce the amount of total carbohydrates being eaten each day which will have an immediate impact on your bodyweight. For each gram of carbohydrate consumed, the body pairs it with 2.7 grams of water. So reducing carbohydrates will definitely cause your body to shed some excess water weight. You may have already noticed the bloating effect of carbs when you ate a huge bowl of spaghetti or splurged on two pieces of chocolate cake at an office party (or maybe both). Then the next day you can't get your wedding ring off to wash your hands because you are so swollen. Usually this is temporary, but if you are accustomed to eating a high-carbohydrate diet all the time, you may be carrying around five to seven pounds of excess water weight. The good news is that the excess water can be easily shed by removing some excess carbohydrate from your diet.

There is adequate scientific evidence to support the efficacy, safety, effectiveness, health benefits and improved satiety of eating a higher protein diet (by percentage of calories). Don't misinterpret what I'm saying. This doesn't mean eating bacon and eggs for breakfast, fried chicken for lunch, and a T-bone steak for dinner. I'm talking about eating high-quality protein from lean sources like chicken, fish, eggs, beans, and supplemental whey and soy. Protein has a higher thermic effect on the body which means it requires more energy to digest and process. Compared to carbohydrates which have only a 4 to 6% thermic effect and fat which has virtually a 0% thermic effect, protein at a 26 to 30% thermic effect is a true value when it comes to calories. To simply illustrate this concept, let's pretend we just ate 100 calories of each macronutrient (protein, carbohydrates, and fat). The body would utilize all 100 calories of fat, about 96 calories of the carbs, but only about 70 calories of the protein (due to its high thermic effect). Just keeping this in mind, if you replace 800 carbohydrate or fat calories in your diet with the equivalent in protein calories (isocaloric modification), you would save a net of about 200 to 240 calories just from the additional thermic effect of the protein.

Again, I must emphasize choosing lean protein sources because most saturated fat comes attached to animal protein. Sure a 16-ounce, beautifully marbled, medium-rare ribeye steak tastes delicious but it comes with about 1,000 calories of pure fat out of the 1,300 total calories. A whopping 77% of the calories are from fat. Remove the fat and you have a reasonable 300 to 350 calories of lean protein. In terms of percentage of total calories, personally I keep my protein intake between 30% and 45%. If I am trying to "lean up" or lose weight, I may take it as high as 55% — essentially eating lean chicken breast, egg whites, and fish paired with green vegetables like broccoli, asparagus, green beans or spinach. By volume, I am eating mostly carbohydrates (ever see what 300 calories of raw spinach looks like?) but since vegetables are mostly fiber and water, they have very little calories but lots of vitamins, minerals, and phytonutrients.

After years of bad-mouthing fat and it's associated health problems, many people associate eating fat with having a heart attack even though it doesn't stop them from eating fried foods and washing them down with full-fat milk shakes or caramel lattes. Some fat is essential to our diet and it is vital to maintaining normal hormonal function and cellular metabolism. Each cell of our bodies has a lipid bilayer that not only protects it but also acts like a bouncer at a night club by determining what gets into the cell. Get the facts when it comes to fat.

So much has been written about fats (saturated, poly- and mono-unsaturated, hydrogenated, trans, etc) that I don't want to belabor the topic anymore than I have to, but be wary of misleading yourself into nutritional complacency. Just because something is labeled "low-fat" or "non-fat" does not necessarily mean it is healthy or low-calorie. I think we have been lulled into a false sense of nutritional security by all the low-fat foods available and as a result, consume far too many calories. We see the low-fat label and quickly rationalize that we can eat more of whatever is in the bag (or the whole bag), because it is healthy. This is an errant way of thinking and can lead us to the fundamental problem of caloric overeating. Low-fat foods are typically "high-carb" foods and we've already addressed the problems with that. Removing the fat also takes away the satiety of some foods. Fat has a low glycemic index so when you remove it from a snack cookie, all you are left with is high-glycemic processed flour, sugar, and artificial flavors. Personally, I would rather have one homemade, full-fat oatmeal cookie then a sleeve of low-fat cookies from the store.

The bottom line with fat is that if you follow my advice (and first nutritional commandment) and eat mostly whole, unprocessed foods consisting of fruits, vegetables, and lean proteins prepared with moderate amounts of olive oil or butter, you will be consuming a low-fat diet representing less than 30% of your total calories. If you have high cholesterol, a family history of heart disease, or have a significant amount of weight to lose, your doctor may want you to get your fat intake down to 20% of total calories. Remove the cooking oil from food preparation and you should be there, assuming you are following the whole food plan.

How many calories should we eat?

The difference between gaining weight and losing weight can come down to as little as 100 calories per day. This is fewer calories than there are in most commercial soft drinks. Consume 100 surplus (more than your body needs) calories per day for a year and you will gain over 10 pounds! The opposite is also true; consume 100 fewer calories than your body burns metabolically and you will lose over 10 pounds during the next year. This is a tremendous simplification of the biochemically complex homeostatic processes that regulate our bodyweight, but it does obey the laws of physics and thermodynamics.

Each day, our bodies create and use energy in many different ways. Some are obvious and others are not. Our biggest energy burner is our metabolism. All the processes necessary to sustain human life (breathing, tissue repair and remodeling, digestion, circulation, heart beats, thinking, etc.) require energy. If you add up the combined energy requirements of these critical processes, you get what is called our resting (or basal) metabolic rate. Surprisingly, this represents 50 to 60% of the total calories we burn each day.

Gaining and maintaining more lean muscle tissue by strength training is one way we can raise our resting metabolic rates. Placing intense physical demands on our bodies with interval training, weight training, or moving all your furniture up three flights of stairs are other ways to temporarily raise your metabolic rate. The thermic effect of food, or TEF for short, is another type of energy requirement. Each time we eat, energy is required to digest and process the food so that our digestive tract can absorb the caloric energy and nutrients. This can contribute up to 10% of the calories we burn each day. Picking high TEF foods like lean protein and eating smaller, more frequent meals can raise our TEF substantially.

Finally, physical activity is the final source of energy metabolism and can represent anywhere from as little as 300 calories per day for a sedentary "couch potato" to 12,000 calories for an ultra-marathon runner. Calories from physical activity are often divided into those from exercise and those from non-exercise activities to illustrate the impact active lifestyle choices can make on caloric requirements. Choosing daily activities that require more energy like walking up stairs, gardening, mowing the lawn, walking a dog, or volunteering for a charity like Habitat for Humanity will promote a calorie-burning lifestyle instead of a sedentary one. Remember all the little things you do can add up to a big difference to your health.

Now that you understand the many different variables which determine how many calories we burn each day, you can clearly see that it can be difficult to estimate how many calories we should consume to meet these energy requirements. On any given day your metabolism, what you eat, and how much physical activity you accumulate can be dramatically different than the next or previous day. That being said, we still need a method to approximate the average caloric needs of our bodies so we can budget how many calories to eat each day. There are several formulas including the Harris Benedict Equation that can be used to estimate caloric intake, but unless you like doing a lot of math...

$655 + (4.3 \text{ x wgt in lbs}) + (4.7 \text{ x ht in inches}) - (4.7 \text{ x age in years}) = \text{BMR}$

BMR x activity factor = Total Calories Needed

Activity factor: 1.2 (sedentary) or 1.55 (moderately active) or 1.725 (highly active)

they can be a little challenging to work with. So I came up with a fairly simple worksheet to help get you in the ballpark of how many calories you should eat each day and I have found it works for most people. I will walk you through the easy six step process to calculate your daily caloric needs. I have also included four real world examples to illustrate the highly variable energy needs we can have depending on our goals, age, gender, and activity levels.

Step 1:   Determine your bodyweight multiple by your gender and goal and write it in "YOU" column.
Ex: A female who wants to lose weight would write 10 in the "You" column

Step 2: Select activity factor in section 2 based on how many days per week you exercise and write it in "You" column. If a negative number is indicated, write the negative integer in front of the number.

Step 3: Determine any applicable special circumstances and add them together (more than one can apply).
Write combined value in "You" column or 0 if nothing is applicable.

Step 4: Determine total caloric multiple by adding positive and subtracting negative values in "You" column and write total in box labeled 'a'.

Step 5: Write current or goal bodyweight (in pounds) in box labeled 'b'.

Step 6: Multiply the number in box *a* by number in box *b* and record in bottom right box. This is your total estimated calories per day to meet your selected goal.

Daily Caloric Intake Worksheet

Select Bodyweight Multiple		Male	Female	*Example 1*	*Example 2*	*Example 3*	*Example 4*	YOU
GOAL	Lose Weight	13	10	10	13			
	Maintain Weight	15	12			12		
	Gain Weight	18	13				18	
then Add / Subtract								
Workout 3 days a week		+1	+1					
OR								
Workout 5 days a week		+2	+1.5	1.5		1.5	1.5	
OR								
Sedentary		-2	-2		-2			
Special Circumstances								
Competitive Athlete		+2	+1.5			1.5	2	
Endurance Athlete		+2.5	+2			2		
Over 200lbs		-1	-1	-1	-1		-1	
Over Age 65		-1	-1			-1		
Under Age 18		+1	+1					
Total Caloric Multiple (a)	*sum of column*			10.5	10	16	20.5	a
Bodyweight in pounds (b)	x			185	220	135	205	b
Calories per day (multiply a x b)				1,943	2,200	2,160	4,203	

calories per day

Example 1:   37 year old, 215 lb female who plans on exercising 5 to 6 days per week plus dieting to lose weight. She has a goal bodyweight of 185 pounds.

Example 2:   43 year old, 220 lb sedentary male. His goal is to lose weight without exercising.

Example 3:   67 year old, 135 lb female competitive triathlete. Her goal is to maintain her bodyweight despite her rigorous training schedule.

Example 4:   27 year old, 205 lb male athlete who exercises 5 days per week. His goal is to gain 10 pounds of lean mass over the next year.

Okay, now you should have a pretty good idea of how many calories you should be eating each day. The next challenge is actually eating that many calories. Most of us haven't a clue about how many calories we eat and if you fall into this category, don't feel bad because even expert dieticians were off by 20% when they were tested in a recent study. This is where the 20% rule comes into play. Take whatever amount of calories you think you are eating and add 20%. If you think you are eating 2,000 calories a day, most likely you are eating 2,400 calories. If you think you are eating 1,500 calories, more than likely you are eating closer to 1,800. If you eat at restaurants frequently, the underestimation factor is closer to 30%.

It isn't realistic for most people including me to measure out their foods on a food scale and specifically determine the gram weights of everything we eat. But knowing your caloric needs and applying the 20% rule may get you closer to where you need to be for health or even weight loss. Take a detailed look at what you eat for a week and add up the total calories (for the week) and divide by seven to get a daily average. Compare this to the amount you determined in the worksheet to see how close you are to your goal. Most people will find that adjustments are necessary. If this seems too complicated, you have my sympathy and understanding. So I came up with some simple nutritional strategies you can follow to improve the quality of your nutrition and painlessly take out some of the caloric fluff in your diet. Read on my friend.

The Ten Commandments of Nutrition

Now it's time to get onto the crème de la crème of this chapter. I've done my best to consolidate 20 years of learning, wisdom, and personal experience to formulate my *Ten Commandments of Nutrition*. Combined, these are a basic philosophical approach I recommend you follow when it comes to nutrition. If you obey these rules, more often than not your bodyweight, energy, health, and vitality will all improve and you will be in great shape nutritionally.

The Ten Commandments of Nutrition

1. Thou shalt eat whole, nutrient-dense, high-fiber foods
2. Thou shalt avoid processed, refined, and/or fried calorie-dense foods
3. Thou shalt prepare thy own food
4. Thou shalt eat *before* you get hungry
5. Thou shalt master portion control
6. Thou shalt eat a good breakfast everyday
7. Thou shalt eat protein with each meal
8. Thou shalt divide restaurant portions in half
9. Thou shalt covet thy neighbor's dessert
10. Thou shalt *not* drink your calories

The First Commandment:
Thou shalt eat whole, unprocessed, nutrient-dense, low-calorie, high-fiber foods

Choose to eat whole, unprocessed foods in their natural state whenever possible. These foods tend to have more nutrients, a lower caloric density, and far more natural fiber. Foods that have been ground, milled, and pulverized into oblivion have higher surface area values. This and their relative lack of fiber make them easier for the body to digest, causing a faster and more pronounced effect on blood sugar levels and a higher resulting insulin response. Chemically and mechanically altered foods and beverages can wreak havoc on the body by increasing cholesterol levels, increasing circulating free radicals, and causing arterial damage. Food processing also removes most of the beneficial nutrients from nature's food which necessitated the practices of artificially fortifying and enriching our foods. Look at the ingredients list of most processed foods and you will see they are "fortified" or "enriched" with the missing nutrients nature gave us in the first place. Whole, complete foods are best!

Unless you live on or near a self-sufficient farm, the easiest way to comply with this commandment is to select foods from the perimeter of the grocery store. This is where you typically find the milk, yogurt, cottage cheese, eggs, lean meat, poultry, fresh fish, fresh fruits, and fresh vegetables — basically all of the whole, unprocessed foods this commandment is dictating. Straying from the perimeter of the store should be minimal but I am a big fan of the *frozen fruits and vegetables aisle*. Studies have shown frozen fruits and veggies maintain more of their nutrients (because they are usually frozen at the peak of freshness) and are less likely to spoil. You can find diced frozen vegetables (like peppers and onions) which can save preparation time for your favorite dishes and frozen strawberries and blueberries to use in homemade protein smoothies. Just don't forget that you have them in the freezer.

The only other aisles I routinely visit on my weekly trip to the grocery store is the *bread aisle*, where I get a loaf of the light (50 calorie per slice) double fiber, whole wheat bread I use for my sandwiches, the *snack aisle* where I get a can of low-salt walnuts or mixed nuts for snacks and peanut butter for my protein shakes, the *cracker aisle* where I get plain whole wheat crackers to eat with homemade hummus or bean dip, and the *canned foods aisle* where I get canned black beans and chick peas (for hummus). Keep in mind, the fewer ingredients on the label the better.

Listed below are the foods included on my weekly shopping list, which for the most part I get at the local grocery store. Lately my wife and I have started buying more of our produce at local farmers markets and produce stands when we have a little extra time to shop. We have concluded without a doubt that the produce is definitely fresher and easier on the checkbook. The weekly produce we typically buy at the grocery store for about 18 to 22 dollars cost us only 12 bucks at a produce stand. It is definitely a win-win situation and I encourage you to explore local farmers markets for yourself.

Grocery Shopping List

1. Hummus
2. Light / Low Fat Cheese Sticks
3. Cottage Cheese (1-2% Fat)
4. Low sugar "Light" Yogurt
5. Plain Greek Yogurt
6. Low-Sugar Pudding Snack Packs
7. Unsweetened Applesauce Snack Packs
8. Light Almond or Soy Milk (no added sugar)
9. Skim or 1% Milk
10. Eggs and Egg Whites

Make Your List and Check It Twice

The best rule of thumb to use when you go grocery shopping is to prepare a list ahead of time when you're not hungry and still thinking intelligently. I prepare mine at home in the kitchen so I can quickly check if I'm short on anything, before I kick myself in the butt for forgetting it later at the store.

11. Sliced Low-Sodium Turkey, Ham, or Roast Beef Sandwich Meats
12. Reduced Fat / Low Sodium Soups
13. Canned Water-Packed Tuna
14. Canned Black Beans and Chickpeas
15. Brown Rice
16. Diced Tomatoes (low salt)
17. Canned Chilies, Onions, and Tomatoes
18. Whole Wheat Crackers
19. Extra Virgin Olive Oil
20. Balsamic Vinegar for Salad
21. Whole Grain High Fiber Cereal
22. Oatmeal (Instant)
23. Oatmeal (Whole Oats)
24. Chicken Breasts
25. Fresh or Frozen Salmon and Tilapia
26. 1 lb Lean Meat or Pork
27. Extra Lean Ground Beef
28. Walnuts
29. Mixed Nuts
30. Sunflower Seeds (for Salad)
31. Peanut Butter
32. Light Whole Wheat Double Fiber Bread (50 Cal per Slice)
33. Fresh and / or Frozen Vegetables - Broccoli, peppers, green beans, cucumbers, asparagus
34. Fresh and /or Frozen Fruit - Apples, blueberries, strawberries, bananas
35. Pre-washed Mixed Salad Greens and Baby Spinach
36. Avocados, Tomatoes, Sweet Potatoes
37. Onions and Garlic (for cooking)
38. Bottled Water

The Second Commandment:
Thou shalt avoid highly-processed, refined, and/or fried calorie-dense foods

Food processing and refining evolved as a necessary evil to extend the shelf life, simplify the packaging, aid in the portability, and most importantly to improve the profitability and availability of our agricultural products. The more something has been processed, however, the less our bodies have to work to digest it. Take a whole grain of wheat for example. By the time you eat it in a cracker, cookie, cereal, or piece of bread, it has been stripped of its bran and husk, with the resulting wheat germ being ground and milled into an ultra-fine, fiberless, low-nutrient, high-glycemic powder we call flour. Because this process of refining flour is so effective of stripping the formerly nutritious grains of wheat of all their vitamins, minerals, and fiber, it became necessary to "enrich" flour by adding some of these nutrients back in. The next time you see enriched flour on the ingredients list of bread, cereal, or box of crackers, you'll know what it means.

White flour is an innovation of the industrial revolution. When mixed with yeast and water, baked, and then consumed as bread, it will raise blood sugar levels higher and faster than an equivalent amount of table sugar, causing the body to overproduce insulin. Insulin is a double-edged sword. It is essential for life and is vital in the process of transporting nutrients into our cells. Unfortunately it is also the fat storage hormone. When our blood sugar rises too quickly from highly processed carbohydrates, too much insulin is released, glucose is converted to triglycerides for storage as fat (driving up blood triglyceride levels) and our blood sugar levels plummet from too much insulin. This is the energy and mood rollercoaster most Americans ride everyday.

When blood sugar levels are low, your body's feedback mechanisms signal you it is time to eat. When your blood sugar gets really low from the insulin-induced, blood-sugar slam dunk I just described, you will crave the quickest fix possible to get it back up...high-sugar, high-glycemic, high-calorie foods; the very foods we should be avoiding. It is a vicious cycle and unless you have the will power of Mahatma Gandhi on a hunger strike, you will be hard-pressed to avoid eating something that will just start the process all over again.

According to recent surveys of the American diet, the majority of our daily calories (over 67%) come from simple sugars and refined carbohydrates. When you consume most of your calories from refined carbohydrates long enough (over a period of many years), ultimately problems will arise with your health. In his book *The Saccharine Disease* published in 1975, T.L. Cleave explains the "Rule of 20 Years." According to Cleave coronary artery disease, high blood pressure, gallbladder disease, type 2 diabetes, peptic ulcers and colitis are all virtually non-existent in any culture until twenty years after refined carbohydrates are introduced into the diet. Want an example? Take a look at the United States. Refined sugar colas and refined flour were introduced into the American diet in the 1890's and twenty years later in 1912, the first case of heart disease was diagnosed. Like I rationalized, you may chalk this up to the juvenile state of medicine in the early 1900's or because better diagnostic tools and methods came along later.

So let's move along in history and look at the Icelandic diet where refined carbohydrates and sugar weren't readily introduced until the 1920's. Guess what? Twenty years later the first cases of modern degenerative diseases started. How about Poland and Yugoslavia where refined foods were introduced in the 1950's? You guessed it, about twenty years later problems like heart disease started to appear. Need even more modern examples? Look at the Chinese and Japanese populations where strong cultural food preferences kept refined foods out of their respective diets until very recently. Heart disease, cancer, type 2 diabetes were extremely rare in China and Japan until they finally succumbed to the international influence of fast, refined foods. Now all the health problems we've been dealing with for almost a century in America are starting to appear in these Far Eastern countries too.

Only in the most primitive and remote cultures of society like the Sardinians, Nicoyans, and elder generation of Okinawans (where whole, unprocessed foods are still consumed as the foundation of the diet) are modern degenerative diseases not an issue. So it doesn't take a PhD in statistics to conclude there is a definite correlation between consuming highly refined carbohydrates and incurring the associated health problems. Few people could argue with this conclusion: The more refined carbohydrates and sugars you consume, the more likely you will have heart disease, stroke, and type 2 diabetes.

Similarly, eating a lot of fried foods isn't a great idea for your health or your waistline either. Frying food was developed as a quick and tasty method of food preparation making most fast food restaurants commercially viable. Unfortunately, you can take an otherwise healthy piece of broccoli, throw it in tempura batter and fry it; turning it into a calorie-dense, high-fat nutritional nightmare. Most fried foods come with a nutritional triple whammy because the batter used to prepare them is made with (drum roll please)… refined flour. So you get added calories, refined carbohydrates, and added fat. Don't forget to throw in the extra salt or sugar typically sprinkled on most fried foods. For long-term health and weight management, I would proceed with extreme caution when it comes to eating fried foods. The added fat from frying foods makes staying within your calorie budget much more difficult.

Finally, highly processed foods also typically have lots of artificial ingredients, flavors, and additives. Let me translate what "artificial" means on a food label. It is telling you that chemicals approved by the Food and Drug Administration (FDA) were added to what you're about to buy and eat. I don't want to beat the panic drum, but a panel of cancer experts appointed by President Obama recently concluded that chemical additives may be responsible for the escalating cancer rates in our country. If obesity, diabetes, heart disease, and stroke weren't enough to worry about from the foods we eat (coupled with our inactivity), now we have to throw cancer in the mix too. Personally I don't want to play Russian roulette with my health so I am going to abide by the first and second commandments whenever possible. As more information is revealed, more and more people will be switching to or demanding organic, whole foods. Until we know more, this is your safest bet.

The Third Commandment:
Thou shalt prepare thy own food

The most basic advice I can give you when it comes to good nutrition is to prepare your own food whenever and wherever possible. Does this require a little effort? It sure does. Putting your clothes on every day requires effort too and I would be willing to bet a lot of money that you don't go to work in the buff. Am I right? If you are already preparing 80% or more of the food you put into your mouth each week, congratulations. For those of you who aren't, can you feel that sudden breeze? That's the winds of change blowin' just for you. If you've been on the restaurant rodeo tour hopping from one restaurant to another, night after night, it's time to step down off your horse and settle into the old homestead at night. Your health, wallet, and waistline will all thank you. Please don't think I dislike restaurants or that I have something against them. I would gladly let someone else prepare my food, serve it to me, and then clean up after me all the time if I thought it was in my best interest.

Eating the right foods can have positive and profound effects on your health, energy levels, mood, bodyweight, and appetite. Eating the wrong foods can have negative, drug-like effects in the body, causing food addictions, moodiness, anxiety and uncontrollable cravings. There is no better way to ensure the quality and quantity of your nutrition than preparing it yourself. Now if you are the fortunate member of your household who eats the fruits of someone else's kitchen labors, then make sure they read this book too. Work on it together, because a team approach is much better for long term success. While you're at it, volunteer to do the dishes every once in awhile if you aren't already… they will certainly appreciate the help in the kitchen.

If you are the person who prepares the food for your family, you are the *nutritional gatekeeper* for the mouths under your watchful care and you bear the responsibility for their stomachs, both inside and out. If my advice seems a little overwhelming in terms of effort, then it may be time to enlist the help of a sous-chef or two by getting other family members involved in food preparation. My mother had me in the kitchen when I was eight and sent me to cooking school when I was 10. We had a lot of mouths to feed in our family and my brothers and I helped our parents whenever we could. Even to this day when I go home, Mom still barks out the directions on what to cut, prep, chop, dice, peel, and slice. Old habits die hard and I'm still happy to help.

Preparing your own food requires a little planning and time on your part. I'm not just talking about dinner either. I'm talking about making a healthy breakfast before you leave the house and packing a lunch to take with you. Having prepared foods and snacks on hand at the office will not

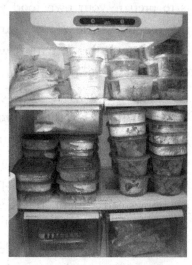

A "prepared" refridgerator

only improve the quality of food you eat, but it will also help you fend off the candy monster that lurks on top of desks and file cabinets across America. If you are already preparing healthy and nutritious meals for dinner, packing a lunch simply requires putting a lunch-size portion of leftovers in a microwaveable container for the next day. I would recommend doing this before you sit down to eat because it serves the secondary purpose of reducing caloric intake at dinner time (when most people overeat). By putting extra food away ahead of time, you will be less likely to have second helpings. If you're not the leftover "Mom's Meatless Meatloaf" type, then you may prefer to make sandwiches or other foods you desire for lunch. The moral of the story is to invest the time necessary to pack a lunch and some healthy snacks to take with you to work on most, if not all, days of the work week.

Before we had the luxury of a microwave where I work, each night I would prepare and baggie two lean meat (chicken, turkey, or ham usually), spinach, and mustard sandwiches on light, double fiber bread and put them in my small travel cooler along with two light cheese sticks, one apple, one snack-size low-fat cottage cheese or yogurt, and one small can of low-sodium vegetable juice. On some days I'd throw in a baggie of carrots or sliced cucumber to snack on. This was my routine for most days of the week until they added a microwave to our break room. Now I can reheat whole foods I prepare at home, which I feel much better about given what we discussed in the previous commandment. I also keep a can of mixed nuts in my locker at the gym so I can grab a handful for a quick snack between clients.

The Fourth Commandment: Thou shalt eat before you get hungry

One of the best ways to fulfill this commandment is by having preplanned, healthy snacks twice a day. If you go long periods of time without eating (a.k.a. skipping breakfast, then eating a big lunch and dinner), it is very likely that you will end up very hungry and have a tendency to overeat. Two to three hours after we eat, our blood sugar level starts to fall and the body sounds the 'time-to-eat' horn. By the five hour point, the horn transitions to an emergency siren and our physiology changes dramatically. We are energy-depleted, moody, irritable, short-tempered, and most likely, extremely famished. When you get to this point, it is going to be extremely difficult, if not impossible, to make a smart food decision. With the siren on, you will crave high-calorie, quick-energy foods and drinks, significantly increasing the likelihood you will overeat.

The key is to avoid this situation by introducing strategic snacks between your breakfast, lunch, and dinner (and between dinner and bedtime for some people). Some of you may be asking: "If I'm trying to lose weight, why should I be snacking?" The answer may surprise you. Strategic snacking will ultimately help you eat less total calories and lose weight more painlessly. Take my father-in-law Robert, for example. Like his daughter (my wife), Bob has a strong appetite. He is a *live to eat* type and before he introduced a strategic snack into his afternoon routine, he would come home famished. Immediately upon entering the house, he would head straight to the fridge and cupboard searching for food like a starving lion searching for its prey. Before dinner, he could easily chow down 300 to 500 extra calories of high-glycemic snacks and still be voracious at dinner time, where he would often have second and third helpings.

After we discussed his desire to lose some weight, we made two simple changes to his daily routine. The first was getting him on a consistent exercise routine, which included both strength training and cardiovascular conditioning. The second was introducing a meal replacement shake after his workouts, which coincidentally is also right before he comes home to dinner. Since Bob is a busy executive and his time is precious, I recommended several types of ready-made protein drinks and he found he really enjoyed MyoPlex Lite by EAS.

What has been the result of these two small changes? Overall he now eats less and has lost the extra 20 pounds he was carrying around. When we talked about it, he told me: "Before I started having the shakes, I would come home with the "shakes." I was starving when I got home and I would have to eat something before dinner. Now I have my shake right after my workout while I'm driving home and it really kills my appetite and I feel normal. I don't snack out of the pantry anymore and I eat less at dinner too." By consuming a 150 - 200 calorie protein drink, Bob no longer eats 300 to 500 calories of snacks and 300 to 500 calories of extra dinner. Do the math: *200 strategic calories save him from the 500 to 1,000 mindless calories he was eating each day.* It is easy to see why he easily lost the weight and now he looks and feels great.

The Fifth Commandment: Thou shalt master portion control

"Eat small, frequent meals." Unless you've been living under a rock, I'm sure you've heard this advice before too. But maybe no one has ever taken the time to explain it to you and how to quickly determine how much of anything to eat. Learning to truly master portion control will make your life easier and promote better health because you will reduce the likelihood of overeating. Every time we eat, we raise our metabolism and provide our bodies with the fuel it needs for work and the raw materials it needs for the repair and remodeling of tissue (primarily muscle). When you eat small, frequent, nutritious meals, each consisting of complex carbohydrates and lean protein, it is like putting your body on an intravenous (I.V.) drip of good nutrition. Your body will maintain a more anabolic state (versus catabolic) which means you will build more lean muscle tissue over time. Having an adequate and constant supply of energy in the body will also keep the "Feed me Now!!!" switch turned off. With this switch in the off position, you will be more in control of what and how much you eat making it less likely you will gain the 4 to 7 pounds most Americans average each year.

The other valuable addition of having smaller meals is actually a subtraction…from your waistline that is. Studies have proven that when you divide the same amount of calories into more frequent meals, you will burn more calories. One study compared two groups consuming 2,000 calories. Group 1 consumed 2,000 calories of food divided into two meals and Group 2 consumed the same 2,000 calories divided into six meals. What do you think the results were? Well the participants in Group 1 *gained* weight on their 2,000 calories while those in Group

2 *lost* weight. It's not as simple as calories in versus calories out. How frequently you divide your calories does make a difference.

I want to give you a ridiculously simple, but effective method of determining how much food to put on your plate at each meal; I call it the "lend a hand" method. For proteins: use the size and thickness of the palm of your outstretched hand without the extended fingers and thumb (don't cut them off, just visualize please!) to match the portion of protein to eat. This portion is relative to the size of the individual and for women will be about four ounces and for men about five or six ounces.

For fruits, desserts, and starchy type foods like corn, sweet peas, all starchy beans (red, black, pinto, lima, etc.), potatoes, bread, sweet potatoes, and foods made from them like grits, mashed potatoes, dumplings, and sweet potato casserole: use the size of a clenched fist to determine the proper portion to have in any one meal and limit yourself to two total portions of fruits, desserts, and starches (in any combination) max per meal, preferably just one. My preferred starch is black beans because of their high fiber and nutrient content. If you are trying to lose weight, it is best to limit yourself to one fist-sized portion of a starchy-type food and one or two servings of fruit per day until you reach your desired weight.

For all the green, red, yellow and other brightly colored cruciferous vegetables: if they are raw or steamed, take both hands and grab as much as you can and fill your plate. In all seriousness, most of your food volume should be from crunchy vegetables and salad greens. These are high-fiber, high-nutrient, high-water-content, low-calorie foods that will fill your stomach but won't fill you out. If a vegetable is put into a calorie-laden dish like green bean casserole, cream of mushroom soup, or broccoli drenched with melted cheddar cheese then all bets are off. Use the fist method to budget a portion of these vegetable dishes. So a simple visual method of portioning your food would be to fill your plate half to three quarters with raw or lightly steamed vegetables and/or salad greens, one quarter with protein, and one quarter (or none) with starch, fruit, or casserole-type dishes.

Here's a 'Pop Quiz' for you. Pretend for a moment you are sitting down to a family style dinner with the following on the table in front of you: a big bowl of "mixed greens" salad (with a choice of blue cheese dressing or a balsamic vinaigrette), a plate of 12-ounce New York strips hot off the grill, a serving dish piled high with steaming mashed potatoes, a platter of corn on the cob bathed with melted butter, a bowl of lightly steamed green beans, and a homemade apple pie warming in the oven. Faced with these choices, how would you best portion and serve the food onto your plate?

I don't know about you, but my mouth is watering and I'm already in a conundrum as to what to do here. For the record, unless I am entertaining guests, I would never put myself into this situation in the first place because I don't have the willpower to not eat something sitting in front of me. But if you follow these rules and let your hand guide you, you could make the most of the situation and put the following portion-controlled meal together. Fill your dinner plate as much as possible with the salad (selecting a small amount of the balsamic vinaigrette) and steamed green beans (and start praying that the potatoes would miraculously disappear). Cut one of the steaks in half (saving the other half for lunch the next day) and put the desired half amongst the plate of green stuff.

Now the big dilemma, what should you do about the two remaining starchy-type foods and the dessert in the oven? Since the corn is a whole food and less calorie-dense than the potatoes, I would recommend having an ear of corn (letting most of the butter drip onto the platter) and a small dollop of the potatoes. Put those two portions together and you have a fist (remember, you're not eating the cob of the corn, just the kernels) — that's two for the price of one! Since mashed potatoes prepared the good old fashioned way with butter, cream, and sometimes cheese are much more calorie-dense than corn on the cob, you would actually save calories by having two ears of corn. But I like to have a variety of foods (variety is the spice of life) and would therefore opt for the small taste of the potatoes so I could have my cake (or apple pie in this case) and eat it too. Limit yourself to a small slice of the pie and even smaller if it was served a la mode. The dessert fist would have to include both the pie and the ice cream.

The Sixth Commandment:
Thou shalt eat a good breakfast everyday

I know this is almost cliché now but since about four out of five people I consult with on nutrition don't eat a decent breakfast, if at all, I know it is still a prevailing problem. The word breakfast means literally "break the fast" and this is why it is so critical. After you have been snoozing for seven or eight hours (if you are getting enough sleep), your body has depleted the energy and nutrients from the last meal you consumed before going to bed. To maintain adequate circulation of essential amino acids and energy (in the form of blood glucose) while sleeping or during prolonged times between meals, your body will break down its own muscle tissue. This process is called catabolism.

Having a healthy breakfast consisting of complex carbohydrates and lean protein will stop muscle catabolism in its tracks. Your breakfast primes your metabolism and sets the nutritional tone for an energetic day. Strive for whole food sources when possible and learn to pair up your carbs and proteins: i.e. low fat cottage cheese and a piece of fruit; whole wheat toast with low fat cheese and Canadian bacon; an egg on sliced tomato; low fat yogurt with sliced fruit and walnuts; or (for my vegetarian friends) tofu topped with black beans, onions, salsa, and fresh cilantro wrapped in a whole wheat tortilla. My personal favorite "power breakfast" is scrambled egg whites (or egg substitute) covered with a half cup of low fat cottage cheese paired with some oatmeal topped with walnuts and sliced banana. I have this meal before any big workout or athletic competition and it gives me the fuel and nutrients to perform my best.

A study of 152 overweight adults conducted at Louisville State University found that the people who ate two eggs for breakfast each day for two months lost 65% more weight than those who ate a lower protein breakfast of the same amount of calories. The researchers concluded that the protein in the eggs increased satiety by 50% which led them to eat 164 fewer calories at lunchtime. Eating protein at breakfast is important because it stops catabolism and jump starts your metabolism. If you delay eating after you get up in the morning (or at night for the shift workers out there), you only prolong this process and cause your body to destroy the calorie-burning machinery you are desperately trying to build with exercise. If you are taking the time to lift weights, it only makes sense to help the body rebuild the tissue you break down. So how do you want your eggs, sunny side up or scrambled?

If you are like many of my clients and are looking for a simpler solution for breakfast, try making a "power shake" to get your day started. On days when I have early morning clients, I make one the night before and put it in the refrigerator to grab as I leave the next morning. This makes having a healthy, nutritious breakfast quick and easy. No more excuses. My basic recipe: 4oz skim, soy, or almond milk; half a banana; half cup of frozen blueberries, strawberries, or raspberries; 1 scoop (20gms) of whey or soy protein; 1 tsp peanut butter; 4 to 6 ounces water or crushed ice. Add ingredients to blender in the order listed (saves time on clean-up) and blend for 30 seconds. Pour into a travel cup and you're out the door with a good breakfast in hand in less than five minutes (including clean-up). Males over 195 pounds and competitive athletes should double this recipe.

The Seventh Commandment: Thou shalt eat protein with each meal

Remember this jingle. "Protein is great, because it will satiate!" Studies and empirical evidence have confirmed the nutritional and hunger-defying benefits of protein. Protein has a low glycemic index which helps keep blood sugar levels more stable and keeps hunger in check. Protein also takes more energy to digest compared to carbohydrates and fat and thus has a higher thermic effect on the body. Protein is digested into amino acids which are the building blocks of all muscle tissue. Without a constant supply of amino acids in the bloodstream, our body will meet its need for amino acids by breaking down existing muscle tissue.

While you cannot completely stop this process of protein turnover, you can significantly influence the rate of turnover in your favor. Studies have shown that keeping a constant supply of amino acids in your blood stream by eating small, frequent portions of protein, can maintain a positive nitrogen balance, spare or create lean mass, and keep your body in a more anabolic (muscle-building) state. And if you remember from our discussion of muscular metabolism in Chapter 1, having more lean mass gives you a bigger metabolic engine that burns more calories each day. In general, high protein diets are more satisfying, have less total calories, and are easier on the pancreas in terms of insulin production. A 2010 study in *Medicine & Science in Sports & Exercise* confirmed that higher protein diets preserve more lean muscle mass when losing weight than higher carbohydrate diets of the same calories.

Don't get this confused with eating a high protein diet that many "nutritional experts" like to criticize. I'm not talking about eating 20 egg whites for breakfast, a pound of turkey for lunch, and a side of beef for dinner. What I'm referring to is about 3 to 4 ounces of protein per meal for women and 4 to 6 ounces per meal for men, on average. At 5 to 6 meals per day, this equates to about 90 to 110 grams of protein a day for women and 150 to 180 grams of protein per day for men. The very people who criticize "high protein" diets fail to realize that most high protein diet advocates like me mean "high" in terms of percentages, not by total grams or calories. Even at the highest recommendation of 180 grams of protein, this only equals 720 calories or 29% of a 2,500 calorie per day diet. Many Americans are already eating more protein by volume then most high protein diets recommend so this recommendation would represent a reduction in total protein consumption. Eating a 16 ounce sirloin would equal about 112 grams of protein, which for one meal is far too many unless you are a 360 pound lineman in the National Football League — and even then it probably isn't a good idea.

Current dietary guidelines call for 0.8 to 1 gram of protein per kilogram of bodyweight which was based on a sedentary, 150 pound adult. Since no one should be sedentary after reading this book, I would say a better recommendation is 0.8 to 1 gram of protein per pound of bodyweight. Not only is the math easier because you don't have to divide your weight by 2.2 to figure it out, but you will feel better, have more energy, be less hungry, and recuperate faster from your workouts and the stresses of life. If you are trying to lose more than 20 pounds of bodyweight, use one gram of protein per pound of lean mass.

To determine your specific protein recommendation, take the *total estimated calories per day* you came up with on the <u>Daily Caloric Intake Worksheet</u> earlier in this chapter and multiply it by 0.3 (or 30% of total calories). This calculation will give you approximately how many protein calories to consume each day. There are 4 calories per gram of protein so divide protein calories by 4 and you will know how many grams of protein this is. For example, if you came up with 2,150 total estimated calories per day, you would calculate your protein requirements like this: 2,150 x 0.3 = 645 (protein calories per day) and 645 / 4 = 161 grams of protein per day. By using 7 grams of protein per ounce of lean meat, chicken, or fish as a guideline, you can quickly figure out how many ounces of protein to eat each day by dividing your grams by 7. Taking our previous example: 161 grams of protein / 7 grams per ounce = 23 ounces of protein (lean meat, chicken, egg whites, or fish). If you eat six meals a day, you would portion out about 4 ounces with each meal. If you prefer to keep track of protein intake by grams that would be about 27 grams of protein per meal (161 / 6 = 26.8).

Remember this is a guideline to shoot for and some meals will have less protein and some will have more. My snacks can have as few as 11 grams of protein and my meals may be as high as 44 grams, but my seven meal average works out to about 33 grams of protein (per meal) to meet the 228 grams a day I target for myself. This represents a reduction from the 250 grams per day I normally eat (when I'm not writing a book and get to exercise two more days per week than I am now). I point this out because I have eaten this way (200 plus grams of protein per day) for over fifteen years now and my annual blood work has always been exceptional according to my doctor. In fact, he gave my blood work an A+ during my physical last year. As I've pointed out previously, consuming excess calories (in any form including protein) and high amounts of refined carbohydrates cause most of the health problems in America today. Having small amounts of protein with each meal will help you eat fewer calories overall and hopefully replace some or all of the refined carbohydrates in your diet.

The Eighth Commandment:
Thou shalt divide restaurant portions in half

Since most people (including me) inevitably eat at restaurants, I feel compelled to give you some advice when it comes to this sometimes necessary and often delicious fact of life. As I pointed out earlier in the chapter, restaurant portions have increased by an average of 30 percent right along with our average weight. If you have ever seen pictures of the typical hamburger and french fries served in the 1960's, you would think you were looking at the "kiddie meals" of today. Due to consumer demand and increasing competition, restaurants started economizing to serve up bigger and bigger portions over the years so consumers would perceive more value for the money. It would be unfair to pick on any particular companies because we live in a supply and demand, market-based economy that dictates whether a business will survive or fail. Since large restaurant chains have financially and geographically expanded by "expanding" their customers' stomachs, it is obvious there was a demand out there.

This "calories per dollar" competition has led to 32-ounce "small size" soft drinks, 1,300-calorie "monster" burgers, and enough super-size French fries in one order to feed three people. The unfortunate consequence of meeting this consumer demand is the two out of three Americans who are now classified as overweight or obese and the associated failing health that comes with it. I don't blame the restaurant companies because they aren't holding a gun to our heads forcing us to eat their food. We do have the freedom of choice and until we have better "calorie smart" restaurants to choose from, I have found the best way to deal with the situation is to divide your restaurant portions in half or share them with another person.

Now admittedly, this takes a little getting used to at first. When we go to a restaurant, we have conditioned ourselves over the years to turn off the calorie-conscious portion of our brains and let our cravings run wild. It's time to take charge of our appetites and the side benefit is that your hard-earned dollar will go farther. You get two meals for the price of one. If you have a spouse, friend, significant other, or family member who shares the same tastes as you, then you can split an entrée with them. Ask your waiter or waitress to divide the meal for you before they serve it. This allows the kitchen staff to present the meal for both of you and is easier than trying to do it yourself. I haven't found a restaurant yet that isn't willing to do this, although some may charge a small fee to do it (but this is very rare).

If you are with someone who doesn't share the same tastes as you or if you are by yourself, then ask your server to have the kitchen box up half the meal before it is served. Like the previous scenario, the kitchen staff will plate up the half portion and chances are you won't miss the extra half. Since we eat with our eyes and by units (i.e. one plate equals one unit), we will still be satisfied with the reduced portion we eat and you get to clean your plate and not feel guilty or overstuffed. Plus you already have another meal ready for lunch or dinner the next day. Again, two meals for the price of one!

When it comes to fast food restaurants, your best bet is to limit how frequently you eat at them and when you do succumb to their convenience, order the smallest items they have on the menu. You could also cut most modern fast food hamburgers and sandwiches in half to share with someone else and have more than enough calories to go around.

The Ninth Commandment:
Thou shalt covet thy neighbor's dessert

You've probably heard that the best kind of boat is someone else's boat. Well dessert works the same way. If you are someone like me who enjoys dessert, then it is best to learn to share with someone else and let them order it (if you are at a restaurant). If you are with a group of four people, one dessert (assuming you can all agree on which one) is plenty for everyone to have a couple of delicious, endorphin-releasing bites to get your dessert "fix." This serves the purpose of rewarding yourself, but at the same time honors the fifth commandment by controlling the amount of calories you eat. Deprivation diets fail, so stick with this policy and you can have your cake and eat it too.

If you are at home and don't have a neighbor (or spouse or child) to share with, then the best policy is to use a very small bowl or plate for your dessert. Some people even use a tumbler-sized glass to have dessert in. Remember, we eat in units and the key is eating a smaller unit by using a smaller serving dish. There are also wide selections of 100 calorie portion-sized desserts that limit the unit size for you. Although these violate the first and second commandments, if you are a must-have-dessert type, then at least we are minimizing the damage.

A better solution is to have fresh fruit for dessert. This takes you out of nutritional purgatory and most fruit already comes in convenient, portion-controlled sizes. The longer you avoid sugary or artificially sweetened foods, the more your taste buds will pick up the natural sweetness in fruit. Try it for two weeks and see what I mean. Fresh and ripe pineapple, grapes, oranges, apples, mangos and strawberries will taste like candy.

The Tenth Commandment:
Thou shalt not drink your calories

One of the easiest ways to lose weight is to stop drinking excess, unnecessary, useless calories. Today, Americans are drinking more calories than ever which may explain why you have gained weight despite eating what you consider a sensible diet. Liquid calories don't register with our hunger mechanism like solid food does which makes it much easier to consume more calories than our bodies are telling us we need. In other words, if you have a milkshake with your

How many calories are we drinking?	
Year	Cal/day
1965	234
1977	284
1989	359
2002	451
2010	?

burger and fries, you won't feel any fuller than if you had water. Since liquid calories empty the stomach faster, you may quickly crave another calorie "fix." Having a whole food snack like an apple or a handful of almonds is a better way to go. The exceptions to this rule are nutrient-balanced, high-protein meal replacement drinks you can have for between-meal snacks or post-workout recovery nutrition and the breakfast "power shake" I described in the Sixth Commandment.

If you are more than 20 pounds overweight and want to lose it, then try to avoid drinking milkshakes and anything that resembles a milk shake (other than a protein smoothie meal replacement). Avoid anything that comes with whip cream on top, is served in a pineapple or coconut, comes with fruit or little umbrellas sticking out of it, or has a name starting with 'frap' or 'mocha' and / or ending in '-arita,' 'uccino' and 'oolata.' Believe it or not, skipping these indulgences can easily save you 300 to 500 calories a day (some "mocha-type" drinks have over 700 calories). Just dropping these extra calories alone can lead to almost a pound of weight loss each week. Maybe you're a little less indulgent, but any excess calories can be detrimental to achieving your goal. Here are some other specific beverages to be wary of:

Soft drinks: Soft drinks offer very little nutritious value. They are essentially carbonated, artificially flavored and colored sugar water that is additionally sweetened with high fructose corn syrup. I'm not trying to criticize the soda manufacturers because I enjoy the "real thing" from time to time, but I don't understand how someone who knowingly must lose weight can stroll into a convenience store and fill up a cup that resembles a grain silo with 1,000 calories of uselessness. Turn on the Discovery Health Channel and watch almost any show on the morbidly obese and the star of the show will inevitably be drinking some type of soda at meal times. It really upsets me when these people share their struggles with weight loss between sips of the cola they are drinking on camera. Either this is ignorance personified or callous, in your face wantonness. It makes me want to give them an enlightening knock on the head with a nutritional encyclopedia. If I'm striking an emotional chord, than I'm playing this song just for you. Learn to replace those empty fluid calories with calorie-less beverages like water, unsweetened tea, and black coffee. Diet sodas haven't proven to help too much if you're trying to lose weight. Studies have shown that diet soda drinkers gain more weight than regular soda drinkers. I have two theories for this. The first is what I call calorie compensation syndrome where people rationalize "Oh, I drink diet soda so I can have the blueberry cobbler with my lunch." The second is a Pavlovian-like response to the sweet taste of the drink which triggers our pancreas to release insulin. Since there is no sugar in the drink, our blood-sugar levels fall and we ultimately crave more sweets or other blood-sugar raising foods — thus eating more.

Sport drinks: My advice with sports drinks is simple. If you aren't doing long-duration, endurance-type exercise for at least 90 minutes, then skip the sports drinks. I know we want to believe there is an athlete in all of us, but the first step to finding your inner athlete is training like one.

Walking around the gym for 30 minutes and then downing a 200 calorie sports drink makes absolutely no sense. I know they taste good but the bottom line is that you are consuming unnecessary sugar-based calories. I had a client who was trying to lose about 40 pounds and he would always show up to our 30 minute sessions with a 200 calorie sport drink; the same amount of calories he was probably burning during the workouts. So essentially he was leaving the gym with a net energy balance of zero when he could have easily created a 200 calorie deficit by switching to water. Fortunately, the manufacturers of sports drinks have caught on and are now making lower calorie and zero calorie sports drinks like Propel, Gatorade G2 and PowerAde Zero. If you can't handle drinking plain water, then at the very least select a low- or no-calorie option.

Fruit Juice and Fruit Drinks: Fruit juices are another sneaky source of sugar in the form of fructose. Eat your fruits in their natural state. Most whole fruits already come in convenient, transportable portion-sized servings. Packaged fruit juices have stripped the fruit of most of its fibrous pulp and when you drink them, it's like mainlining sugar…a quick high, then you crash and burn. In fact, I have seen how fast drinking juice can restore someone about to pass out with low blood sugar (hypoglycemia). It takes literally seconds. People who don't eat a nutritious meal before an intense workout can quickly end up hypoglycemic and I always keep some orange juice or apple juice on hand to bring them back. Drinking a four ounce glass with breakfast can be incorporated into your meal plan, as long as you can spare the calories and are washing down an egg white and veggie omelet. Dr Arthur Agaston, author of *The South Beach Diet* calls fruit juices "a big source of trouble." He goes on to say: "They do carry nutrients, especially freshly made juices. But they also bring with them high levels of fructose, which can be the undoing of any effort to lose weight."

Alcohol: If your primary goal is weight loss, I would recommend putting the wine away and locking up the liquor cabinet until you reach your goal. When you consume alcohol, the fat burning process (fatty acid oxidation) is inhibited while your liver switches priorities to alcohol detoxification. The consensus of most diet plans I've reviewed is to restrict or severely limit alcohol, not only because of the extra calories, but primarily because of this inhibiting effect on fat burning. We are trying to stoke the fat-burning furnace and drinking alcohol is like dousing the metabolic flames with water. This is why I put alcohol on the "red" (avoid) list of my *Nutrition Traffic Light* I discuss in the next chapter.

The other problem with alcohol is it turns off our common sense switch. Suddenly, stopping for a double cheeseburger, fries, and a milkshake at two in the morning can make perfectly good sense after a few alcoholic beverages. I can speak of this firsthand because I've looked for the golden arches or ran for the border myself a few times after a good night on the town. I have also heard the countless stories from my normally self-disciplined clients who couldn't resist the high-calorie temptations of fast food after a few drinks. Even though we worked our butt off in the gym and did our best all week to maintain good nutritional habits, we can throw our weekly caloric deficit out the window after one alcohol-induced binge eating episode.

Even just one drink with dinner can influence your ability to exercise good judgment when it comes to how much food to eat. Alcohol can be a potent appetite stimulant requiring more will power than you or I possess. Unless you are the rare exception, I guarantee you will eat less at mealtimes when you don't drink alcohol. I had a client who lost 20 pounds in six weeks simply by eliminating the two to three glasses of wine he had with dinner each night. Since the total calories required to lose that amount of weight were far more than the calories in two glasses of wine per night, I can only deduce he ate less food overall too.

Try it for yourself…the best advice I can offer you is to limit alcohol to one drink per night (moderation) and avoid alcohol completely when you are trying to lose weight. Save the champagne for your victory celebration!

Some final tips on nutrition

Savor the flavor of your foods. One of the easiest ways to eat smarter is to slow the process down and learn to savor the flavor of each bite of food or sip of drink we take. In our rush, rush, rush society, it is very easy to wolf down our food and get onto the next task at hand. If you consciously interrupt this lifetime of food programming and slow things down when you eat, inevitably you will eat less, have less indigestion, and feel better. There are just two simple rules to follow: 1) Chew each bite you take 15 to 20 times and 2) Put your fork or spoon (or sandwich) down between each bite. If you follow these rules, you will be amazed with what happens to the whole eating process. While I was a freshman at the Air Force Academy, it was a disciplinary ritual to ground our forks after each bite and then chew each bite 21 times. At the time it felt like torture, but now in hindsight, it makes a lot of sense. By eating slower, you give your brain a chance to perceive fullness and by chewing food completely, you improve digestion. Another added benefit of slow, deliberate eating is less gas in the tailpipe (so to speak) because you aren't gulping down air with each bite. These new habits will take a little time to get used to at first, but will definitely pay off in the long run.

Eat without distractions. Another simple strategy to incorporate into your eating habits is to eat without distractions and make meal times more of a conscious behavior. When we eat while driving, watching TV, watching a movie, or surfing the internet, our brains have less opportunity to get involved in the eating process. Suddenly eating becomes an unconscious or mindless activity and we lose track of what and how much we eat. The most obvious illustration of unconscious eating is the popcorn we eat at movie theaters. The small microwaveable bags seem to be more than enough to feed two people at home, but put us in front of a big screen action adventure movie and suddenly we can eat a grocery bag full of popcorn non-stop for two hours. The same is true when you sit down in front of the TV with a bag of chips…hand to bag to mouth, hand to bag to mouth, repeating over and over again until the bag is empty. If you absolutely must eat with some kind of distraction, then at least be aware of the food portions you take with you to the couch or computer desk. Take a bowl or plate with an appropriate serving and put the rest away. You will be amazed at how many calories you will save. If you want to learn some fascinating information on this topic, I highly recommend you read Brian Wansink's book *Mindless Eating*.

Drink lots of water. I'm sure you've heard this before so I am not going to beat a dead horse over and over but you should be aware of a few important points regarding proper hydration. Most people are chronically dehydrated and when we are even a little dehydrated, we have less energy, our metabolism slows, and we are hungrier. We counter the energy drain by drinking caffeine and eating sugar when in reality, all we have to do is stay adequately hydrated.

If you don't believe me, try this experiment for one week: Each day, drink 20 ounces of cool water when you first get up and then another 20 ounces before you eat your lunch. Pay attention to your appetite and how you feel. Most people will notice a significant difference — eating less at lunch and maybe even skipping their afternoon "pick-me-up" beverage. Drink another 20 ounces of water while you exercise and with only a little modification to your daily routine, you will be consuming 60 ounces of pure water. For most people this will be enough to prevent dehydration when you combine it with other fluids typically consumed. If you want to take it a step further, the golden rule I try to follow is drinking 100 ounces of water a day. Admittedly I don't accomplish this every day, but on the days that I do I notice a big difference in my energy levels and feel a lot better. Finally, if you follow my *eat green to be lean* philosophy I cover in the next chapter, you will be eating high volume, low-calorie foods that have a lot of water content. This will not only help fill you up, but will also support your quest to stay properly hydrated too.

Applied knowledge is power

I hope you will put the information in this chapter to good use and follow the Nutritional Ten Commandments as best you can. You now know how many calories a day you should be eating and how to use the glycemic index to make wise food choices. Be wary of the low-nutrition, calorie-dense foods that sneak their way onto our plates and into our cups and then ultimately into our mouths. In the next chapter, we will learn how to use nutrition to lose weight and keep it off successfully. Even if you don't need to lose any weight, the principles can still be beneficial and you may know someone you can help.

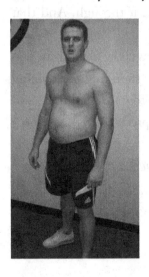
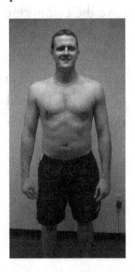

Jim
Age: 25
Project Manager

In 6 weeks, I lost 20lbs, lowered my bodyfat by 5%, and dropped 5 inches off my waist. Most importantly, I lowered my cholesterol level and risk factors for heart disease.

"I had high cholesterol and was also at risk for heart disease given the amount of belly fat I was walking around with. Being able to lose 5 inches off my waist and lower my cholesterol has given me a new appreciation for my body and well-being. Working with a trainer like Matt has not only helped me physically, but also mentally. I was definitely naive and somewhat ignorant when it came to my health. During the past six weeks, I learned not only about the importance of strength training but also about nutrition and how to balance my diet. I now apply everything I learned into everyday life. I no longer eat only three big meals a day. I try to cut down on portion size and eat between 5 and 6 times a day. I also learned how to push myself more in the gym because complacency is what got me overweight in the first place.

I always told myself that I could lose my excess weight if I wanted to, but it was a case of finding the motivation and time to do so. Matt taught me how to set motivational goals which helped me to prioritize my activities and energy. I proved to myself that if I want something I have the commitment and determination to see it through. And that is a great feeling!

Working out with Matt was amazing! He knows how to motivate you and get that 'little extra' out of you without ever sounding patronizing or arrogant. I would definitely recommend his program, seminars, and training. Thanks for your help mate, I really appreciate it."

- Jim Rowe

CHAPTER EIGHT:

Reduce Yourself

"People who are unable to motivate themselves must be content with mediocrity, no matter how impressive their other talents."

Andrew Carnegie

The Time Tested Strategies of Losing Weight

Since the year 2000 Americans have spent more than 119 billion dollars (yes billion) annually on obesity-related medical costs. Each year over 40 billion dollars are spent by the weight loss industry on marketing. At last count, there are over 25,000 books related to weight loss and many of them offer contradictory information. Google the word 'diet" and you will get over 160 million responses. There are so many books, clinics, and programs available, yet less than 10 percent of the people trying to lose weight have long-term success on any diet plan. As a fitness professional, I have been my own guinea pig and personally tried many of the popular diet plans myself. I have a fairly regimented dietary protocol so it is always interesting to see how a particular eating plan or nutritional philosophy will affect me (my weight, energy levels, mood, productivity, etc.). As a personal trainer over the past 12 years, I have witnessed my clients try every conceivable weight loss program...The South Beach Diet, Atkins, Jenny Craig, Weight Watchers, medical weight loss programs, even something called the "Cookie Diet." You name it and chances are, I've tried it or have seen someone try it and monitored the results.

The bottom line from my personal experience and that of my clients is this: to lose weight you must have an effective system for governing caloric intake, you must have a daily nutritional plan, and you must increase your physical activity. I don't care if it is eating high fiber cookies all day or having microwaveable meals for breakfast, lunch, and dinner, the people who lose weight exercise and know how many calories they are eating and it always works. In a nutshell: *move more and eat less.* Simple rules. Incredible results!

But you don't have to take my word for it. In 1994 the National Weight Control Registry was established by Rena Wing, Ph.D. and James O. Hill, Ph.D. to monitor people who are successful at long-term weight loss. Over 5,000 people are being followed who have lost an average of 66 pounds and kept it off for at least five years. Researchers have investigated the behaviors of these individuals and found that 78% eat breakfast, 75% weigh themselves at least once per week, 62% watch less than 10 hours of television per week, and a whopping 90% exercise for at least an hour a day. They say imitation is the ultimate form of flattery and if you are trying to lose weight, I would highly encourage you to imitate the habits of the many people who have been successful at losing weight and more importantly, successful at keeping the weight off. The following list provides a summary of the most common behaviors identified by the National Weight Control Registry (NWCR) for weight loss and weight maintenance.

Secrets to successful weight loss and maintenance (from NWCR website)
- Consumption of a low calorie, low-fat diet
  - 1,300-1,680 calories per day (25% fat)
- Consistent food intake each day
- Eat 4 to 5 times per day
- Consistent consumption of breakfast
- Physical Activity for 60-90 minutes per day (on avg)
- TV viewing was less than 10 hours per week

- Weekly or daily weigh-ins
- Immediate corrective action taken with even a small amount of weight regain

If losing weight is one of your goals, benchmark these practices and incorporate them into your own life. Everybody has the ability to lose weight. Have you ever watched the CBS show Survivor? Every single person without regard to race, body type, nationality, or gender all lose weight while participating on the show. Why? During the show, they are in a highly active environment and eat a reduced amount of calories (of mostly unpleasant foods). You may be thinking: "I exercise and watch what I eat, but my body stays the same." Your genes and your parents aren't to blame. Genes can certainly influence your appetite, basal metabolism, rate of caloric burn during exercise, speed of weight loss or gain, and your set point range, but they won't prevent you from losing weight. The reality is anyone can lose weight and if you have some extra pounds hanging around, hopefully you will find this information useful. The program outlined in this chapter, coupled with the exercise advocated throughout this book will help you maximize your metabolism, lose weight successfully, and keep it off reliably and comfortably without starving yourself.

Why is America Fat and getting even fatter?

The average American female during the 1800's could eat a whopping 3,800 calories each day and not gain any weight. Today, women can gain weight eating a miniscule 1,800 calories a day. Why? Thanks to the industrial revolution and modern technology, our foods take less energy to prepare and digest and more importantly, we are much less active than we used to be. Technology makes things easier on us physically, financially, and mentally. Instead of plowing the fields, planting, and then harvesting our own food or at least trekking over to our neighbor's house a couple miles down the trail to borrow some molasses or a couple of eggs, now our food comes to us by delivery or we sit down in our cars and go to it. And the foods we do eat are so highly processed that even our digestive systems have to do less work now too. With the increasing urbanization of our country, we are now confined to smaller and smaller areas. If you now have a quarter acre patch of land you call home, consider yourself lucky. Urbanization, industrialization, mechanization and the sedentary lifestyle all contribute to the surplus calories being stored on the collective waistlines of America.

Fast food restaurants have become permanent fixtures on real estate near highly traveled intersections in almost every town in America (and now across the globe too). They lure us in like fish, baiting us with their neon signs, 24-hour drive-thru windows, and super value menus. Many of us are now "hooked" on the fast food lifestyle and unless we cut the line by changing our food selection habits, we will continue to be reeled in. Like our genes and last names, poor nutritional habits are passed along from generation to generation. This is why obese parents are now passing on their habits to their children and we are seeing childhood obesity and all of its health consequences on an epidemic rise. If you fall into this category, you have been a product of a bad environment and you must do something about it — for yourself and for your children.

Be wary of the false allure of a "low-fat" lifestyle. Studies with hogs show that when high carbohydrate, low fat, low protein feed is constantly available to them, hogs will eat until their stomachs almost explode, pass out for 90 minutes, then wake-up and eat again; repeating the cycle over and over. Farmers have known this for centuries and it is common practice for fattening hogs for slaughter. Interestingly enough, experiments found that when fat was added to the feed, the rate of eating and the total amount of calories the hogs ate, went down. When the feed was 45% fat by calorie content, the hogs actually stopped gaining weight.

I think it would be safe to say Americans are also fattening themselves for slaughter with the only difference being the method of death (heart disease, stroke, type 2 diabetes, obesity and all related complications). In our age of convenience, we have food constantly available and for most of us, it is the wrong foods; foods which are highly processed and calorie-dense with fat, flour, corn, potatoes, salt, and sugar heading the ingredients list (much like donuts, pastries, fries, pizza, chips, and cookies). The National Health and Nutrition Examination Survey (NHANES) found the "top three" food categories where Americans get the majority of their calories are:

1. White bread, rolls, crackers
2. Doughnuts, bagels, cookies, and cake
3. Alcoholic beverages

Hopefully we can work together and find a simple solution that will help you on your weight-loss journey. The secret to weight loss or maintaining a healthy weight is learning to avoid the blood-sugar rollercoaster ride by eating the right balance of nutrient-dense, high fiber, calorie-portioned foods and it really is not as hard as you may think. In addition to the *Ten Commandments of Nutrition* I covered in the previous chapter, I have devised a system to help you plan your meals each day. The more you plan ahead, the more successful you will be. Research has proven this over and over. Go into any restaurant without a clue of what you are going to eat and before you know it you're slamming a huge fried onion down your throat...and that's just to kill the time before you're 20 ounce side of beef arrives. The bottom line: Don't plan and you will be much more likely to order something with way more calories than you need. Plan what you are going to have beforehand and you will make much better food decisions when confronted with the inevitable temptations on the menu. I advise my clients to decide what they are going to order before they even get to a restaurant or see its menu. Remember, you have to get rid of the excuses and take ownership of your eating.

At the very end of this chapter, I will share with you the system I have used to help people lose thousands of pounds of unwanted bodyfat. If you are currently struggling to lose weight, you are not alone and I hope you will read this chapter and use the tools I give you. Weight loss is never easy and can be even more challenging for some, but you have to believe it is possible — beliefs create reality. If a lifelong smoker can quit "cold turkey," you can immediately change your food habits too. Like nicotine patches can help a smoker quit, you will need the support of your friends and family to help you quit the foods and beverages that have caused you to gain weight.

Ultimately the key is calorie control and you must have a realistic and sustainable system to get you in the right caloric range. If you completed the *Daily Caloric Intake Worksheet* in the previous chapter, then you already have an idea of how many calories you need to eat each day to lose weight. If you didn't, I would strongly encourage you to do it now. I would also recommend you buy a small spiral bound notebook to use for journaling your food. The simple act of writing down what you eat each day is probably the single-most important thing you can do to ensure you successfully lose weight. Studies and my personal experience with clients have proven this over and over. Journaling food intake adds a layer of accountability and turns mindless eating into a more conscious behavior. Once you understand your caloric needs and which foods will help you stay in your "calorie zone," weight loss becomes fairly simple.

Dieting – What's old is new?

During the past few years, my insatiable curiosity for health and fitness related information has led me to read and review older books, studies, and research...some dating back to the late 1800's. It is fascinating to me to see information concerning weight loss and I mean the true essence and principles associated with it, haven't changed all that much over the past 100 years. Like I said at the beginning of this chapter, it's simple: *move more and eat less*. The marketing of different approaches to the concept seem to rotate in a cyclical pattern much like the real estate and stock markets move up and down over time. Many new, hot off the presses, "state-of-the-art" books on dieting and nutrition have essentially regurgitated the same information and marketing fads over and over.

Low-fat diets were popular in the 1930's and again the late 1980's and 1990's. In fact, America developed its fat phobia from all the negative marketing about fat. The idea of a "low-carb diet" was introduced in the 1920's, again in the 1950's, and I'm sure you are aware of the low-carb craze we are now enduring from the marketing moguls who attempt to shape our daily food decisions. High-fat diets first became popular in the 1940's and then again in the 1990's, championed by Dr Atkins and his *New Diet Revolution*. Not so new after all.

If you are trying to lose weight with high protein diets, sugar-busting diets, cookie diets, WeightWatchers', Nutrisystem', South Beach Diet', Atkins", Pritikin, The Zone", or Jenny Craig', there is one fundamental principle any successful "diet" must have in order to illicit weight loss — it must create a caloric deficit. Every aspiring diet author is attempting to create a system to accomplish this with the least amount of pain, discomfort, and inconvenience to the prospective dieter. Any plan that states you can eat whenever and whatever you want without a bold caveat acknowledging the fact that you must burn more calories then you consume is inherently misleading you. Success in any endeavor isn't always easy or without sacrifice. Losing weight is no different.

It was learned over 60 years ago in studies conducted by Dr Robert W. Keetan, that it didn't matter what type of macronutrients (protein, carbs, or fats) were eaten or in what proportion, as long as the calories were the same, weight was lost at the same rate in a caloric deficit. What we also know, however, is that certain foods are more satiating or satisfying for a longer period of time, increasing the likelihood that you won't overeat. On the flip side, certain foods have a much shorter satiation time and can make you hungrier than before you ate them. This obviously increases the likelihood you will feel hungry and have the overwhelming desire to snack on a bag of potato chips or piece of candy.

Like I mentioned previously, farmers have known for centuries that when they want to fatten a pig for slaughter, they remove the fat and protein from the hogs' corn-based feed. This turns the hogs into gluttonous carboholics. With our sugary drinks and high-carb snacks, are we Americans any different than the fattened hogs? Eating a bag of corn puffs is eerily similar to the fattening of a hog. The good news is that even a hog will refuse food when the right amount of fat is included in the food available to them. If fat can satiate the virtually insatiable appetite of a hog, then employing the use of fat in our nutritional strategy can certainly be helpful in controlling our own appetites too. This isn't a license to eat a tub of bacon grease, but it does illustrate the importance of incorporating healthy fats into your overall nutritional plan.

In 1938 a federally funded inpatient study was conducted involving obese patients weighing between 295 and 350 pounds (yes there were obese people in the 1930's too and it is not a recent phenomenon, just the overwhelming prevalence of obesity now is). In the study, the patients were admitted into a controlled hospital environment, where everything they ate and drank was carefully monitored and weighed and even the food they left on their plate was accounted for so those calories could be deducted from their consumption totals. Initially, the patient volunteers were given personal choice for their food and drink and virtually all of them chose a moderate protein, high carbohydrate, and extremely low-fat diet. Hmmm... Even in 1938 people thought "fat makes you fat" and it seems today this myth is philosophically ingrained into our dietary thinking, as well. Just like more and more people are becoming obese now, this philosophy didn't help these volunteers either and they continued to gain weight.

What the researchers eventually determined through this study was a "reducing" diet (dieting was called reducing back then) of 1,300 calories containing 50 grams of carbohydrates, 70 grams of protein, and 90 grams of fat led to the most consistent weight loss. The study participants ate a breakfast consisting of two eggs with bacon, ham, or sausage, 2 ounces of fruit juice, and coffee or tea with cream. For lunch and dinner, they had a 3 ounce portion of meat, chicken, or fish, a vegetable with butter, a salad with salad dressing, a glass of milk, and a small serving of fresh fruit for dessert. They took supplemental B vitamins in the form of brewer's yeast tablets. That's it, a very basic and simple eating plan.

What were the results? All the volunteers lost an average of 10 pounds per month and most interesting of all, almost all of them reported they were comfortable and satisfied with the amount of food they were getting and some didn't even finish all of it. One of the participants, an 18 year old girl who started at a weight of 295 pounds, lost 158 pounds over two years on this plan, most of it on her own when she returned home. When the desired weight was achieved, participants added a piece of whole wheat toast to their breakfast meal and a small dessert to dinner or a snack in the afternoon. If their weight started creeping back up, they eliminated the extras (toast and small dessert) until the weight was lost again. So if you want a proven method to effectively lose weight, try it for yourself. That seems simple enough to me. How about you?

My point in bringing this up is the fat we eat doesn't cause the health problems we have in America, being fat does. And people get fat by eating too many calories, pure and simple. It has been proven that the most comfortable method of losing weight is to include a moderate amount of healthy fats. Fat is the great satiator of your stomach's hunger pangs. Gastric emptying studies with barium and x-ray imagery have shown that fat empties out of the stomach slowly. When food is present in the stomach, a feedback signal is sent to the brain saying "Hey, we're ok down here. No need to eat right now."

Unfortunately, most of us either ignore this signal by stuffing food in our mouths too fast or by distracting our brain by eating in front of the television, while driving, or reading a newspaper. I'm not saying these things are inherently wrong, just that your brain is less likely to hear the feedback from the stomach saying "it really is ok to put the second half of the foot long sandwich down," because you're no longer hungry. Unless you are an Olympic swimmer in training or a professional football player during two-a-day preseason practices, you most likely don't need the extra calories either.

Compared with protein and fat, highly processed and refined carbohydrates are easily digested and empty the stomach rapidly. This not only causes a rapid rise in blood sugar and a subsequent insulin surge, but also lets the stomach tell the brain "hey I'm empty down here and it's time to eat again." This message, coupled with the low blood-sugar rebound after the insulin surge, are two powerful, drug-like effects of eating the wrong foods or combination of foods. You will be unable to fight these hunger signals and getting another "carb fix" will become the most predominant thought on your mind. Unless you learn to change what you eat, this process will become a daily ritual, just like a junkie who needs to get their drug fix. Don't be a junkie, learn to avoid the "junk" foods and select only those foods which satisfy you longer.

Today, people are more apt to play the blame game and say they watch what they eat, even as they continue to gain weight. I'm not saying whether this is right or wrong, but until we accept full responsibility for our lives, weight loss will be much more difficult. While there is some truth to metabolic resistance by the body, 100 out of 100 people will lose weight when they eat the appropriate amount of calories. Why? The laws of the universe tell us so. The Law of Conservation of Energy states that energy is neither created nor destroyed and the 1st Law of Thermodynamics states energy can be converted from one form to another.

In this case, we're talking about calories. If you are overweight, you are an energy storage unit. The universe has taken the energy of the sun and converted it into plants or algae, which either you ate or some animal or fish lower on the food chain ate before you had them for supper. Follow me so far? If you are losing weight, you are converting stored energy into heat via the mitochondria in your cells and releasing it back into the universe. This is an acceptable form of global warming, by the way. So when I say you want to be a fat-burning machine, essentially I'm saying you want to be a heat producer instead of an energy hoarder. Give it back to the universe and your body will thank you.

Each pound of bodyfat you have equals 3,500 calories of stored energy. Therefore, to lose this stored energy, you have to create an energy deficit to force your metabolic machinery to tap into this energy reserve and convert it to biomechanical energy and heat. For most people, one to two pounds of weight loss are acceptable and achievable each week. For one pound of fat loss a week, you would need to burn 500 more calories each day than you put in your mouth and swallow (500/day x 7 days = 3,500). For two pounds a week, simply double this to a 1,000 calorie deficit per day. If you want to be extremely aggressive, you could bump it up to a 1,500 calorie daily deficit average and lose three pounds of bodyfat each week; although for most people this would be extremely challenging (but not impossible).

Now that you conceptually understand the formula for weight loss you are probably wondering: what's the best way to achieve the appropriate caloric deficit to lose weight? The wrong way is to starve yourself each day. This is definitely no fun and a lot harder in the long run, because of metabolic resistance. Studies have found that when you reduce your calories by over 30%, the body will shut down many of its non-critical functions and use available energy for things like breathing and heart beats. With too little calories, your body even cannibalizes its own muscle tissue to release essential amino acids into the bloodstream. This effectively gives you a smaller engine to burn the fuel you're trying to get rid of. Your body slows its metabolic rate to compensate for the drastic calorie reduction and the moment you resume eating a normal amount of calories, your body will very efficiently store the now excess calories as fat. Then you are right back where you started. Therefore, a smarter and more successful approach would be a 10 to 15 percent reduction in total calories consumed and increasing physical activity to widen the caloric deficit. Learn to frequently eat the right foods and you essentially keep stoking the metabolic furnace.

Basal Metabolic Rate

Our basal metabolic rate (BMR) and resting metabolic rate (RMR), what we commonly refer to as our metabolism, in terms of fuel (energy) consumption is like the idle setting on our own internal combustion engines. As your metabolism goes up by exercising regularly, increasing lean mass (skeletal muscle tissue), eating small, frequent meals, and staying adequately hydrated, the idle gets turned up by signals from the hypothalamus in your brain and you start to operate at higher RPMs (rotations per minute) causing you to burn more fuel (fat and sugar). Keeping a high metabolism will help you lose weight faster or allow you to eat more calories while you're maintaining your weight.

Each day, it takes only two to six calories to sustain a pound of bodyfat whereas a pound of muscle (lean mass) takes 50 calories to sustain. This means for every pound of lean mass you put on your body, you will burn an extra 50 calories per day. With proper strength training and sound nutrition, most people can add 6 to 10 pounds of lean mass over the course of a year. With 10 extra pounds of muscle working for you, you'll be burning 500 extra calories each day. This is the essence of how strength training can raise your body's RPMs around the clock and help you lose weight. Once you settle into a healthy weight and maintain it with diet and exercise, your metabolism will learn to become your ally instead of your foe. When you "yo-yo" diet and severely restrict calories for extended periods of time, your metabolism slows down to compensate and you end up fighting a losing battle. There is a better way.

Besides adding muscle to boost metabolism, you can manipulate your caloric intake to do it too. You may have read, heard, or seen recommendations to periodically spike or confuse your metabolism by eating more calories than normal on one or two days per week. Some people call it carbohydrate cycling and some people call it "cheat meals" (as opposed to the "clean meals"). Regardless of what you call it, your body strives to maintain homeostasis (your set point) and therefore when you fall off the wagon and gorge on a pizza or inhale a fast food combo meal, your metabolism will compensate for the extra calories by turning up the idle. This is assuming that you are maintaining a 500 to 1000 calorie deficit on at least five days of the week. Having one or two days each week to take a mini-vacation from your diet can actually be beneficial. Notice I said "mini" vacation because I'm not talking about taking a dietary cruise around the world. Rather, I'm saying you can add in a dessert or a slice of pizza to give your diet some pizzazz once or twice a week. Personally, I plan for 300 to 500 extra calories on Wednesdays and Sundays each week to keep my metabolism guessing and cranked up. I will adjust the days if there is a special occasion on a different day of the week, but it all is part of a weekly plan. If you are disciplined with your food intake and perform a sufficient amount of exercise each week, the higher calorie days will help you maintain a higher overall metabolism.

Essentially, your body burns off the excess calories by creating a mini fever. An actual fever is your body's defensive immune response to an infection and by revving up metabolism, heat is produced and the body temperature begins to rise. Viruses cannot live at temperatures over 100 degrees Fahrenheit and begin to die off. Most people lose weight when they have a fever, some of it due to fluid loss from sweating, but a lot of the weight is from additional calories burned producing the fever. It is not uncommon to see two to three pounds of weight loss from a fever. Don't worry, I'm not recommending you go out and drink an influenza milkshake or eat an E coli sandwich. That wouldn't be the best way to lose weight. But it illustrates my point about the mini-spikes in metabolism your body is capable of.

Do you know what your metabolism is doing? I recently tested my own resting metabolic rate with a BodyGem, indirect calorimeter (manufactured by Microlife) and it was estimated at 2,600 calories per day. Add to this the 900 calories I burn from exercise and physical activity and I can essentially eat around 3,500 calories a day without gaining weight. If I decided to lose weight, I could reduce my calories down to 3,000 calories a day and expect to lose about a pound of fat a week (500 calorie deficit per day for seven days equals 3,500 calories; the amount contained in one pound of fat). The calories you calculated for your daily caloric intake already account for your goal of losing weight and need not be adjusted. Only if you follow the calorie intake for two weeks without any weight loss would I recommend adjusting the number down by 250 calories or a better solution would be to add 250 more calories of activity (about 30 minutes for most people).

The nice thing about having a higher metabolism and maintaining my 193 pounds with diet and exercise is the occasional food holidays I allow myself (see my moderation mantra in Chapter 9). I can have a 4,500 calorie day celebrating with family and friends or watching sports with the fellas, and other than my sheets getting damp from my body cranking up the heat that night, I have no ill effects or weight gain. Now keep in mind I couldn't do this all the time either because my body would start saying "I guess we're in feast mode now" and the calories would start being stored for the future famine our bodies expect when we are in feast mode all the time…"feast or famine." Unfortunately, most Americans are constantly in feast mode periodically interspersed with brief, self-induced famines while they attempt starvation diets.

When you start eating plain salad for breakfast, lunch, and dinner thinking you are going to lose weight, your metabolism actually heads in the wrong direction. When you severely restrict calories your body says: "Hey dude, what's up? How come we aren't having fried chicken tonight? What's with the celery and carrots? No donuts with the coffee? You're killing me!" In response to the drastic calorie reduction, the hypothalamus signals the throttle to slow down the idle and conserve fuel. Indy car racers actually have a switch they can activate to conserve fuel in latter laps of a race. The upside is they may skip a fuel stop and be in position to win the race. The downside is, like your body at a lower metabolism, the engine produces less power and they can get passed by the cars behind them and end up losing. When you don't eat enough calories, your engine slows down, produces less power, and conserves fuel.

Most people like to start diets aggressively and go from eating 2,500 calories a day to just 1,000. Are you like most people? Even though you may be eating 1,000 calories or even 1,500 calories less than you're accustomed to, and you think the pounds should be falling off of you like clothes at a nudist colony, your body has other plans. Since it thinks you're in famine mode and calories must be conserved until the next hunt, your metabolism slows to a crawl. Your engine is now running on one or two cylinders, at low RPMs, and with little power. Instead of having a basal metabolism of say 1,800 calories, it plummets to 1,000 calories, sabotaging 800 of the 1,000 calories you're not eating. And since you have little energy or power, your activity level slows down and you conserve the other 200 calories and *BAM!!!*, your weight stays the same. Extreme suffering for extreme disappointment. Unfortunately, it happens all the time.

Learn to use your metabolism as your ally instead of your enemy. If you're trying to lose weight, start by reducing your caloric intake by 200 to 500 calories per day and increase your activity level by burning 200 to 500 additional calories with physical activity each day. With a decent amount of food still coming in, your metabolism won't slow down and the combined caloric deficit will range between 400 and 1,000 calories a day. This range will cause about one to two pounds of fat loss per week. Any more than this, not only will you lose muscle in addition to fat, but your metabolism will slow down and most likely you will feel terrible, have little energy, and be a moody bear no one wants to be around. There is a right way and a wrong way to do weight loss and I hope this helps you understand both.

Exercise complements nutrition for weight loss

Exercise should be an integral part of any weight loss plan. Losing weight by dieting alone will inevitably end up in failure because you lose unwanted bodyfat, but you also lose calorie-burning muscle. Not good. Both exercise and lean muscle tissue help keep metabolism high and make weight loss attempts more successful. Be wary of situations where you decrease your overall level of activity or exercise. As job situations change, we may find ourselves moving around less. Going from a high-activity position stocking trucks to a low-activity position driving the trucks or going from a foreman position on the line to a management position behind a desk are classic examples where your activity levels can suddenly go down. This can cause the pounds to sneak back on and like the old ball and chain, they slow you down even more.

I know of someone who experienced this firsthand. He had been consistently exercising five days per week and eating a fairly nutritious diet for over 15 years, allowing him to maintain a trim and athletic 193 pounds on about 3,000 calories a day. Then he was promoted to a stressful, time-consuming position sitting behind a desk and had to reduce his exercise in time (30 minutes instead of an hour) and frequency (from five times per week to just two times per week). Despite reducing his food intake by 500 calories a day, in just three months his weight shot up seven pounds and during the subsequent three months, he gained an additional four pounds — a total of 11 pounds gained in just six months of eating *less*. When his 17" x 33" dress shirts wouldn't fit in the neck and he got to the last hole on his miraculously shrinking belt, he realized this was a losing game and something had to be done.

I know this person all too well, because that person was me. I was trading my health, happiness, free time, and waistline for the opportunity to make a high income and let me tell you, money doesn't buy happiness. If nothing else, this served as a powerful lesson to me on the importance of exercise and strength training as it relates to bodyweight. By exercising more now as compared to then, I can eat more calories and still keep my weight the same. While I was working 12-hour days crunching numbers and managing a sales force, I fell into the two meals-a-day habit (lunch and dinner) and despite eating fewer calories than I do now, I gained weight. Fortunately, life and circumstances pushed me into a new direction. I was able to lose the weight with exercise and return to my true passion working in preventive medicine as a personal trainer. Experience is a wonderful teacher.

Calorie Compensation Syndrome

Exercisers who are trying to maintain their weight and especially those trying to lose weight must be wary of what I call "calorie compensation syndrome." This is the psychological phenomenon that convinces many people who exercise they can eat whatever they want. Just because you put in an hour at the gym doesn't mean you can go to your favorite restaurant and inhale a 20-ounce T-bone, loaded baked potato, bottle of wine (for the resveratrol of course), and dessert every night of the week. I'm exaggerating of course, but the point must be made because it happens oh too frequently. And yes, it is the pot calling the kettle black because I've suffered from this syndrome and so have many of my clients. I think there is a little voice in people's heads that says "Hey, you worked out hard today. Go ahead and eat the mountain-sized piece of chocolate cake."

Unfortunately, exercise doesn't give you carte blanche on eating and drinking. You still have to pay attention to what goes in your stomach and have a reasonable understanding of how many calories you consume versus how many calories you burn by exercise, your daily activity level, and your basal metabolism. If they don't sync up favorably, then you will gain weight. Therefore, to prevent calorie compensation syndrome, create an exercise and nutrition plan and stick to it *at least* 80% of the time; the old 80/20 rule. If you are eating the recommended five to six meals a day, this means that for 32 meals a week you are strictly following your nutrition plan and for the other five to eight meals a week you can drift off the reservation a bit. When you rationalize your indulgences, think in terms of mouthfuls, shared desserts, 12-ounce sirloins, and two glasses of wine. This will keep you out of trouble and hold your waistline in check.

Jim
Age: 36
Industrial Engineer

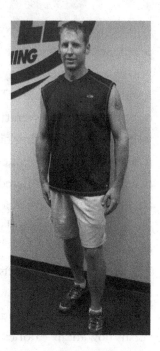

THE FACTS:
In 42 days…
- Lost 11.62 pounds of body fat
- Gained 2.42 pounds of muscle
- Lowered body fat by 5.7%
- Increased strength by 40 pounds on bench press and 85 pounds on squat
- Lost over 2 inches off his waist

"Following a structured exercise and nutrition program has helped me become a stronger and more confident person. I now have the determination and perseverance to work through anything. I've won my health back and what I've learned will carry me through the rest of my life. I would recommend Matt's nutritional approach and high intensity training to everyone. It is a body and life changing experience."

The Secret to losing weight
Want to know the common denominator to any successful diet, nutrition plan, or weight loss success story? It always boils down to this: the amount of calories consumed is controlled. I know I already mentioned this, but if you don't have a pretty accurate grasp of how many calories you eat and drink each day, you are doomed. And if you don't, trust me, you are not alone. Studies have proven that people underestimate the calories they eat by 30 to 40%. That's 400 to 700 calories for most people, which is more than enough to add weight quickly. So if you think you are eating about 2,000 calories each day, you are actually eating closer to 2,700 calories. The unfortunate reality is that we only

have to eat about 20 to 30 surplus calories a day to gain the two to thee extra pounds Americans average each year.

What follows is my essential formula for bodyweight change, boiled down to the rudimentary essence of weight gain for most people. Keep in mind it is extremely simplified and does not account for gains in lean mass (which come at about 1,500 calories per pound of muscle due to its high water content).

The Essential Formula for Bodyweight Change

Net Energy Equation: $E_{in} - E_{out} = E_{net}$ **(in calories)**

Bodyweight Change: $\Delta BWT = E_{net} / 3500$ **(in pounds)**

The food and drinks we consume are a form of energy expressed in kilocalories (kcals), the universally accepted system to determine how much energy something we eat actually has. Let's call this *energy in* which is expressed as E_{in} in my Net Energy Equation. The amount of energy we burn for maintenance of all our bodily functions (your basal or resting metabolic rate) combined with the calories we burn for all daily activity and exercise we'll collectively call *energy out*. This is expressed as E_{out} in my Net Energy Equation. E_{out} is the energy we release in the form of heat through biochemical enzymatic reactions and the liberated energy used for biomechanical movement and vital functions.

When E_{in} is equal to E_{out}, E_{net} = O and we maintain our weight. This is called homeostasis or a set point. According to set point theory, our bodies want to maintain a set point and the longer we stay at a certain set point, the harder the body will manipulate hormones and metabolism to maintain it. Unfortunately, most people never give their bodies this option because they continually move less and eat more, causing surplus energy to be stored as bodyfat.

If E_{in} is greater than E_{out}, then you create a positive E_{net} which represents a calorie surplus. If you average a 200 calorie surplus each day for a month you will have a monthly E_{net} of 6,000 calories. Put this into the formula for Bodyweight Change and you can calculate the monthly impact to your weight: 6,000 / 3,500 = 1.71 pounds. If you want to lose weight, than you have to create a negative E_{net} by having E_{out} exceed E_{in}. Averaging a 500 calorie daily deficit for a week will give you a negative E_{net} of 3,500 calories. That's enough to lose a pound of fat for each week you achieve it (-3,500 / 3,500 = -1 pound). Averaging a 1,000 calorie daily deficit through diet and exercise will help you lose two pounds of fat per week (-7,000 / 3,500 = -2 pounds).

A Typical Example – Cindy goes to college

Let's look at a typical example like Cindy. Cindy is a young woman in her late twenties who has settled down with a family to take care of, a professional career to manage, and a husband's affection to maintain. Despite being a 125-pound soccer player and very active in high school, when she went to college she put on the so called "freshman fifteen" as activity was replaced with studying and partying. By the time she graduated, she weighed 150 pounds, at a height of 5' 4" and went on to gain another 20 pounds after settling into married life and giving birth to two wonderful children. Now Cindy is 29 years of age, weighs 170 pounds and is facing the reality that she is overweight and doesn't like the person in the mirror anymore. How does this happen to her and so many more people in America?

It is simple math. When Cindy went to college, during her freshman year she continued to eat the same 2,000 calories (E_{in}) she did in high school when she was more active and her body was growing. Without these demands her metabolism slows a little and other than walking across campus, Cindy gets no real physical activity. Her resting metabolic rate accounts for about 1,450 calories a day and her daily movement and walks across campus burn an additional 380 calories, for a total energy out (E_{out}) of 1,830 calories. Using the Net Energy equation, 2,000 calories (E_{in}) minus 1,830 calories (E_{out}) = a positive net energy balance of 170 calories per day. This expressed formulaically would look like:

$$2000_{kcals} - 1830_{kcals} = 170_{kcals/day} \text{ (surplus)}$$

Wow, that's not too bad you might think. She is less than a candy bar away from losing weight, right? Well, let's take a look at the impact of having just a 170 calorie surplus (daily average) for Cindy.

$$170_{kcals/day} \times 365_{days/year} = 62,050_{kcals/year}$$

It takes approximately 3,500 surplus calories to create one pound of stored bodyfat. Cindy's 62,050 surplus calories in her freshman year divided by 3,500 calories per pound of bodyfat equals 17.73 pounds!!! "Holy Hotcakes Batman, that's the evil freshman fifteen!" Robin would exclaim.

$$\textbf{Bodyweight Change} = E_{net} / 3,500_{kcals/lb}$$

$$= 62,050_{kcals} / 3,500_{kcals/lb}$$

$$= 17.73 \text{ pounds (gained)}$$

So for her sophomore year Cindy gets smart. She cuts out the french fries or bag of potato chips she has almost everyday at the snack bar and pays more attention to what she eats. Excitedly and much to the chagrin of her parents checkbook, she moves off campus and starts driving to class. This cuts down the only activity she was getting on her walks across campus and drops her *energy out* by about 150 calories per day. So despite saving almost 300 calories per day on the fries and chips, her weight essentially stays the same during her second year of college because her *energy net* is around zero.

$$1,700 \text{ kcals}_{in} - 1,700 \text{ kcals}_{out} = 0_{net}$$

Then in her junior and senior years, Cindy turns 21 and discovers beer and the college party scene. She and her sorority friends have three or four beers on Thursday, Friday, and Saturday nights and even though she drinks light beer (rationalizing that she is saving calories), Cindy is now consuming an average of 174 to 218 calories per day in light beer (102 calories per beer multiplied by 12 to 15 beers a week = 1,224 to 1,530 beer calories per week divided by seven days per week equals 174 to 219 calories on average per day).

Cindy likes the fact she maintained her weight during her sophomore year and wants to combat the additional calories she is drinking. She learns in her health class that exercise burns calories, so she starts going to the campus gym and walks on the treadmill for 30 minutes three to four times per week. She burns an additional 250 calories each time she does this, and assuming she goes four times a week, Cindy will burn 1,000 calories each week with exercise or an average of 143 extra *calories out* per day (1,000 divided by 7).

What is the impact of these decisions on Cindy's weight? Let's go back to the Net Energy equation and assume her resting metabolism hasn't changed and we won't even account for the negative impact alcohol can have on fat metabolism in the body. So her daily *energy out* goes up by 143 calories to 1,843 calories (1,700 + 143) and her *energy in* is adjusted accordingly: 1,700 calories previous daily E_{in} + 174 average calories per day drank in beer equals 1,874 *calories in*. Thus:

$$1{,}874 \text{ kcals } (E_{in}) - 1{,}843 \text{ kcals } (E_{out}) = 31 \text{ kcals } (E_{net})$$

Now Cindy is doing much better with the Law of Conservation of Energy than she did during her freshman year, but the 31 surplus calories equates to an additional 3 pounds of bodyfat on her body each year for her junior and senior years.

$$31_{kcals/day} \text{ x } 365_{days/year} = 11{,}315_{kcals/year}$$

$$11{,}315_{kcals/year} \text{ divided by } 3{,}500_{kcals/lb} = 3.23\text{lbs per year}$$

The four years Cindy spends in college can be summed up like this:

Starting weight:	**125 pounds**
Freshman year:	+ 17 pounds
Sophomore year:	no change
Junior Year:	+ 3.2 pounds
Senior Year:	+ 3.2 pounds
Graduation weight:	**148.4 pounds**

This pattern of weight gain continues with the start of her career, marriage, pregnancy, raising two children, unsuccessful attempts at dieting and by the time she has her 29th birthday, Cindy has gained another 20 pounds. Put all this together and you'll find Cindy close to the 170 unhealthy pounds she is at today. And that my friends, is how it happens. Without us even realizing it sometimes, the weight keeps sneaking on each year like Cindy's did. Since two out of every three Americans are now classified as overweight or obese, this pattern is probably familiar to many people. It may be more or less weight, or the circumstances of how it is gained may be different, but the basic formula never changes. If you're putting more calories into your body then you are burning with your metabolism, exercise and daily activity, you will gain weight — pure and simple.

Fortunately, the formula for losing the weight is the same and we have to create a negative energy balance on most or all days of the week. Just like the weight came on, the weight will also come off. Is it easy? Let's just say that success comes easier for some people, but most things worth having don't come easy. Working with hundreds of different people, I have found that losing weight doesn't have to be difficult and can actually be enjoyable for some with the right approach, personal outlook, mental attitude, and support of your family and friends. From my research and decade of experience working with clients trying to lose weight, I determined there are five critical steps of weight loss in addition to creating a sustainable caloric deficit. They are listed below and then subsequently explained:

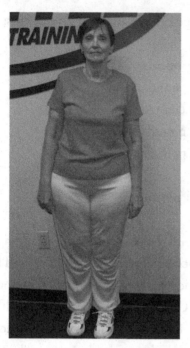 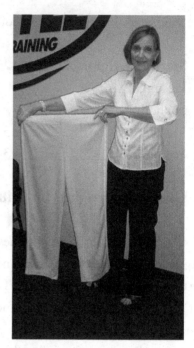

Karen lost over 30 pounds following these steps

The Five Critical Steps of Weight Loss
1. Don't play the blame game
2. Make lifestyle type changes
3. Form healthy habits
4. Get the support of your family and friends
5. Change your environment

1. Don't play the "Blame Game"

If you seriously want to commit to a successful weight loss plan, first and foremost, you have to acknowledge that the weight you're trying to lose was not completely your fault. There is nothing positive that will come from blaming yourself or anyone else for anything in life. Operating from this perspective means you have an external locus of control and often feel like you are the victim of your circumstances. Playing the blame game only increases stressful feelings of guilt and failure which subsequently causes the emotional eating habits that contribute to the problem. Eating for emotional pleasure or reward will only temporarily relieve or mask the pain, but can definitely cause additional weight gain and even more feelings of failure — thus perpetuating a negative cycle. The past is the past and it is time to move on in a more positive direction. Where you decide to go from here is what really matters. Weight gain is typically a product of the environment we spend the most time in, how we were raised and our own unintentional ignorance when it comes to eating and exercise. After reading this book, you are no longer a victim of ignorance. You control your own destiny!

2. Make some "Lifestyle" changes

You *must* acknowledge that you are going to make some changes to your lifestyle. This goes without saying (even though I said it) because whatever you are doing now is not working. We should all know the definition of insanity by now: Doing the same things over and over and expecting different results. Successful weight loss is not going to happen unless we change the process we use (no more yo-yo famine dieting) and change the thinking patterns that got us there in the first place. When I look back at my own success and the success stories of my clients, it is apparent we all made lifestyle changes as part of the process. These should not be perceived as sacrifices, because the rewards are so worth it and you won't miss the old lifestyle at all.

Incorporating exercise and healthy eating habits must be viewed as a long-term lifestyle change, not a quick fix. Go into the process with this mentality and you will prevent the disappointment many people experience when they realize the weight doesn't fall off overnight. Just like preventive maintenance will keep your car running longer, a healthy lifestyle will keep your body running longer too.

3. Form healthy habits

You *must* form new and better habits of food selection, eating, and exercise. We can blame the food industry for developing, marketing and distributing the foods we can't seem to live without or we can take personal responsibility for our own actions and step up to the accountability plate and decide to make a positive change. When it comes to food, we are own worst enemies. We leave snacks and treats around the house with the excuse that they're "for the kids." We are kidding ourselves with this one. First of all, the kids don't need to eat sugary, fatty foods and second of all, neither do you.

Another form of rationalization is when there are numerically enticing specials at the grocery or large box stores for foods we don't need, sucking us in like a moth to a light… "Wow! They have five for five dollars on snacky sweet cakes! What a deal. We must buy them." If they offered you five for five dollars on arsenic apple pies would you buy those too? You must learn to recognize the things which influence your decisions and learn to counter them with your own food strategies. We Americans too often serve our families of three or four enough food to feed 12 people and brainwash our kids with the idea that they must clean their plate because of the starving children in Africa who would love to have the food.

Last month I tried to get to the origin of the "clean your plate" mentality most of us grew up with, so I talked to my grandma, who is 97, figuring she goes a way back. I asked her: "Did you tell my mom to clean her plate when she was growing up?" And she replied with: "You bet I did!" I then asked her if her parents told her to clean her plate when she was growing up and she said they did. Being curious, I asked for her insight. "What do you think that mentality comes from?" She grew up in the 1920's and said "It comes from the mentality of lack or being without. Food wasn't always as plentiful as it is today and so you never knew how much you were going to get to eat in future meals." Thanks to modern agricultural and food processing methods, this does not seem to be a likely problem anytime soon. Maybe it's time to change this mentality and decide that it is ok to leave some food on our plates.

4. Get the help and support of your family and friends

If you want any chance of being successful on your weight loss journey, you *must* get the support of your family and friends. Have you ever seen the Discovery Channel shows on climbing Mt. Everest or read the book *Into Thin Air* by Jon Krakauer? Climbing the world's highest peak is an extreme challenge and would be impossible without the help of experienced guides and sherpas to help you on your journey. Losing weight is also a challenge and to get to the top of the metaphorical weight loss mountain, you will also need the help and support of your family and friends. I can't emphasize this enough.

If you don't get everyone close to you "on board" your weight loss train and have them acknowledge to you in person, face to face, that they will help you in any way they can, then you are far more likely to fail. Without your request for support, your spouse, your family, and your friends can unknowingly become your worst weight loss enemies. If you don't involve them consciously in the process, they may sabotage your efforts with their requests to order pizza and dessert, telling you to "skip the gym today" or surrounding you with other food temptations. Human beings can be selfish creatures and will serve their own best interests and desires unless you remind them of your need for support. Make helping you their selfish interest and getting you to your goal will help them achieve their goal of helping someone else.

5. Change your environment

The final step and one that warrants a lengthy discussion is you *must* change your environment. A 32-year study published in the *New England Journal of Medicine* linked obesity with our social networks. It concluded that if your closest friends are obese, you are far more likely to be obese too. This correlation also applies to close family members and spouses too. So you either have to change your family and friends or what would be much better and more realistic, get them involved with you. If you have a group of people at work who want to lose weight, collectively pool some money for a trip or something enticing (make it a significant prize) and have a weight loss contest. This will help improve everyone's participation, motivation, compliance, and ultimate results. Everyone share their success strategies with each other and in the long run, someone gets a nice prize, but everyone wins!

Regardless, if you make the decision to change for yourself, you have to be willing to let some friendships go or even risk altering the relationship with your spouse. If he or she is not willing to join you or support you, then they are either extremely selfish or more than likely, they are scared. They are scared that you will lose weight and leave them or scared that you will succeed where they have failed. These are completely normal feelings and ones you will need to discuss and be prepared to deal with. This is definitely a controversial "gray area" but I leave it up to you to decide. If someone doesn't make the effort to take care of themselves, you will eventually lose them prematurely anyway.

What I have seen in my professional experience in the situation where one person in a relationship takes action without the support or participation of the other, is the success of the participant ultimately serves as motivation for the other to get started. I want to warn you that this is not always the case. But if one person makes the sacrifice and it even costs them their relationship, in the long run they are better served and especially if there are children involved. Having one parent alive past 50 is better than having two dead ones or worse, the children having to take care of both parents because of the avoidable complications of obesity. I honestly have a lot of sympathy for people suffering with excess weight, but I hope what I am trying to say makes sense too. I really want to help people who have at least a glimmer of light inside showing them the way to a better life. But I know it can be a long, difficult process and even with help, it can and will be challenging.

We need to be aware of our personal environment, or in other words, the environments in which we live, work, play, and eat. Studies have conclusively proven that our environment can have a profound impact on us unless you are consciously aware of this relationship. Through the study of human psychology, we have learned how we can unconsciously link the events of our circumstances and environment to both pain and pleasure. This is called cognitive linking, where we can link one thing to another. An unfortunate, but common example is a married woman in an abusive relationship who is repeatedly taunted with "I will kill you if you divorce me" threats from her husband. If she ever builds the courage to get out of the relationship, she will forever link marriage with death or bodily harm in her subconscious mind. This will inevitably sabotage her future relationships unless she becomes aware of this connection and breaks the link. When it comes to weight loss, you may have someone in your life who tells you that you will always be fat. Hear it enough and you may start to believe it. You may even start linking your own name with being fat. This mental abuse is criminal in my opinion and is just as damaging as physical abuse, just less obvious. If you're in a situation where someone is constantly putting you down, please seek some professional help and either change the relationship or get out of it.

I have a client I'll call Nicole. Nicole's 52-year-old mother Samantha is now living with her own mother (my client's grandmother) who is debilitated with advanced age and the effects of nerve damage in her feet. Nicole's grandmother uses a motorized scooter to get around. After a year in this environment, Nicole's mom Samantha now thinks she needs a scooter too. Remember she is only 52! She is trying to justify her need for a scooter with the aches and pains caused by her sedentary lifestyle. Fortunately, Nicole let her know (in a not so subtle way) that demobilizing herself will only make things worse. Samantha's muscles, which are already starving for some attention, will atrophy at an accelerated rate by moving even less by riding around in a scooter. Living with her feeble mom is programming her thinking in the wrong direction. She needs to change her environment a little and get in one where she is surrounded by people who exercise and take a more proactive approach to their health and well-being. This doesn't mean she needs to move out or abandon her mother, but it does mean she needs to find a more physically active environment to spend some time in each day.

It is often said in financial self-help books that you can predict how much you will be earning in three years by looking at the average income of the five people you spend the most time with. The weight on your body is the same. Epidemiological studies have proven a definitive link between obesity and social networks. If you spend most of your time with an overweight spouse, overweight friends and overweight family members, then you are more likely to be overweight yourself. In your mind, you are linking fun, friends, and good times to being overweight. I'm not saying to abandon your friends, but you need to be aware of this relationship. Successful weight loss is contagious because when you are successful losing weight, you will be happier, feel better, look better, and live longer. Your friends and family will link your success with exercise and will want to do what you do too.

It can work the opposite way too, which is why I'm discussing the cognitive linking process with you. Many people are unwittingly linking failure or pain to exercise. If you have ever attempted to lose weight on your own (without proper guidance, counseling, and instruction) by going to the gym and attacking the treadmill everyday for 50 minutes like a raging banshee with an attitude problem then ambiguously pushing some weights around the gym for 30 minutes and after one week you jump on the scale and say: "Why is it not moving?" This applies to you. You are programming your mind with "exercise equals failure and pain." It is time to change your thinking and understand the process of successful weight loss.

Losing weight is a process

If you are planning to start an exercise program to lose weight, it is critical that you are aware of the entire process. Your excess weight did not suddenly slip under your sheets in the cover of darkness and slap itself on your belly and thighs overnight did it? Similarly, the weight doesn't miraculously fall off your belly and thighs overnight either. Gaining weight is a process like Cindy's example I explained earlier. Losing weight is a process too which takes time, effort, a little self-discipline, and lots of patience. With proper guidance, accountability, instruction, motivation, and monitoring, you will learn to set incremental, realistic goals and celebrate each milestone along the way to your ultimate goal.

I'm sure you've heard the question: "How do you eat an elephant?"... and the answer: "One bite at a time." You have to approach weight loss the same way and set yourself up mentally for realistic success through constant progress. Otherwise, you may end up linking failure to your attempts to do something great for yourself and develop an aversion to exercise. Ever throw up drinking too much tequila on college spring break then later find yourself gagging at even the smell of it? (Or did that just happen to me?) Similarly, if you find yourself getting nauseous at the thought of sweating in the gym, you have an aversion to exercise and we will need to reprogram your mind. Try to befriend someone who is passionate about exercise and just like a virus, their attitude can infect your thinking too. Before you know it, you will be passionate about exercise too.

People who do succeed with weight loss have a *daily plan* and this plan generally includes the following:
1. Calorie control
2. Cardiovascular exercise
3. Resistance exercise
4. Dietary support
5. Personal help and assistance

One of the most difficult aspects of being a personal trainer and working with clients trying to lose weight is compliance. I invest a tremendous amount of time, energy, and compassion into each client and give them a road map and all the written directions they need to take them exactly where they want to go in the shortest amount of time possible. Then some of them throw out the map, drive off the road, turn around and go backwards, and continue to be lost. Even people who have the best intentions when they begin can easily slip back into their old habits. Some people are unwilling to make the simple changes necessary to develop lifelong habits required to achieve a healthy lifestyle. This is where you, the individual, have to take ownership of the direction you are heading and follow the map. There is no need for guess work or trial and error. The method is simple in concept but evidently, challenging in its execution.

I tell all my clients that I will help get them in the best shape of their lives; that much I can guarantee. But what they end up bodyweight wise is completely up to them. I push my clients hard and their muscles, heart, lungs, and arteries will all get in better shape very quickly. On a good workout day, they can burn 400 to 600 calories if they are female or 500 to 700 calories, if they are a male. Over the course of a week, this can lead to 1,200 to 2,100 additional calories burned from our workouts (three hour-long workouts a week). But they can easily negate this caloric effort in just five mindless minutes at a fast food restaurant or by having additional alcoholic drinks or dessert throughout the week using the internal rationalization (calorie compensation syndrome) that they workout hard, so they can indulge themselves. We are our own worst enemies and I have to constantly remind even myself that I have to watch what and how much I eat.

I put a lot of pressure on myself to help my clients get results and fortunately, a lot of them do. When they try to thank me because they achieved their weight loss goal, I always tell them to thank themselves because I can't take credit for it. I will tell them: "I am only the navigator; you are the captain of your ship." And it's true. They make all the daily decisions leading to their success, I can only help steer them in the right direction and try to correct them if they get off course. The same will be true for you. You control your destiny and the last two chapters of this book can help you reprogram your mind and set goals that you will achieve.

The Best Diet in the World

The best diet in the world is the one you don't know you're on. Diet comes from a Latin word meaning "way of life." Genetics, environment, and behavior are all factors which can influence our waistlines, our health, and our happiness. There are literally thousands and thousands of diet books trying to convince us of a unique way to lose weight. The problem is that anything which makes people feel deprived will ultimately fail. This is why most diet books and weight loss infomercials include the marketing headline: "Eat whatever you want!" Okinawans have the largest percentage of centenarians in the world. They have a philosophy called Hari Hachi Bu which means *eat until you are 80% full*. Another approach is the "30% rule" which states: throw 30% of your food away or even better, save it for later. We were taught by our parents to "clean your plate" and we have to deprogram ourselves from this conditioned thinking.

So the best diet secret is learning to eat higher volumes of the right foods and lower volumes of the wrong foods which cause most of the weight gain. The 80/20 rule applies to weight gain because 20% of the foods we eat and drink will cause 80% of the weight gain. By reengineering the way we eat by moderating those 20% foods, we can solve 80% of our problems. I have come up with a simple way for you to identify the foods which fit into this category and modify what you eat a little without sacrificing food volume — what Barbara Rolls calls "volumetrics" in her book of the same name.

What follows is my philosophy for planning meals each day, week in and week out. Hopefully, you can learn to use it in some capacity to manage your weight and help control blood sugar levels. You will have more energy to accomplish your goals each and every day, whether they are fitness related or being the CEO of your own company or most importantly, being the best parent you can be. The first system I explain to anyone trying to lose weight involves three simple steps.

1. **Control or eliminate the "White Carbs"**
   a. Sugar, white bread, pasta, potatoes, and white rice
2. **Eat the right portions**
   a. Protein: use the size and thickness of your palm (without fingers)
   b. Starch or fruit: limit to the size of your fist
   c. Cruciferous, fibrous "green" vegetables: unlimited (within reason)

3. Eat 5 to 6 small lean protein and fibrous vegetable meals every 3 to 4 waking hours

That's it; it is a very basic approach that works remarkably well for most people. Once someone understands and incorporates this system they are ready to take their nutrition to the next level. Even the best drivers in the world would get lost or crash if it weren't for traffic signs and traffic lights. In our modern society, we need help and guidance to get where we want to go. This is especially true when it comes to eating and weight loss.

What follows is my ultimate food selection guide that will help anyone who wants to lose weight and have more healthy energy each day. After reading book after book on dieting and nutrition, I wanted to devise a system that made food selection simple and easy to understand. If you are like most of my clients and friends who don't have time to read volumes of information on what to eat, this guide will be your ally in understanding how to eat. It will not only help you lose weight, it can also help you lower your cholesterol levels, lower your blood pressure, and increase your energy levels. It may not be perfect or full-proof, but I guarantee you it works!

The Nutrition Traffic Light

Like modern traffic lights guide how we drive each day, the *Nutrition Traffic Light* will guide how you eat each day. It follows the simple premise that red means *stop*, yellow means *caution*, and green means *go*. The "red foods" (and beverages) are the most calorie-dense, carb-addicting, high-glycemic, fat-storing types of foods that must be consumed in very limited quantities if you are trying to lose weight. The "yellow foods" are less calorie-dense foods (than the red foods) but still should be eaten in moderation; paying particular attention to portion sizes. The "green foods" are what you should be eating at most or all of your meals. I tell my clients: *to get lean you have to go green* and refer them to the foods on the green list. Even if you aren't trying to lose weight, for your health and longevity you can't go wrong staying "in the green." If you are a visual person, highlight each category with its respective color and post it on your refrigerator at home and your desk, dashboard, or computer monitor at work.

How do you best use the Nutrition Traffic Light? Simple…you pair a four to six ounce portion of protein from the *Lean proteins* list with a fruit or vegetable from their respective lists at each of your five or six small meals each day. For one or two of your meals each day, you can have a small fist-sized portion (four to six ounces) of a food or a cup (four to six ounces) of a drink on the yellow list. Once or twice a week max, you can indulge yourself with a food or beverage on the red list. Even so, try to limit yourself to one small fist-sized portion or one eight-ounce beverage or ten ounces of meat, whichever is appropriate. If you are in the process of losing a decent amount of weight, this is not the time to have an 800 calorie milkshake or a half dozen donuts. Get the smallest size possible of the shake or opt for a few donut holes if that's what you really want. Keep in mind this list is not all-inclusive but does include the most popular choices in each category. Use your own judgment when deciding which color category something not on the list belongs. Follow this system along with the *Ten Commandments of Nutrition* from Chapter 7 and you will feel great and undoubtedly lose weight.

"Red Foods" = Avoid (1 - 2 Servings <u>Per Week</u> Max *if any*)

White carbs	*Anything fried*	Cheese fries	Jams and jellies
White flour	Fried Chicken	Cheese sauces	Mashed potatoes
White potatoes	Fried fish	Cinnamon rolls	Milk shakes
White rice	Fried hamburgers	Cookies	Muffins
White sugar	Fried potatoes	Corn syrup	Onion rings
White pasta	Dessert pies	Crackers	Pancakes
Fatty meats	*Alcoholic beverages*	Dinner rolls	Pork gravy
Brisket	*Calorie-dense beverages*	Donuts	Potato chips
Liver	*Calorie-dense foods*	Fast food	Pretzels
Beef ribs	Bagels	French fries	Sodas, colas
Pork ribs	Beef gravy	Frozen yogurt	Sweetened cereals
Ribeye steaks	Brownies	Fruit juice	Tortilla chips
Pulled pork	Cake	Fudge	Waffles
Sausage	Candy	Ice cream	White bread

"Yellow Foods" = Moderate (1 - 2 Servings <u>Per Day</u> *combined total*)

Whole grains	*Cereal grains*	*Dairy*	*Starches*
Whole wheat bread	Bran flakes	4oz Milk (1%)	Beans (all)
Whole wheat crackers	Shredded Wheat	4oz Milk (skim)	Brown rice
Whole wheat pasta	All-Bran˚, Fiber One˚	4oz Soy Milk (Light)	Chickpeas
Barley	Cream of wheat	1oz Cheese (reduced fat)	Corn
Couscous	Oatmeal (low sugar)	4oz Yogurt (low sugar)	Hummus
Quinoa	Kashi˜, Smart Start˚	4oz Pudding (low sugar)	Lima Beans
Wild Rice	*Nuts*		Peas
	2oz Walnuts, almonds,		Sweet
	peanut butter		potatoes

"Green Foods" = Enjoy (3 - 5 Servings <u>Per Day</u> *of each category*)

Vegetables		*Lean proteins*	*Fruits*
Alfalfa sprouts	Lettuce	Beef sirloin	Apples
Arugula	Mushrooms	Beef tenderloin	Apricots
Asparagus	Mustard greens	Beef top round	Bananas
Bean sprouts	Okra	Canadian bacon	Blackberries
Beets	Onions	Chicken breast	Blueberries
Bell peppers	Peppers (all)	Cottage cheese (1-2% fat)	Cantaloupe
Broccoli	Pumpkin	Egg Beaters˚	Cherries
Brussel sprouts	Radicchio	Egg whites	Grapefruit
Cabbage	Radish	Ham	Grapes
Carrots	Salad greens	Lean ground beef	Honeydew
Cauliflower	Snow peas	Pork tenderloin	Kiwi
Celery	Spinach	Salmon	Mango
Collard greens	Squash	Shellfish	Oranges
Cucumber	String beans	Soy protein (20 grams)	Papaya
Egg plant	Sugar snap peas	Tofu	Peaches
Endive	Tomatoes	Tuna	Pears
Green beans	Turnip greens	Turkey bacon	Pineapple
Kale	Watercress	Turkey breast	Plums
Leeks	Zucchini	Whey protein (20 grams)	Rasberries
			Strawberries

To illustrate an example of how this comes together in the real world, one of my clients named Hope put together the following meal plan and used it to lose 53 pounds in six months. Her story is featured at the end of this chapter and I encourage you to read it.

<u>**Meal 1**</u>
½ cup Oats (dry measure)
20gm Whey protein
20oz Water

<u>**Meal 5**</u>
5 oz Chicken Breast
2 cups Broccoli
12oz Water

<u>**Meal 2**</u>
6 egg whites, 1 yolk
½ cup Onions
½ cup Green peppers
1 cup Broccoli
12oz Water

<u>**Meal 6**</u>
6 egg whites, 1 yolk
½ cup Onions
½ cup Green peppers
1 cup Green beans
20oz Water

<u>**Meal 3**</u>
5 oz Chicken breast
1 cup Spinach
20oz Water

<u>**Meal 7**</u>
1 sc Meal replacement powder
1 tbsp Natural Peanut Butter
12oz Water

<u>**Meal 4**</u>
20gm Whey protein
1 tbsp Natural Peanut Butter
12oz Water

Listed below is how Hope's meal plan breaks down by macronutrient, calories, and percentage of total calories.

	<u>Grams</u>	<u>Calories</u>	<u>% of total</u>
Protein:	240	960	49%
Carbohydrate *(42grams are fiber)*:	127	508	26%
Fat:	48	486	25%
Totals:	**415**	**1,954**	**100%**

That's a lot of food by volume, but not a lot of calories. Keep in mind Hope started her weight loss at well over 200 pounds and was exercising over an hour a day, six days a week. She followed this nutritional plan Monday through Friday with an occasional fist-sized portion of a starchy carbohydrate (like brown rice or sweet potato) two days a week (carbohydrate cycling) and allowed herself a little leeway on the weekends for a restaurant meal or a food holiday. By following this plan, she obeyed all the *Ten Commandments of Nutrition* and was in the green on the *Nutrition Traffic Light*. Come up with your own plan and stick with it. The results are worth it.

Hope's Story

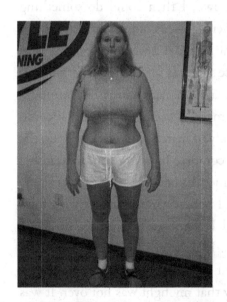

I remember very clearly the day my life was changed forever. I was in my mid 20's, my two children were playing quietly in their room, and I was feeling sorry for myself. I had once again failed on a strict diet I put myself on and this time I was nearly in tears. I had told myself I was going to compete in figure competitions and I would workout and diet hard until I reached my goal.

But here I lie in bed, having skipped my workout and eating the very junk food I said I would avoid. In the past, I had always blamed circumstances for my dietary failures: "My family took us to dinner, I couldn't be rude!" or "The car broke down, the kids are fussy, the bills are due and I'm stressed, what point is a diet right now?" Even excuses like, "It was sweet, my husband brought me home my favorite candy and I ate it to show my appreciation..."

The reasons went on and on. But this time I was crying because I knew I had no one to blame but myself. I had just given up. I made the decision and I blew my diet. But a strange thing happened while I was feeling sorry for myself. While lying there a revelation hit me. I realized that my previous excuses were just that; excuses, and my weight problem was not anyone else's fault. I was the one that picked up the fork and put it in my mouth. I chose to sit on the couch and skip the gym. I pressed snooze on my alarm instead of getting up for my morning workout. The responsibility lied squarely on my shoulders. But with that revelation, the tears stopped, my face dried and a new sense of strength began to well within me.

Why? Because when I entrusted the responsibility for my health with others, I was powerless to change. When I realized my health was no one else's responsibility but my own, I then could do something about it. This revelation was empowering — a completely new idea to me and I didn't want to forget it. The next day I went and got my very first tattoo. I chose to get the Chinese symbols for "Determination" put on my right shoulder blade. I wanted a permanent and visible reminder of my revelation and the decision I made. I *would* change my life and become healthy! I *would* train my body to match who I felt I was on the inside and I *would* get on stage and compete in figure competitions!

Now I wish I could say that six months later I was in perfect shape and ready to get on stage, but in all honesty my struggles with food were not over. But never again did I blame circumstances or create other excuses for my lack of results. I could not forget the promise I made to myself. Even when I was put on bed rest because of a difficult pregnancy with my son, I still knew that my fight was not over. It was simply delayed.

In November of 2007, after relocating to Florida and settling into the home I wanted to stay in forever, I knew the time had come to make good on my promise to myself. I was 90 pounds overweight, but that reminder tattooed on my shoulder was still there beckoning me not to give up on my dream. I joined a gym and started the process of eating healthy and training hard. I was relieved to see the weight begin to release its grip on me. By exercising regularly and eliminating most of the junk food I had been eating, I lost about 30 pounds over the next four months.

Then in February of 2008 I told the front desk staff at my health club that I was looking for a trainer who could help me get in shape to compete in a female figure competition. Since I was still a good 60 pounds above anything that could be described as bikini shape, I am not sure they took me seriously. But I was more determined than ever so I persisted in my requests. I was eventually introduced to Matt O'Brien who became my trainer and friend for the biggest and final part of my journey. Matt quickly explained to me that setting and writing down a goal was extremely important and would largely dictate my success or failure. Even though I felt like I was seemingly years away from my goal of being onstage in a figure competition, he wanted me to pick an actual show within the next eight months. Although a bit apprehensive, I picked the show and the date and we began working toward the goal. Having that future date written on my calendar solidified in my heart and mind a reason to keep working hard even when I felt like giving up.

During my first session with Matt, I told him I would give 100% effort and not complain about anything he asked me to do. I said to him: "I hired you to help me and if you say do it and it's not physically impossible, then I will do it." I laugh now because I remember there were many moments when I regretted making that promise...pain is Matt's middle name. But when I was asked by him to do more than I thought I could and I wanted to stop or throw up, I remembered that looming date and I kept going.

I sit here today at a healthy weight, with a strong body, and having completed the goal I made so many years ago. The date I set with Matt was indeed the day I got onstage for my very first competition. It was a very emotional time for me and I shed many tears backstage as I saw my dream coming to life in front of me. I failed at my goals so many times before, but the dream did not die and setting goals (and some good training, nutritional advice and an occasional kick in the tail) got me there.

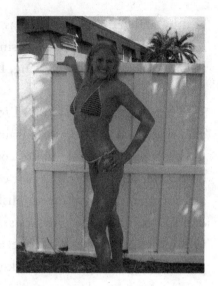

Thank you Matt for taking this special journey with me. You believed in me even though I was so far away from my goal and pushed me to heights I never thought possible. You helped me see how strong I was on the inside and for that reason you will always have a special place in my heart.

- Hope Christoff

CHAPTER NINE:

Supplement Yourself

"You don't have to put an age limit on your dreams."
Dara Torres
2008 Olympic Champion

Live Longer and Perform Better

According to the U.S. Food and Drug Administration on their website at www.fda.gov, a dietary supplement is defined as: "a product taken by mouth that contains a 'dietary ingredient' intended to supplement the diet. The 'dietary ingredients' in these products may include: vitamins, minerals, herbs or other botanicals, amino acids, and substances such as enzymes, organ tissues, glandulars, and metabolites. Dietary supplements can also be extracts or concentrates, and may be found in many forms such as tablets, capsules, softgels, gelcaps, liquids, or powders." Are supplements right for you? Can they help you live longer, feel better, and lose weight? Are they a waste of money? These are the questions I will attempt to answer in this chapter and I hope to alleviate some of the confusion that I know exists in most people's minds. I will present you with some research-backed conclusions about which supplements can help you with your general health and some that can help you with weight loss and some that can improve your performance on the track, in the water, on your bike, or even in the gym.

The use of supplements is arguably a highly controversial subject. If you ever want to stimulate a great debate, or more realistically a one-sided lecture, just ask almost any physician what they think about nutritional supplements. I tried this with my personal doctor and he simply said: "If you eat a balanced diet, they probably are a waste of money. But then again, they probably won't hurt you either." With such convincing advice (insert sarcastic tone here), what's someone to do?

The reality of the matter with regard to nutritional supplements is that due to conflicting reports in the media and lackluster support from the medical profession, most people are rightfully confused. Recently I attended a nutritional medicine lecture presented by Dr Ray D. Strand (author of 7 books on nutritional medicine including *What Your Doctor Doesn't Know About Nutritional Medicine May Be Killing You*). He pointed out that physicians are disease and drug oriented because of the educational emphasis placed on the diagnosis and treatment of disease during medical school. Dr Strand said: "Very little time in medical school is devoted to disease prevention or nutrition." With that in mind and considering the billion-dollar marketing power of the large drug manufacturers, he concludes doctors are generally biased against nutritional supplementation. When it comes to the media, whether it is the 5 o'clock news, newspaper and magazine articles, or radio "breaking news" reports, you have to realize that pharmaceutical companies represent a significant portion of the advertising dollars for these "for-profit" companies. Thus, knowingly and unknowingly, they may be quick to point out the "bad" or inconclusive studies regarding nutritional supplements and hesitate to report the "good" or positive ones.

Personally I believe the tide is finally turning as more definitive research on the health benefits of specific supplements is now available. Many successful doctors are adding nutritional medicine to their practices and finding the results are beneficial for their patients and their businesses. Even some of the large drug manufacturers are getting into the supplement business by developing prescription formulations of natural products and acquiring some of the more successful supplement companies. I guess they figured: "If you can't beat 'em, join 'em."

For the past 18 years or so, I have followed the latest scientific developments dealing with supplements both as an athlete and as a former owner of a sports nutrition business. Personally, I have always looked for natural ways to improve my strength, conditioning, and athletic performance, but more importantly, I have always wanted to know what I can do to live a long, high-quality life. When it comes to nutritional supplementation, these are two different animals. Performance-enhancing supplements are called ergogenic aids and life-extending, health-promoting supplements are often called nutraceuticals because of their medicinal effects on the body. I have always used the results of double-blind, placebo-controlled studies to guide my decisions on what supplements to take and will share some of what I've learned with you.

Safety and effectiveness

The first two things that must be considered before you take any supplement are its safety and effectiveness. Pharmaceutical companies can legitimately argue that supplement manufacturers aren't regulated by the Food and Drug Administration (FDA) the same way prescription drugs are. But does regulation equate to safety? The reality of the matter is that prescription drugs are responsible for more American deaths than traffic accidents, violent crimes, and plane crashes combined. In fact, adverse reactions to prescription drugs are the third leading cause of death for Americans (and many celebrities it seems lately). Even though prescription drugs are highly regulated and have to go through rigorous clinical studies, this doesn't necessarily make them safe. The safety of many drugs (or lack of safety) is often discovered after it becomes available to the public.

Supplements on the other hand don't have to go through a rigorous FDA approval process and the onus is on the manufacturer to ensure a product is safe before it is marketed. Maybe this doesn't give you the same kind of warm and fuzzy feeling that a 100-million-dollar clinical trial does, but I would argue that we are better protected from supplements than we are from prescription drugs. Because the FDA has the authority to force a supplement manufacturer to recall any supplement with reported adverse effects and the fact that we live in the information age where we have access to immediate information from around the world, most dangerous supplements are withdrawn from the market before they do any significant harm. The FDA is much more likely to pull the regulatory trigger on a supplement than they would on any prescription drug because of the money tied up in research and the political lobbying efforts of the drug manufacturers. With millions and millions of dollars spent in the research and development of their drugs and demanding shareholders to answer to, drug manufacturers will fight long and hard to ensure the profitability of their companies. Deaths from a dangerous supplement are usually less than ten people where deaths from a "FDA approved" prescription drug can be in the hundreds or thousands before anything is done. So I will leave the question of product safety up to your own best judgment, but generally speaking supplements are in fact safe.

Effectiveness is a completely different issue and if you are like me, I'm sure you would hate to waste your hard-earned money on a useless, ineffective, or unnecessary product. Thanks to the Dietary Supplement Health and Education Act (DSHEA) passed in 1994 by Congress, today we have access to a virtually limitless supply of "performance-enhancing," "life-extending," and "fat-burning" supplements. The best advice I can give you when it comes to the effectiveness of any supplement is to be wary of the marketing hype. Supplement companies collectively spend hundreds of millions of dollars marketing their products and in many cases, the product had very little to do with the results they claim. All too often, it is the hard work and discipline of the testimonial subjects that led to the dramatic results pictured in the ad. I have worked as a consultant on weight loss testimonials and let me tell you there is a whole lot more that goes into weight loss than popping any supplemental pill. That being said, I do believe that supplements do have a valuable place in our lives and there are many additional benefits you can get from safe and effective supplements.

United States Pharmacopoeia guidelines

Make sure any supplemental pill, tablet, or capsule you take meets the U.S. Pharmacopoeia (USP) guidelines — primarily meaning that they will completely dissolve when you take them and the ingredients listed on the label are accurate. The USP is a non-governmental, not-for-profit public health organization aiming to ensure quality and safety standards of medicines and supplements. It has recently started a voluntary program for supplement manufacturers to have their products verified for quality, potency, and processing methods. If you want peace of mind, look for the "USP Verified" mark on the labels of the supplements you use. A list of verified supplements is available on their website at www.usp.org.

In general, if you take a supplement in powder, soft-gel, gel capsule, or liquid form you can be assured that you are at least absorbing what's in the pill. If you are taking a caplet or tablet, I would recommend that you grind it up (I use a mortar and pestle) and add it to a beverage or protein shake. I have seen enough evidence to believe many of the vitamin tablets on the market are compressed under so much pressure that they pass through the digestive track like a small stone and exit the body undigested. You can have the best ingredients in the world in a tablet, but if it isn't broken down while in the body and absorbed into the bloodstream, it is worthless.

The Supplement Trilogy

There are three supplements I believe can be beneficial for all people (unless contraindicated by any medication you are taking — check with your doctor or pharmacist): 1. a high-quality, high-antioxidant multivitamin and multimineral formula; 2. Green tea extract; and 3. Fish oil. I call this the "supplement trilogy" because of the tremendous benefits available to anyone who takes them regularly. More and more scientific research is pointing towards nutrient deficiencies and circulating free radicals as the underlying cause of many modern diseases like Alzheimer's and Parkinson's. Even though I invest my time and energy into taking care of myself physically and nutritionally, I view supplementation as an insurance policy to add additional protection to my overall health. Let's take a look at each one individually and learn what they can do to support our health and longevity. *NOTE: If you are currently using any prescription drugs, consult with your doctor or pharmacist for any possible contraindications or drug interactions before you begin taking any supplements.*

1. High-quality, high-antioxidant multivitamin and multimineral formula: With regard to our health, which in the big picture of life I consider more important than the short-term focus of performance enhancement, living a long, functional, disease-free life is likely a common goal. As medical research constantly pursues the causes and treatments of modern diseases, more and more studies are linking most of the chronic degenerative diseases like heart disease, cancer, stroke, diabetes, Alzheimer's, and Parkinson's to uncontrolled oxidative stress and inflammation.

Living in the modern, mechanized world, we are constantly exposed to more environmental, emotional, and chemical stressors than any other time in history. Combine that with the ever-decreasing nutrient-density of our foods caused by the increasingly industrialized farming of our soil and we are putting are bodies into a losing battle — the war within. Smoking, sunlight, medications, pollutants, pesticides, radiation, and even excessive amounts of exercise increases production of "free radicals" in our bodies from oxidation. Free radicals are oxygen molecules with highly reactive unpaired electrons that can rust our bodies from the inside out if they aren't effectively neutralized with antioxidants.

Dr Kenneth Cooper published *The Antioxidant Revolution* in the mid-1990s and can be given some credit to popularizing the benefits of taking supplemental antioxidants. Just like a good coat of Rust-Oleum® paint can prevent your bike or patio furniture from rusting in the outside elements, taking the right combination of antioxidant vitamins and minerals can help your body mitigate some of the oxidative stress in our bodies. In his book *BIONUTRITION,* Dr Ray D. Strand tells us that the body is its own best defense against developing chronic degenerative diseases and it is up to us to properly equip it with the right nutrients to do so.

When the Recommended Dietary Allowances (RDAs) were established in 1980, they identified the amounts of vitamins and minerals to prevent deficiency diseases like scurvy, rickets, and pellagra. The problem with chronic degenerative diseases is not deficiency, but rather oxidative stress. Therefore more optimal levels of key vitamins, minerals, and micronutrients are needed by the body to combat oxidative damage. For example, the RDAs for Vitamin E and Vitamin C are 30 IU (international units) and 60 mg (milligrams) respectively but research has concluded that 400 IU of Vitamin E and 1,000 mg of Vitamin C are the optimal amounts to provide a health benefit.

So which of the micronutrients and in what amounts are most beneficial to optimize are health? Based on my research and the general conclusions of medical experts willing to make recommendations, everyone should take a high-quality, pharmaceutical grade, complete and balanced multivitamin and multimineral formula. Even the prestigious *Journal of the American Medical Association* reversed its long stand against supplements in August of 2002 and now advises all adults to take at least one multivitamin pill each day. To list specific recommendations would be beyond the scope of this book, but I'll provide a quick summary of what to look for in a quality multivitamin and multimineral supplement and the suggested optimum dosages for each nutrient.

Multivitamin / antioxidant complex: Vitamin C (500 - 1000 mg), vitamin E (400 - 800 IU), vitamin D (500 – 1,500 IU), vitamin K (50 – 120 mcg), CoQ_{10} (20 – 50 mg) and alpha-lipoic acid (250 - 500 mg); **carotenoids** like beta-carotene (5,000 - 10,000 IU), lycopene (2 mg), and lutein (5 - 10 mg); **bioflavanoids** like quercetin (500 mg), rutin (250 mg) and grape seed extract (50 – 100 mg).

B vitamin cofactors including B_1 - thiamin (1 - 5 mg), B_2 - riboflavin (5 - 25 mg), B_3 - niacin (20 - 40 mg), B_5 - pantothenic acid (50 - 125 mg), B_6 - pyroxidine (10 - 35 mg), B_{12} - cobalamin (50 - 200 mcg), biotin (100 - 500 mcg), and folic acid (400 - 800 mcg).

Multimineral complex: Calcium (800 – 1,200 mg), chromium (100 - 250 mcg), copper (2 mg), magnesium (250 - 500 mg), manganese (2 - 5 mg), selenium (100 - 200 mcg), vanadium (50 mcg), and zinc (10 - 25 mg).

2. Green tea extract (315 mg of ECGC each day): If you don't drink seven to eight cups of green tea every day, then supplementation with green tea extract is a fantastic way to reap its many health benefits. Green tea has been a popular beverage in Japan and China for centuries. Epidemiological studies in these cultures have found that catechins found in green tea are very potent antioxidants and have anti-carcinogenic, anti-inflammatory, anti-atherogenic, thermogenic, and antimicrobial effects on the body. In common language this means green tea extract can protect you against cancer, reduce inflammation, protect your arteries, help you burn extra calories, and kill bacteria, fungi, and viruses living in the body. Sounds good to me, pass the tea bags!

Green tea leaves have polyphenolic substances call catechins which are classified as flavonoids. Epigallocatechin gallate (EGCG) is the most abundant and potent of the green tea catechins and is typically found in most green tea extract supplements. Scientific research hasn't completely unveiled the biochemical mechanisms at work, but numerous studies have confirmed green tea protection against many forms of cancer and cardiovascular disease. Researchers have also found thermogenic properties of green tea which can promote fat oxidation. Because of this effect, many supplement manufacturers add green tea extract into their fat burning, weight loss formulas. More recent research has found green tea and green tea extracts may protect against neurodegenerative diseases like Alzheimer's disease.

With all of it many purported health benefits it makes sense that we should be consuming green tea in some form each day. I would recommend trying to consume green tea by drinking it the old fashioned way whenever you can and by taking a green tea extract supplement every day. Green tea extract supplements are available at most health food stores and drug stores. Look for at least 200 to 350 milligrams of catechins like ECGC listed on the label. Personally I take 315 milligrams of ECGC once a day around lunch time.

3. Fish oil (2 grams per day): To complete your optimal health supplementation, there is a large body of evidence promoting the health benefits of taking two grams (2,000 mg) of omega-3 fatty acids either in the form of fish oil or cold-pressed flaxseed oil per day. The two most studied omega-3 fatty acids are eicosapentaenoic acid (EPA) and docosahexaenoic acid (DHA). Omega-3 fatty acids have been found to lower blood triglyceride levels, reduce inflammation, increase fat burning, improve and protect brain function, and may even protect against cancer. In 2000, the Food and Drug Administration approved the following health claim regarding dietary supplements containing omega-3 fatty acids: "Supportive but not conclusive research shows that consumption of EPA and DHA omega-3 fatty acids may reduce the risk of coronary heart disease." Fish oils supplements are derived from lipids found in oily, coldwater fish like salmon, tuna, sardines, and herring which are rich sources of these omega-3 fatty acids.

Research has found that supplementing with fish oil can lower triglyceride levels by inhibiting lipogenesis (converting blood sugar to fatty acids) and by increasing fatty acid oxidation in the liver. Since there is a definitive link between high triglyceride levels and cardiovascular disease, anything that can help lower triglyceride levels is obviously a good thing. One seven week study found that daily supplementation with either 3.8 grams of EPA or 3.6 grams of DHA lowered triglyceride levels by 21 to 26 percent compared to 4 grams of corn oil (which served as the placebo in the study). Combine those benefits with the triglyceride-lowering effect of exercise and you have a very powerful protocol for protecting yourself against heart disease and stroke.

When it comes to heart disease prevention, a review of 17 different studies found that supplementation with three or more grams of fish oil per day significantly lowered systolic and diastolic blood pressure in people with hypertension. When it comes to weight loss, or more specifically losing fat from our bodies, fish oil seems to help too. One study found that people who replaced six grams of fat in their diets with 6 grams of fish oil lost two pounds of fat in just three weeks. Some preliminary research has found that fish oil may also reduce joint pain in people with rheumatoid arthritis, protect the brain against the early stages of Alzheimer's disease, and help clear up psoriasis.

With so many possible benefits and no reported negative side effects, it makes sense to take a fish oil supplement each day. Fish oil supplements typically come in soft-gels or in bottles of oil you take with a spoon. You can find them in drugstores, pharmacies, health food stores, and even the vitamin isle of your local grocery store. Look for supplements that have at least 800 milligrams per serving of either EPA or DHA (or some combination of both). Some people have found that fish oil supplements can cause unpleasant "fish burps" so many companies have developed formulations that eliminate the problem. Look for "no fish burp" or something similar on the label. In 2005, the FDA even approved a prescription omega-3 supplement called Lovaza for lowering high triglyceride levels. If you want a pharmaceutical grade fish oil supplement, talk to your doctor.

Performance Enhancement

Now we turn our attention to the ergogenic or performance-enhancing side of supplementation. Ever since human beings started competing with each other, people began looking for an "edge" to help them be more competitive. For some elite athletes, a three to five percent performance improvement could be the difference between first place and last place. With so many products competing for our attention and hard-earned money, how do we know which ones will work for us? So far, there have been just two proven ergogenic aids that have stood the safety and performance enhancement tests of time: caffeine and creatine.

Caffeine picks you up

Caffeine is undoubtedly the most widely used ergogenic aid by people around the globe. Many people like caffeine because it makes them feel more alert, gives them more energy, improves their mood, and makes them more productive. Whether you are aiming to improve your 10K time in a weekend race, trying to speed fat loss during exercise, or just need an afternoon "pick me up," a little jolt of caffeine is an inexpensive way to improve performance...and improve performance it does. Studies have found that caffeine increases power production, time to exhaustion, total energy expenditure, and fatty acid oxidation. In fact, a 1.3 milligram per pound (of bodyweight) dose of caffeine can increase VO_2 max by 3.26%. For a 150-pound athlete that would be around 200 milligrams of caffeine or the amount found in about two cups of brewed coffee.

Caffeine works to improve performance in several ways. Like other xanthine derivatives, caffeine is a non-selective adenosine receptor antagonist which has a stimulant effect on the central nervous system. By revving up the body's fat burning machinery, caffeine can help you tap into fat stores during prolonged endurance-type events and competition. Since caffeine also acts on the adenosine receptors in the brain, it can increase alertness and focus as well as increase beta (β) endorphin release during exercise. These psychotropic effects of caffeine decrease pain perception which makes it possible to exercise longer and harder on the track or in the gym.

Most competitive athletes use caffeine in some form or another and the International Olympic Committee took it off its list of banned substances in January 2005. If you are worried about the diuretic effect of caffeine, worry no more because recent studies have found that it does not negatively effect fluid or electrolyte balance in routine consumers. If you want to use caffeine somewhat scientifically to improve performance then it is recommended you take a three milligram per kilogram (3mg/kg = 1.36mg/lb) dose 60 minutes prior to training or competition. There is about 100 mg of caffeine in a normal cup of coffee, about 45 mg in a can of diet coke, and God only knows how much is in the proprietary formulas of most energy drinks. It would be wise to experiment with different forms of caffeine during practice and training to find out which works best for you prior to trying it in competition or at an event.

Creatine builds you up

Over the past 15 years, creatine has been the most studied ergogenic supplement available to the public. Thousands of studies have proven the safety and efficacy of creatine, so even its harshest critics have quieted down to a dull roar. Creatine is a non-protein amino acid synthesized in the liver, kidneys, and pancreas and then transported to the muscles, heart, and brain where it is metabolized and stored as creatine phosphate. Taking supplemental forms of creatine increases the amount of creatine phosphate being stored in muscle tissue which can increase short-term energy production during anaerobic exercise. In other words, a muscle cell saturated with creatine will be a stronger muscle cell capable of more contractions. Creatine supplementation has been proven to increase muscular strength, power, and endurance (number of repetitions performed) by five to 10 percent and increase muscle gains (lean mass) by up to five pounds during 12 weeks of resistance-based training. The current theory on creatine is that creatine loading hyperhydrates muscle cells which subsequently increases nitrogen balance. Maintaining a positive nitrogen balance leads to increased protein synthesis and decreased muscle degradation. Both these actions equate to enhanced recovery from exercise and an additional muscle-building response to resistance training.

Most current research on creatine has shifted focus to its "brain benefits" and it will be interesting to learn what medical science will reveal in the coming years. Studies have already found that creatine supplementation may protect the tissues of the brain and heart, as well as improve brain function. A 1999 study published in the *American Journal of Physiology* found that supplementing with 20 grams of creatine monohydrate for 28 days increased brain creatine phosphate levels by 8.7% which led to decreased mental fatigue, improved memory and intelligence scoring during testing, and improved cognitive functions. So if you want to compose poetry while pushing some weights, you might want to give creatine a try.

How do you supplement with creatine? There are countless creatine products that claim to have a better "transport system" for getting creatine into your body. Don't believe the hype! Most of these products come loaded with sugar-based, high-glycemic carbohydrates to stimulate an insulin release which is purported to facilitate creatine transport and uptake into muscle cells. If you can afford the extra calories and the extra cost of these highly-marketed products, then knock yourself out. A better idea is to buy a pure creatine monohydrate powder (a white, odorless, tasteless powder) and add it to the meal replacement protein shakes or recovery drinks you already should be drinking every day.

I personally spoke "off the record" with two of the world's top authorities on creatine supplementation at the 2008 Annual Meeting of the American College of Sports Medicine. They informed me in no uncertain terms that most heavily-marketed creatine formulations and creatine transport products are a waste of money and calories when you consider that maximum cellular creatine saturation can be achieved with the inexpensive form of creatine: pure creatine monohydrate. Instead of spending 30 to 50 dollars a month for these products, you can pay 10 to 15 dollars for the plain powder. They recommended brands with the Creapure˚ symbol because it is manufactured in Germany compared with most of the creatine on the market which comes from China (where currently there is less quality control).

To get maximum results from creatine supplementation, take 20 grams of creatine monohydrate per day in divided doses for the first week (loading phase) then continue with a single dose of 5 to 10 grams each day thereafter. Studies of chronic users for 10 years or more have found no ill-effects of long-term creatine use, but personally I use it for two to three months at a time then "cycle" off for two to three months. The most common anecdotal criticism of creatine is that it causes "bloating." I always chuckle when I hear someone in the gym tell me: "I tried creatine before, but I don't use it because I bloat up." Rest assured faithful reader that creatine monohydrate powder, in its pure form, will not cause any bloating or distended bellies. In reality, it is the high-glycemic carbohydrates (usually added sugars) in creatine formulations that cause this undesirable effect. Just like I don't recommend eating high-glycemic carbohydrates in your foods, I wouldn't advise drinking them with your supplements either. Stick to the pure powdered form of creatine monohydrate and you and your waistline will be fine.

Use "Nutrient Timing" to get better results

The final performance nutrition strategy I want to talk about is what I call performance nutrition. Taking in the right macronutrients (protein, carbs, and fat) in the right ratios at the right time relative to your workouts is what John Ivy calls "nutrient timing" (which is also the title of his book). In his often cited research, he found that consuming 30 to 70 grams of simple carbohydrates and 11 to 22 grams of protein in a relative ratio of three to one immediately after training enhances recovery and improves subsequent performance. If you are looking for a quick and easy solution, this 3:1 ratio of carbs to protein is found in low-fat chocolate milk. If you would rather pay for something a little more scientifically formulated, most sports nutrition companies have developed pre/post training "RTD's" (ready to drink) to make nutrient timing more convenient. The two downsides of RTD's are the cost ($1.50 to $4 per serving) and the additives included to preserve taste and shelf life. If you want to save a few bucks and also have more control over what you consume, make your recovery protein drinks yourself. There are many delicious tasting protein-only and meal replacement powders available and you can either mix them in a blender or get a shaker bottle and shake your way into sports nutrition.

Hundreds of studies have proven the effectiveness of using supplemental protein to improve the training response to resistance-based strength training. By consuming 15 to 25 grams of supplemental whey or soy protein 30 minutes before or immediately after your resistance-based workouts you can improve your 12-week lean mass gains by 22 – 26% compared to someone who does not. Mark Verstegen, CSCS author of the popular *Core Performance* series of books calls these timely doses of protein "shooters" and recommends them to all the elite athletes he trains at his Athletes Performance training facilities.

The bonus in using supplemental protein drinks is they provide lots of nutrition with relatively few calories when compared to whole foods and you can include them as part of your five to six meals a day. Because of this benefit, many supplement companies call their products meal replacement powders (MRP's). One study demonstrated that people who used meal replacements drinks lost six times the amount of weight when compared to food only groups. The researchers concluded the additional weight loss was most likely achieved because of better calorie control afforded by the meal replacement drinks. Another study asked 43 registered dieticians (RD's) to compose meal plans to get 100% of the Recommended Dietary Allowances (RDA) in macro and micronutrients and the lowest amount of calories any of them could come up with was 2,400. Unfortunately, most American women will gain weight eating anything over 1,800 calories a day. So you either get on the supplement train to meet your RDA's without additional calories or you can get your RDA's with food and gain weight. I think most people would agree that skipping the weight gaining option would be best.

Individual needs vary

I have one final note on supplements. Each individual has different needs when it comes to sports nutrition, nutrient timing, and athletic performance. I would encourage you to consult a qualified trainer, registered dietician, or sports nutritionist to get a more specific and customized recommendation. For more comprehensive information on supplementation, complete product information, and lists of ingredients, I recommend you get the latest *PDR* for *Nutritional Supplements*™. At the time of this writing, the 2nd Edition published in 2008 is the most current edition.

Stephen
Age: 37
Network Engineer

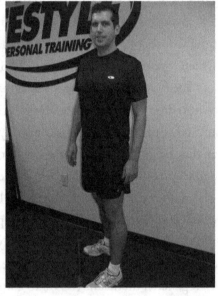

THE FACTS:
In 40 days…
- Lost over 24 pounds!
- Lowered his body fat by 9.5%
- Increased strength and cardiovascular endurance
- Lost over 3 inches off his waist and dropped over 2 pant sizes

"I definitely have more energy now. I do not feel like sitting on the couch, I want to get up and be active. Once you make it a habit it is in not scary anymore. I am healthier; I have lost weight but still gained muscle. I feel better and I have more confidence. Matt really knows his stuff; he gets you to work hard because he shows you the benefits of achieving your goals."

PART THREE:

ACTION
The Path to Success

CHAPTER TEN:

Moderate Yourself

"It is better to rise from life as from a banquet
— neither thirsty nor drunken."
Aristotle

"Eat not to dullness; drink not to elevation."
Benjamin Franklin

"Moderation in temper is always a virtue;
but moderation in principle is always a vice."
Thomas Paine

Matt's Moderation Mantra

If you carefully consider the words of Aristotle, Benjamin Franklin, Thomas Paine, and especially the biblical teachings on moderation (see Proverbs 25:16 as an example), you will quickly surmise that too much of a good thing can be a bad thing. Unfortunately in our consumption-based society, too much has become the norm. We live in the "land of plenty," but unless we learn how to control ourselves, this will come to mean plenty of problems. There is a significant difference between eating for pleasurable nourishment and gluttony. There is also a significant difference between having a glass of wine with dinner and drunkenness. That being said, if you want to find the happy medium between indulgence and deprivation, I offer the following mantra to apply to your life and how you live it:

Everything in moderation, including moderation.

If you subscribe to conspiracy theory or have read any of Kevin Trudeau's books, then you probably believe cooking with non-stick pans causes cancer and will kill any parakeets hanging out by the stove, microwaving alters the energetic force field of the food you're cooking, artificial sweeteners rot your brain and cause cancer, chewing gum (if swallowed) stays in your intestines for 12 years, pouring cola on meat makes worms come out, living near power lines changes our DNA, talking on a cell phone microwaves your brain, and we are being sabotaged intentionally by a coalition of the food and drug industries to make us sick, fat, and unhealthy. In this case, too much information can be bad for our peace of mind.

Like most of Americans, you're probably confused about what is good and bad for us to eat, drink, wear, watch, hear, or touch and it's easy to see why. Everyday we are barraged by advertisements, articles, "breaking news" reports, internet blogs, consumer advocacy groups, industry watchdogs, special reports, emails, "tweets," books, billboards, and something one of our friends heard from old so-and-so. Each one cites industry experts, research studies from everywhere around the planet, anecdotal tales of miraculous healing, or a tragic calamity of epic proportions. All make a convincing argument to influence our decisions. We have been told milk is bad for us then new research shows people who drink milk are healthier and weigh less than non-drinkers. Caffeine is bad for us, caffeine is good for us. The sun causes cancer and you must wear sunscreen. Now vigilant sunscreen users are getting illnesses like osteoporosis associated with Vitamin D deficiencies from a lack of sunlight. Research concludes one finding then contradicts itself in the next study. It is absolutely confusing and caused by what T. Colin Campbell calls "scientific reductionism" in his book *The China Study*. What, who, when, and why should we believe?

The reality of the matter is this…Nobody knows everything for certain. Anybody who says or believes otherwise is living a life of delusionary grandeur and needs to take a seat at the nearest 24 hour diner to savor a nice big slice of humble pie. Some people may even need a whole pie. Even though I have spent thousands upon thousands of hours over the past 15 years reviewing research studies; reading diet, nutrition, and exercise books; and attending seminars and lectures on all topics related to health, I'm not going to pretend I have all the answers. The only constant in life is change and the more things change, the more they stay the same. Learn to separate the fundamental truths from the "half-baked" flavors of the day. Ultimately, you are the captain of your ship and must decide the fate of your vessel (and blood vessels too). Apply a little moderation to your own life and you will avoid most of the troubled waters that the sea of life can have in store for us.

Life is precious and short

There is no need for us to live in perpetual fear and trepidation about each morsel of food we put into our mouths, how we prepare it, and what we drink with it. Try not to get caught up in all the journalistic hype, sensationalistic marketing, or miraculous capabilities of any one thing. This is where a little common sense and moderation must reign supreme. Are plants on Earth for us to eat as they are in their natural state? Or were they put here for us to invent ways to alter their structure, strip them of their nutrients, cram them with preservatives, add artificial flavors, sweeteners, and colors, put them into boxes and cans with 20 years of shelf life so we can conveniently binge on them like a starving wolf on a caribou carcass anytime we please? Or graze on them like the grass free-range cattle munch on throughout the day? These questions could generate some great discussion at a debate or in a philosophy class, but we need to exercise our own good judgment about what we eat and drink, which pills we take, and how we treat our bodies.

Besides what we put into our mouths to eat or drink, we must even moderate the amount of exercise we do. As an exercise advocate who loves to workout that was hard for me to say. My hat goes off to the marathon runners, Ironman, triathletes, and ultra distance competitors out there, but these events come with a price. It takes the human body about two months to completely recover from the damage inflicted on the body from a marathon (26.2 miles). Putting the time, effort, and energy into preparation and training, plus the events themselves, will take a long-term toll on the body. I experienced this firsthand when I jogged and walked for 40 miles on my 40th birthday. I was in a world of hurt for days afterward and it took a couple of weeks for the phlegm in my lungs to go away completely. You have to ask yourself: *Is the reward worth the cost?*

Honestly, the psychological reward, sense of accomplishment, and self-esteem boost of completing a marathon or any other long-distance event may be worth it for some people. Just be aware that if your primary goal is living a long, functional, and pain-free life, you may have to moderate the high impact activities you subject your muscles and joints to. Looking at it from a lifetime perspective, it may mean you train and compete in a few of these events throughout your adult life or for a set period of time, cycle in and out of competing in these events. Maybe it means doing shorter distance events like 5K and 10K runs or Olympic or Sprint distance triathlons. Just make sure you are aware that doing anything in excess, even exercise, comes with a price.

Enough is enough, but how much exercise is too much?

A study of 17,000 Harvard male alumni with similar demographics sought to answer how much exercise is too much. The results may surprise you.

Exercise amount (hours per week)	Death rate
Little to none	highest
3 – 5 hours	22% decrease
5 – 10 hours	**54% decrease**
More than 10 hours per week	38% decrease

According to this study, exercising for more than ten hours a week would put you in the grave sooner than exercising for five to ten hours a week. In terms of longevity (how long you'll live), the optimum amount of exercise is five to ten hours per week on average. More is not always better, once again proving the merits of my moderation mantra.

Just recently, a man named Robert Kraft was profiled on ESPN's show *Outside the Lines*. Robert, who is nicknamed "The Raven" because of his ever-present black attire, has ran 8 miles every single day (rain or shine...or even hurricanes) dating back to 1975. By early 2009, he crossed the 100,000 mile mark for total miles run over 34 plus years. While I applaud his unique discipline, miraculous consistency, and relentless effort, the point of telling you his story relates to moderation or the lack of it in this case. Despite running all of his miles on the softer than pavement sands of Miami Beach, Robert's cumulative miles have taken their toll on his body. In his own words, he is in a lot of pain every day and has trouble getting out of bed each morning. Doctor's have advised him to quit and his body has obviously relayed the same message, yet he persists on running his 8 miles each day. I wish him the best of health and many more miles.

For you the reader, I say seek balance in lieu of compulsiveness, impulsiveness, or obsessiveness. Exercise enough in duration, frequency, and intensity for the benefits, but not so much to overburden and overstress the body. Learn to disperse high-impact types of exercise like running throughout the years of your life. Choose to focus on running for awhile, even train for and run a marathon if you want, but if you are in it for the long-haul like me, you have to budget the miles you put on your body wisely. When planning your weekly exercise, alternate or space out your running days with weight training, cross-training, or other non-impact type activities. This will give your muscles and joints a chance to recover from the high impact days.

Like long-distance running, training with insanely heavy weights can also take a long-term toll on the body. This is why I would recommend spreading out high-intensity strength training activities throughout your lifetime as well. There is no need to train for maximum strength unless you are entering a powerlifting competition or competing as an Olympic weightlifter. You can still achieve plenty of intensity by training in the eight to twelve repetition range without the stress of one or two rep maximum lifts. Like a professional athlete gives his body time to heal after the competitive season is over, you too have to give your body time to heal after you train for an intense event like a marathon, triathlon, or powerlifting competition. For all you workout junkies out there (and I'm one of them), schedule one week breaks from training periodically throughout the year. This will give your body the chance to completely heal any minor injuries and muscle damage, as well as rejuvenate your enthusiasm for exercise.

Highly competitive and intense, adrenaline-producing sports and activities can also take their long-term toll on your body. Before you enviously dismiss the high salaries of professional athletes as undeserved or unfair, realize these gifted individuals are trading some of the future quality and duration of their lives for their current fame and fortune. Longevity studies of professional football players, for instance, have found they live shorter, more painful lives than average Americans. The violent collisions current professional football players subject themselves to have been equated to the impact forces in a 35 mph head-on collision in a car. They endure this time and time again during their often short careers. Because of this fundamental understanding, I believe hardworking athletes we pay to watch and love to criticize, earn every penny they make. There are many other ways to earn a living that don't require sacrificing long-term health, like writing books for instance.

We are blessed with an incredibly complex working system of cells and we need to be careful not to abuse the recuperative powers we have. Overtraining your body (too much exercise stress with too little recovery time) can be extremely counterproductive. It decreases the muscle-building hormones testosterone and growth hormone, increases production of the stress hormone cortisol, decreases dopamine levels in the brain, impairs hypothalamic function, and decreases immune function. Most people have the opposite problem called "zerotraining." Just be cautious when you catch the exercise bug and find yourself overdoing it. Follow the moderation mantra (Everything in moderation, including moderation) and you'll probably turn out just fine.

Hedge your bets in life. Take some occasional long-shot chances like completing an IRONMAN. triathlon or eating indulgences like prime rib, fettuccini alfredo, ice cream sundaes, and fried chicken, but keep a strong portfolio of blue chip stocks like exercising for an hour, 5 days a week and eating whole, unprocessed foods and drinking plenty of water. I like to tell my clients: "You can have a piece of cake, just don't eat the whole cake."

How do I apply this mantra into my own life?

Food: Like I've said previously, I enjoy food and love to eat. Using the moderation mantra keeps me out of trouble while still allowing me to enjoy the "excess" foods I love from time to time. I typically have pizza 4 to 5 times per year (moderation) and when I do, I'll have 2-3 slices of thin crust with vegetable toppings (moderation) or make a whole wheat crust pizza with fresh ingredients. But every now and then, I will enjoy what I truly love: a few pieces of meaty, cheesy, gooey, Chicago-style pizza (moderation in moderation). Some other indulgences I enjoy from time to time are: two pieces of fried chicken; a rich, peanut butter and chocolate ice cream sundae; or my all-time favorite food in life…a delicious, grilled rib-eye steak.

These would qualify as moderation in moderation, but I do this moderately. Confused? Put it this way. During the past three years, I had deep-dish pizza six times, fried chicken twice, ice cream sundaes five times, and about seven rib-eye steaks. So I enjoy food in moderation, but let my diet stumble completely off the reservation once or twice a month at the most. Most of the time, I counter some of the additional calories with an extra hour of exercise. This way I feel like I am healthy but not giving up the things I love completely. You learn to truly appreciate and savor each morsel of these foods when the opportunity presents itself, but find I don't miss them either because I truly enjoy healthier foods almost as much.

Put yourself to the test. Can you remember and count how many times you've had indulgent high-calorie, high-fat, and high-sugar foods during the past year? If you can't remember because they are too frequent or numerous, then it might be time to suck down a moderation milkshake.

Alcohol: Personally I enjoy having a glass of red wine, or a "dirty" vodka martini, or a glass of champagne, or a blended scotch whiskey from time to time. Using the moderation mantra means I can enjoy a glass or two of a nice cabernet or pinot noir with dinner once or twice a week, a dirty vodka martini with my wife if we go to one of our favorite "hot spots," or a glass of champagne when I feel like celebrating (I love to celebrate life). And I especially enjoy a glass of 12 year old scotch whenever I get to meet up with my conversational friends. Over the course of a week, I will have three to five drinks total and on some weeks I find myself having none at all. *(Note: If you are trying to lose weight, limit alcohol consumption to one or two drinks total per week max. See Chapter 8 for more details.)* Applying the moderation in moderation principle means I may splurge on the expense and smoothness of a 25 year old scotch one or two times a year or drink a glass of each of my favorites during a casual evening with friends once a month. We make transportation arrangements ahead of time or take a cab home. My waistline and liver (and fellow drivers) seem to thank me for this philosophy.

Exercise: Yes, I even apply the mantra to exercise too. Unless you're a competitive athlete training in a specific sport which requires prolonged training, there is no need to exercise for more than seven hours a week. A 1977 study of Harvard graduates found that minor athletes lived longer than both major athletes in highly competitive sports and non-athletes. The way I see it, too much exercise and competitive stress puts excessive wear and tear on the body and I want mine to be alive and functional for as long as possible. Even though I love the adrenaline surge of sports competition, I know the subsequent price and risk of injury that comes with it. Over the past 20 years I have tapered down the amount of sports I compete or participate in each year.

The key to cardio-based workouts is to primarily select low-impact or non-impact activities for the majority (80% or more) of your total training time. Examples would include: cycling, rowing, elliptical-type machines, swimming, and walking outside or on a treadmill. I have seen the cumulative crippling effects of distance running on too many people to advise doing it for too long, too many miles, or too often. With that in mind, I exercise four to six times a week for about an hour. (Note: While I was writing this book, I typically exercised three times a week which was sufficient to maintain the health benefits accrued in years past.) I alternate my cardiovascular training between low-impact, longer-duration activity and high-intensity, short-duration intervals. I lift heavy weights but do not perform single-rep maximums. I think this philosophy is the best of both worlds and at over 40 years of age, my strength, endurance, and capacity to perform are holding up fine so far. Most importantly, I live pain free other than the short-term soreness I get from my weight training workouts.

In six weeks, I lost 12 pounds, lowered my bodyfat by 4%, and lost inches all over my body. I lost 3 inches off my waist, 4 inches off my hips, and would have lost more if I wasn't sick for a week during the program.

"Matt's *Magic Pill* approach and moderation mantra helped me develop a new attitude towards weight loss and exercise. Everything I learned I now apply to my everyday life and it is so easy! Weight loss and the loss of bodyfat are just some of the benefits. Overall my health has improved as well as my outlook on life.

Working with Matt is awesome. He inspired me to reach my goal and did everything he could to keep me going and stay positive about reaching my goal. I now have an 'I can do it' attitude instead of 'I can't' which used to hold me back in the past. Intense exercise is very challenging, but it can also be fun, and it definitely makes a difference. Matt and I have now set a new goal and I am already well on my way to achieving it. Day by day, pound by pound, inch by inch, I will achieve what I once thought was an impossible dream."

- Donna Davenport

CHAPTER ELEVEN

Assist Yourself

"People are anxious to improve their circumstances, but are unwilling to improve themselves. They therefore remain bound."

James Allen

Getting Some Help: Hire a Personal Trainer!

Would you buy a car if you weren't allowed to ever drive it? Would you buy a book if you weren't allowed to read it? Would you spend 60 bucks at a fine restaurant if you weren't allowed to eat the food you paid for? Spending time in the gym without getting any results is kind of the same thing. Having a trainer show you how to properly exercise and construct an effective training plan will substantially increase the likelihood that you will get results from your investment of time, energy, and money. A great trainer is like getting a performance upgrade for your car. You can go further and faster while improving your physiological gas mileage. For some people new to exercise altogether, having a trainer can transform your 1980's Cutlass Supreme into a modern day Corvette…leaner, sleeker, faster, more powerful, sexier, and even more fuel efficient.

Hiring a good personal trainer is one of the best decisions you could ever make in your life. Granted, I'm a little biased, but consider the facts and possibilities. Most successful company turnarounds in corporate America were orchestrated, masterminded and implemented by a charismatic leader. Every successful sports team, whether it is the World

301

Series champion New York Yankees, Super Bowl champion Pittsburg Steelers, or NBA champion Los Angeles Lakers, has a strong coach to push the players to their best possible performance. Even the most elite athletes competing in individual sports like golf, mixed martial arts, cycling, and Olympic events like sprinting and swimming have a coach, and in some cases a team of coaches, to help them achieve competitive success. Ask Tiger Woods, George St Pierre, Lance Armstrong, Usain Bolt, and Michael Phelps about their preparation for competition and inevitably they will give credit to their coaches who helped them bring out their best.

A personal trainer can serve this purpose and help you achieve the best possible results in the least amount of time. Having the accountability of a person watching over you, if nothing else, will ensure you get those last two reps and show up for your workout in the first place. Furthermore, exercise adherence is considered a primary health care issue because 50% of people who start exercise programs quit within 6 months. You only reap the benefits of exercise if you put in the time and effort. Any good personal trainer worth their weight in spandex will no doubt increase the likelihood that you will consistently make it to the gym.

A 2008 study published in the *Journal of Strength and Conditioning Research* proved the value of having a personal trainer for women who exercise. The researchers concluded that women who exercise *without a trainer* self-select intensities (40-52% of max intensity) far below what is required to produce a training response. To get physiological results from exercise, you have to exercise at an intensity level above 60%. The women in the study who worked *with a trainer* exercised at far greater intensities (65 – 70% plus) and thus achieved better results from their time in the gym. If you don't exercise at intensity levels high enough to get a training response, you are "walking in the gym" and essentially turning your back on all the metabolism-boosting benefits of strength training. I do want to point out that any type of exercise (at any intensity level) is better than nothing. But if you are eager for body-changing results than more intensity and effort are necessary. Women often fear they will grow big "bulky" muscles when they "pump iron." This is a myth. As more and more scientific and anecdotal evidence is presented to the public, I truthfully see this common misconception losing its grip on women's attitudes towards resistance training. There is no better way for women to maintain their youthful muscle-tone than lifting weights.

Men can be their own worst enemies too errantly thinking it's my way or the highway. Just like we don't like to stop and ask for directions, men often think they know where they're going in the gym too. Far too many men are lost! A recent study proved that men who worked out *with a personal trainer* progressed more quickly in strength and achieved results much faster than those working on their own. The study found that only seven percent of the men exercising *without a trainer* were training at sufficient intensity to get physiological results. If you're not good with percentages, that equates to less than one person out of every ten. I was at a presentation in May of 2008 which discussed the training of Olympic athletes and even the most elite athletes in the world train at much lower intensities on their own compared with when they work with a coach or trainer. Without this assistance and motivation, these athletes, just like you, would never reach their true potential.

The Role of the Personal Trainer

A personal trainer can serve many roles…coach, motivator, exercise physiologist, research scientist, nutritionist, counselor and friend. Personal trainers design resistance and endurance training programs and prescribe intensity, volume, frequency, workout structure, exercise order, exercise selection, rest intervals, repetition speed, and choreograph all of these variables into a progressive training plan. Even if you can do all of this on your own, a trainer can help you do it better, faster, safer, and with much more intensity and motivation.

A good trainer will take the guesswork out of the fitness process and your only responsibilities are to show up on time (fueled up and warmed up) and be ready to work hard. Your results will be measured and monitored so you will continually progress, which will also help you stay motivated. Having measurable results is extremely important because you will see the numbers start to change far sooner than you will notice the visible changes to your body.

Whenever I start working with a new client, I always do a follow-up assessment after four weeks. They are always amazed when they see the results of their efforts in black and white. "Wow! I've lost four pounds of fat and gained two pounds of muscle. I had no idea." Some of my clients even said they were frustrated because their weight hadn't changed until I show them with a bodyfat analysis that their body had actually changed. It is all too easy to get hung up on what the scale tells us when in fact, your actual body composition (percent fat and percent lean mass) is so much more important to understand. Most personal trainers will track your body composition for you and adjust your training plan, if necessary, to maximize your results.

Applied knowledge and exercise experience are the invaluable traits of a good personal trainer. The results of a focus group of personal trainers were presented at the 2008 American College of Sports Medicine Annual Meeting. The group determined that an exercise professional should have adequate knowledge in the following areas (core competencies): anatomy, biomechanics, exercise physiology, lifestyle and health, chronic disease, cardiovascular disease, exercise programming, program management, health behavior modification, and nutritional planning. Credibility, reliability, and trustworthiness are also very important considerations.

How much does personal training cost?

Most people can afford a personal trainer. You should not view having a personal trainer as a luxury for only the rich and famous. View personal training as a necessity that you can work into your budget. It doesn't cost an arm and a leg to hire a personal trainer and if you are on a tight budget, there are several ways you can incorporate personal training into your fitness regime. I have clients that spend as little as 22 dollars a week or 47 dollars a month to have me on their team. I want to help you learn more so you can reap the benefits of having a coach on your team too.

Most personal training is priced by the session and offered in both half hour and hour-long increments. Fitness companies and health clubs often offer discounts for buying sessions in bulk or as a "package," which will usually include a fitness assessment and some form of bodyfat analysis. Average prices depend on: the location (large cities have higher demand and overhead which equals higher rates); the experience level of the trainer (more experienced trainers usually command higher rates); and special package promotions being offered. Half hour sessions average between $25 and $45, but I have seen them as low as $15 and as high as $85. Hour sessions cost anywhere between $45 and $90 with the obvious exceptions, as well. Pay for your training with an airline miles credit card and earn reward miles while you get in shape. Use the miles to get a ticket to a tropical destination so you can show off the beach body you will have!

Some health clubs also offer "boot camps," matrix training programs (small groups), and semi-personal training (two to three people) where you can work with one or more personal trainers as part of a group or team. This can substantially reduce the cost of training to as little as $10 to $20 a session which should make it affordable for almost anyone. Prices for these programs can vary depending on the location and trainers involved. If cost is a primary concern of yours, then definitely ask about these types of programs at your local health club. If your budget is even more limited, than take advantage of the best deal going in training — group fitness classes. Most health clubs offer a variety of group exercise classes led by trained instructors. While they don't have the individualized approach of personal training, you will still get more benefits than exercising on your own. More often than not, the classes are included with your membership dues…meaning there is no additional cost to participate. If money is tight (and who's isn't), than find a health club that offers them.

If you are new to exercise, have a lot of weight to lose, have special needs or circumstances, have a specific goal you are working towards, or want fast and safe results, hiring a personal trainer is an absolute must. Health clubs and independent trainers will work with you and your budget to get you started and then typically workout a pay-as-you-go plan. Initially, I would recommend getting the most sessions you can afford to jump start your training and exercise results. If you have to make a decision between a month of hour sessions and two months of half hour sessions, go with the half hours and have your trainer instruct you on what to do for the other half hour you should be exercising. Try to get the most volume of sessions when you first start, because having the accountability factor is very important to ensure you get into the exercise habit. The dropout rate for people trying to exercise on their own is dismal…25% within the first month and more than 65% by six months. Having a trainer working with you will reduce the likelihood of dropout to almost zero!

Keep a Lifeline

After you establish good exercise habits, learn proper form and technique, and feel comfortable exercising on your own, one of the best values in fitness is to train with a trainer once a week and have them structure your other workouts for that week. You get the accountability and monitoring of having a trainer and you get a fresh workout routine each week. You could even train with a trainer every other week or stretch it to one time a month, although your results and motivation may suffer a bit. I have several clients (high school students, teachers, retirees, single moms) who meet with me once a week or even every other week and they fare so much better than my clients who disconnect and try to do it on their own. Maintaining this relationship with a personal trainer is your exercise lifeline.

It is always hard for me to see people come in excited, guns a' blazing, ready to conquer the world. They buy three to six sessions to get started, because as they say: "I'm confident I can do this on my own." We have fun, they learn as much as I can teach them, they see their body start to change, I develop a program for them to follow on their own and then they disappear once the lifeline is cut. The reality for most people is it is very hard to exercise on your own. Unless you have developed daily exercise habits for at least two consecutive months and learned a safe, fun and effective exercise program to follow each week, I would recommend you keep an exercise lifeline. At the very least, I would encourage you to buddy up with someone reliable to exercise with once you get started on your own.

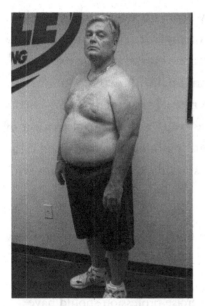 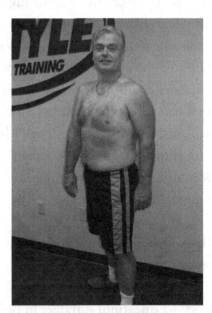

Akos lost 60 pounds in three months keeping an exercise lifeline

Learning to exercise properly is like learning a foreign language. It takes time, persistence, practice and a good teacher. Just like you wouldn't expect to speak Mandarin Chinese fluently overnight, you shouldn't expect to become a fitness expert overnight either. Get some good training and instruction early, and it will definitely keep you from getting lost or misdirected. It is critical to start on the right foot and lay down a strong (literally and figuratively) foundation for you to build on.

How do you hire a personal trainer?

I always tell my prospective clients and people who are referred to me to approach hiring a trainer like a job interview. I tell them: "You are the boss and you are hiring me. Interview me like you would any other new hire or job applicant." Have your questions written down ahead of time and don't be afraid to interview more than one trainer at the same gym. This approach will help you find the right fit for your personality and goals you are trying to achieve. Most good trainers are humble enough to know they work for their clients even though they get the pleasure of torturing them during the workout sessions. My clients like to yell out: "He's crazy; I can't believe I am paying him to do this to me!" To which I always reply: "It's the pain you love to hate and you keep coming back for more — so who is the crazy one?" It is usually during the most intense and painful final repetitions of a set when I instruct them to "do two more!" that many of my clients will inadvertently scream out "I hate you!" For this exclamation of pain intolerance I always reply: "Hate me now, love me later!" The bottom line is we have fun and you should expect to have fun with your trainer too.

I have identified several criteria for you to consider during the interview process.

- **Education:** A trainer in the exercise profession should have an undergraduate education from an accredited institution of higher education, although I wouldn't necessarily limit my selection to only those who have degrees. It is more and more common to see undergraduate degrees and even advanced education in a trainer's credentials, but it is a fairly recent trend. I'm sure that some of the most experienced trainers may not have any formal education, so if experience is most important to you, you might not want to exclude someone because they don't have a PhD in Kinesiology from Harvard.

308

I'd like to think most successful trainers who truly value their clients, have what I call a "real world PhD. "

That being said, I personally believe it definitely helps to have a scientific education and background. The most beneficial education would be a four-year degree in biology or exercise science and I'm not just saying it because I have my degree in biology. I'm saying it because it provides the trainer with the skill set to acquire additional knowledge and understand the scientific principles behind industry-related research. To be successful as a personal trainer, like many other professions, it is critical to constantly pursue continuing education opportunities in training methods, exercise programming, health benefits of exercise, human motivation, and nutritional science. Most credible certifications in personal training have continuing education requirements which have to be met every two to three years to maintain the certification.

Personally, I spend thousands of dollars each year on workshops, trade shows, the American College of Sports Medicine (ACSM) Annual Meeting, and the National Strength and Conditioning Association (NSCA) National Conference because I want to have the most current and valuable information at my fingertips. This helps me serve my clients needs by designing the most efficient and effective nutrition and exercise programs to get them to their goals. It also helps me learn and grow professionally, which is one of my personal goals.

- **Certifications:** There are currently 19 different organizations (and growing) offering personal training certifications. To keep you on the path to success when picking a personal trainer, look for at least one current, credible certification from organizations like the American College of Sports Medicine (ACSM), National Academy of Sports Medicine

(NASM), National Strength and Conditioning Association (NSCA), American Council on Exercise (ACE), American Fitness and Aerobics Association (AFAA), National Federation of Professional Trainers (NFPT), International Sports Sciences Association (ISSA) or International Fitness Professionals Association (IFPA).

While this is not a comprehensive list and there are many other good organizations, the ones I listed are generally considered the most credible and have been around the longest. Most of these organizations have directories of their certified personal trainers on their respective web sites to help you locate a trainer in your area or to ensure your prospective trainer's certification is current.

If you have specific athletic goals, there are several sports performance certifications like the Certified Strength and Conditioning Specialist (CSCS) from the NSCA and the Performance Enhancement Specialist (PES) from NASM that you can look for to get a more educated approach. If you have issues with specific joints or problems with normal movement, you may want to consider looking for a trainer with the Corrective Exercise Specialist (CES) certification from NASM. If you want a highly educated, integrated approach to exercise and health, then look for someone with the Health/Fitness Instructor (HFI) certification from ACSM. If you want assistance putting together a sports nutrition program to maximize your results on the field, track, road course, water, or simply in the gym, ISSA has a Specialist in Performance Nutrition certification you can seek out but personally, I would recommend hiring a Certified Sports Nutritionist (CISSN) from the International Society of Sports Nutrition (ISSN) which requires a 4-year degree in an exercise science and successful completion of a comprehensive certification exam.

A final note on certifications: A trainer can have all the certifications in the world and still be a bad trainer. Applied knowledge is always the best rule of thumb. Look for someone who has been down the same road you want to travel because they will be a better guide for you. Use certifications only as a prerequisite when you're selecting your trainer, not the sole criteria for your decision.

- **Experience and Longevity:** How long a trainer has been training professionally should be one of the first things you determine when selecting a trainer. Being a dedicated personal trainer is physically hard but rewarding work, with long hours spent at the gym morning, noon, and night, when others are out having fun. Unfortunately, this leads to a lot of turnover as budding trainers discover they have other priorities or can't get up every day at 5AM.

  Anybody who has been a personal trainer professionally for at least three years must be doing something right, has a decent amount of "real world" experience and is usually in the business to serve, not to be served. Thus, I would use three years of experience as a benchmark when deciding between trainers, but make sure they still have enough enthusiasm left in their game to keep you motivated too.

  One caveat: All good trainers have to get started at some point and as long as they're competent, enthusiastic, and dedicated, it may be worth your while to give them a chance. You can always change trainers if it doesn't work out and a new trainer's per session rate is typically a lot less then someone with years of experience. You may stumble on a bargain this way.

- **Client Testimonials and References:** During the interview process, ask for testimonials or references from clients the trainer has worked with in the past. Most experienced trainers should have at least a handful of "success stories" to share with you. Some health clubs will even post these testimonials on the wall or on their web sites for you to read. Look for a testimonial of someone who you can relate to and if you have any doubts, ask to speak to the person and get their take on their experience working with the trainer.

Honestly, my clients are my best source of advertising and I have only worked off of referrals for the past several years. I love when someone asks to speak to my clients, because they can sell me better than I can. If a trainer is hesitant to share any testimonials with you, they are either brand new to the profession or haven't kept someone's attention and motivation long enough to get them marketable results. If this is the case, proceed with caution or better yet, proceed to another trainer.

- **Personality and Personal Appearance:** You will definitely want to work with someone whom you can get along with and someone who looks the part. As a trainer I believe *your body is your billboard* and how a trainer presents himself or herself is the easiest way to see if they practice what they preach. I'm sure when someone tells you "do as I say, not as I do" you are less likely to value the advice they are giving you and you may even resent them for telling you to do something they themselves don't value enough to do.

  This doesn't mean you should hire a fitness model with three percent bodyfat either. Oftentimes, these trainers are egocentric, cake-eating, genetic freaks who value partying more than showing up to early morning sessions with their clients. This obviously isn't always the case, but get a reference of their reliability just to be safe.

Considering all these criteria, do your best to find the right trainer for you. It will never be a perfect fit, but getting you safe, fun, and fast results should be the trainer's number one priority. It never hurts to ask the front desk or operations staff: "Who is the most dedicated trainer?" and you should get a pretty honest answer. If you ask them who the "best trainer" is, they may give you a recommendation for a friend or someone they like personally, which is obviously biased.

Your health should be one of your top priorities, because without it, you can't earn a living, can't hug your spouse, can't see your kids grow up, can't enjoy the free time you have, and won't live long enough to enjoy the prosperity you have worked so hard for. So invest in yourself and hire a personal trainer. You'll be thanking me soon enough.

For most people in our skeptical, opinionated, and ever-changing world seeing is believing. For this reason, I want to share with you a remarkable "real world" success story of how personal training can pay off. About three years ago I was approached by one of our long-standing gym members named Greg. Greg was a permanent fixture at our gym in terms of his consistency and effort so I was initially surprised. He asked me some general questions about exercise, but what he was really looking for was results. By shaking up his diet and exercise routine, dialing up his intensity, and adding the motivational power of a goal, I was able to help Greg move in the right direction. Greg went from a tired-looking, overweight, and unhealthy man, looking much older than his chronological age, to a confident, energetic, young-looking stallion ready for almost any physical challenge…and he did it in six short weeks. Greg proved to me, his wife, his friends, and most importantly himself, what proper training, nutrition, and commitment can achieve in a very short period of time. Dreams can move mountains when you harness the power of faith! I hope Greg's example will inspire you, build your own faith and take you to the destination of your dreams.

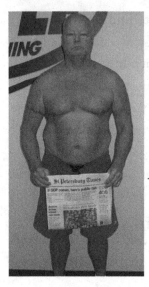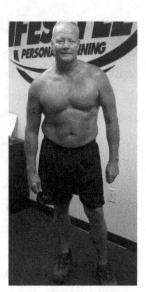

Greg
Age: 56
Retired Police Officer

I lost over 36 pounds in just 41 days!!! I lowered my bodyfat by 10%, lost 5 inches off my waist, my total cholesterol dropped from 208 to 154, and I lowered my resting heart rate by 18 beats a minute. Anything is possible!

"They say a picture is worth a thousand words, but I would say my before and after pictures tell a much longer story. I can't believe how much you can change your body and your whole life, in just six short weeks. As a former athlete and retired police PE instructor, I didn't think I would benefit from a trainer. But after being stuck overweight for years trying to do it on my own, I decided I needed a push and boy did I get it. After my first three sessions with Matt, I was so convinced by his expertise, motivational shills, and professionalism, I hired him to train my wife as well.

I feel so much better physically and mentally. My strength, stamina, weight, blood pressure, and cholesterol have all improved! I thought I was in decent shape, but after Matt showed me what intensity really is, I learned my true potential. My recovery heart rate dropped from 101 to 83 and I have so much more energy and vitality. Because Matt helped me find my youth again, I even decided to start competing in mountain bike adventure races. It feels great to be able to do the things I thought were lost to my age and condition. I'm writing a new chapter in my life now and I have Matt to thank. I would recommend personal training to anyone who wants to positively change not only their body, but their life too."

- Greg Crays

CHAPTER TWELVE

Empower Yourself

> *"You only lose energy when life becomes dull in your mind. Get interested in something. Get absolutely enthralled in something. Throw yourself into it with abandon. If you're not getting into good causes, no wonder you're tired. You're disintegrating. You're deteriorating. You're dying on the vine. The more you lose yourself in something bigger than yourself, the more energy you will have."*
>
> Norman Vincent Peale,
> *The Power of Positive Thinking*, 1952

The Power of the Mind

Each of our brains has more capabilities than the most powerful supercomputer. How we learn to use our brain can determine our successes and failures in life, jobs, relationships and even how we perceive reality. Unfortunately, many of us are guilty of letting our human potential go untapped and people end up stuck in a quagmire of negative emotions, feelings of uselessness, and states of depression. Teaching you how to flood your mind and body with positive emotions may be the greatest purpose I can serve. Exercise has always been the vehicle I use to take me from whatever emotional state I'm in to a more positive one. If you feel like your life is out of control, one area where you most definitely can gain control is your health. This gives us hope! I know firsthand that having hope is a powerful way to keep the stress and monotony of life in check.

Believe it or not, you can learn to control and manipulate your emotions. As Tony Robbins likes to say "emotion is created by motion" or in other words, motion creates emotion! To change your mental state or psychology, you have to change your physiology; how you sit, stand, breathe, speak, and move. Studies have proven this over and over. Don't believe me? Try smiling for the next few minutes. Give me a big smile. Go ahead, show those pearly whites and cute dimples. Notice how you feel now...happier! You can use this simple technique to feel better anytime you want. In this chapter I hope to give you the tools, knowledge, and motivation to use your mind to propel you in a positive direction.

The mind is extremely powerful at controlling all aspects of our lives. If you learn to harness its power, you will have limitless opportunities during your lifetime. In the fairly recent book *The Secret* by Rhonda Byrne, she discloses the timeless Law of Attraction which dictates that you will attract that which you think about...good or bad. The Law of Attraction is either the central premise or one of the fundamental principles of practically every self-help book ever written and dates back to centuries-old wisdom. Napoleon Hill's *Think and Grow Rich* is considered by many to be the first true self-help book. This best seller was published back in 1936 and even its title illustrates the Law of Attraction. Whatever and wherever your thoughts are will determine your destiny in life. Norman Vincent Peale was an amazing man and he liked to say "faith power works wonders." I like to say "beliefs create reality" and whether it is making more money, getting in shape or not getting sick, as long as you truly believe it, God, the universe, infinite intelligence (or whatever you choose to call it) will ultimately lay the manifestation of your predominate thoughts at your feet. Let me repeat that for more emphasis. The universe will lay the manifestation of your predominant thoughts at your feet.

"The greatest achievement was at first and for a time a dream. The oak sleeps in the acorn, the bird waits in the egg, and in the highest vision of the soul a waking angel stirs. Dreams are the seedlings of realities." —James Allen

Beliefs create reality!

You are probably familiar with the placebo effect and how people in "double-blind, placebo-controlled" studies experience medicinal effects from sugar pills 20 – 30% of the time. If a medication does not show better results than the placebo it's compared with, then FDA approval is obviously out of the question. Why do we get the placebo effect? Is it because of some miraculous power of sugar? No, it is because of the power of the mind. Studies have been done on the placebo effect and they have found a direct correlation between the type of placebo given and its perceived effects — the more powerful a drug the participants perceived they were getting the higher likelihood of an associated effect. For instance, a small, white pill will deliver the placebo effect 30% of the time, while a red pill will be closer to 50%. Give someone an injection of saline solution (salt water) and tell them it is a powerful drug and the placebo effect can climb to 87%. It's all from the power of the mind.

In fact, a voluntary study was conducted on Harvard medical students to determine what is more powerful, someone's expectation of what a drug will do or what the drug is actually intended to do (its pharmacology). Researchers gave half of the student participants a barbiturate (central nervous system depressant) but told them it was an amphetamine and gave the other half of the students an amphetamine (stimulant) but told them it was a depressant. Essentially the students were given either a stimulant or a depressant but were told they were getting the opposite. What do you think happened? The study concluded the mind, in the form of our expectations, is more powerful than the pharmacology of the drugs because over 80% of the time the students experienced the effects of the drug they *believed* they were taking. If the students were given speed, but *believed* they were getting sleeping pills, they got tired. The students given the sedatives actually became wide awake with their hearts racing, because this is what they *believed* they would experience. This is why I like to say "beliefs create reality!"

Let this be a lesson in the power of expectations and I hope you will start applying it to your life. Expect great things and you will experience great things. Expect lousy things and you will get lousy things. It's the power of choice and we all have it. Learn to use this power by focusing on positive thoughts and the achievements you seek will become fulfilled as your destiny in life. Faith power works wonders!

Don't be afraid of failure either. I know this is easier said than done. Personally, it took me many years to overcome my own personal fear of failure and I still have to constantly train my mind with positive thoughts and expectations to keep it in check. There is a Japanese proverb that translates to mean: "Fear is only as deep as the mind allows." Like the muscles in your body will expand from demand, your life, confidence, and self-esteem will too. I like to tell my clients that "failure begets success in the gym and in life." You probably know that Thomas Edison failed thousands of times before he successfully invented the light bulb and Abraham Lincoln had personal and political failures time and time again before he became one the greatest leaders in our nation's history. Every failure is one step closer to success and you must have the conviction to keep moving forward. Don't be paralyzed by fear, learn to embrace it!

Be aware of "Defensive Thinking"

Speaking of fear, are you in self-preservation mode? Are you saving your ego with defensive thinking techniques? Maybe you don't even realize it, but I see people do it all the time. We don't want to admit to ourselves that we made a mistake or that maybe someone doesn't like us. Or we trick ourselves into thoughts, behaviors and actions we know with our intellectual mind are bad for us. Psychologists call this process cognitive dissonance. When presented with an internal conflict like smoking cigarettes for example, one part of a smoker's brain says "smoking is bad for me, can cause lung cancer and lead to premature death." Another part of their brain says "I get tremendous pleasure from smoking, it relaxes me, keeps my weight in check, and I feel better." These two sides are incongruent because they don't agree with each other. Typically, the brain justifies the bad behavior by focusing on the reassuring thoughts.

This effectively shifts the mental balance of power towards whatever gives us the most pleasure.

It is human nature to move away from pain and towards pleasure. The problem with this philosophy is that most short-term pleasures like eating sugary foods, smoking, drinking mind-altering amounts of alcohol, or using illegal drugs can lead to long-term pain. And vice-versa, the short-term pain of exercise that people avoid, can lead to the long-term pleasure of lasting health, mobility, and independence. Learn to sew the seeds of good habits and you will harvest a positive self-image and reap lasting rewards. Self-image guru and bestselling author of *Psycho-Cybernetics: A New Way to Get More Living out of Life* Dr Maxwell Maltz said: "Our self-image and habits tend to go together. Change one and you will automatically change the other." Shift your thinking towards what you wisely know is best for you by using pain and pleasure to your advantage but also be wary of the following defensive mechanisms we commonly use to get around bad behaviors.

1. **Rationalization:** *Unconsciously justifying unacceptable behaviors with logic.* This is the process which leads us to eat unnecessary extra helpings of food at a friend's house because we rationalize to ourselves that it is better to eat a lot instead of possibly offending the cook. Or justifying to yourself that you earned that five pound piece of cheesecake because you closed a big deal or had a rough day. Or the very common rationalization that you are tired from a long day and will go to the gym tomorrow because you probably wouldn't have enough energy to workout anyway. Or when a smoker rationalizes that quitting would cause weight gain which is unhealthy, so I better keep smoking. Learn to recognize the irrational side of rationalization and you will be much better off.

2. **Repression:** *Pushing information out of your head when it doesn't support your current reality.* This is an overwhelming dynamic

affecting Americans today because most people have heard about the benefits of exercise, but repress these thoughts so they don't have to make a change in their life. Unfortunately, many people will repress the information in this book because it requires effort and energy to move in a new direction. Because of the Law of Inertia, an object at rest tends to stay at rest and an object in motion tends to stay in motion. In other words, it takes more energy to get started in a new direction and many people will repress the knowledge of what exercise can do for them rather than invest the energy it takes to get started. American entrepreneur Victor Kiam said: "Procrastination is the natural assassin of opportunity." Take heart with the fact that it takes less energy to maintain new habits once they get started.

3. **Transference / Displacement:** *Displacing unresolved aggression and conflict onto someone or something else.* Ever get a ticket on the way home because you were actually speeding, then snap at your spouse when you get home because he or she forgot to take out the garbage? This is a classic example of transference and if you learn to recognize it before it happens, then you will save someone else the grief of your negative transfer of emotion. Mistakes happen, so what? Accept it and move on. Fortunately, transference can work for positive energy too and in this case, it can be a good thing. When something good happens, your mood is elevated and this can be transferred to someone else. Keep this in mind when you're meeting with someone face to face or coming home to your spouse and family. Put yourself in a positive mood so you can set a happy tone and transfer it. People tend to be attracted to positive people, so the key is to find a source of positive energy each day. Exercise, for most people, can be this source. I have never met anyone who felt worse after exercising than before they started. I can't tell you how many times I've heard my clients exclaim: "Wow, I felt like garbage before I got here today. I was

even gonna call you to cancel but I'm glad I didn't…I feel great!" Inevitably, they will share this positive energy with the people they encounter later that day, paying it forward so to speak. What kind of energy do you want to transfer?

4. **Projection:** *Casting failures, unacceptable thoughts, or unwanted emotions onto someone else.* If you spend a lot of time around someone who is negative, angry, unethical, or verbally abusive, it is far more likely these traits will be projected onto you and then, in turn, onto the other people you encounter. Likewise, if you spend time around positive, uplifting, caring, happy, giving, and trusting people, it is very likely these character traits will rub off on you. So the moral of this story is to be selective about who you spend time with. Be conscious about the influence your spouse, friends, supervisor, coworkers, and family can have on you and how you project this influence. Also be aware of this influence on your children if you have any. Invest the time and energy to seek out people with the traits you desire and avoid people with the traits you least desire (as much as possible). If you are trying to lose weight and begin an exercise program, hanging out with a non-exercising cynic is probably the worst thing you could do. It only takes one bad apple to ruin the bunch, so get rid of the bad apples in your life and your inner strength will ripen to its true potential.

5. **Denial:** *An unconscious attempt to resolve internal emotional conflicts by refusing to believe our external reality.* When you refuse to accept reality, you are in denial. If you are 5'5" and weigh 250 pounds and refuse to accept the possibility that you just might have a tiny little weight problem, than you are drinking from the fountain of denial. Guys who come into the gym thinking they know all there is to know about working out from their vast amount of exercise knowledge learned back in high school

20 years ago are also in denial. If you think you know all there is to know about anything, your cup is in the fountain too. Pour out the delusional Kool-Aid and accept reality. Whether you're dealing with weight control, exercise programs, work performance or relationship issues, get the honest opinion of a professional or friend you trust. Don't seek out the people who tell you what you want to hear, because not only are they in denial too, but it is highly likely they will unconsciously (and sometimes consciously) want to sabotage your results so they won't have to deal with the reality of their own failures. Misery loves company, so be careful where your advice comes from. The same Tony Robbins I launched this chapter talking about said: "If you don't set a baseline standard for what you'll accept in life, you'll find it's easy to slip into behaviors and attitudes or a quality of life that's far below what you deserve."

These are all very common mechanisms we use in our lives to get us through the day and most of us use a combination of all of them. I'm simply making you aware of them in hope that you will learn to incorporate a positive approach to your overall plan. Acknowledge that you are truly in control of your life, because even the smallest steps, when taken consistently, add up to miles of progress.

Your body can do it if your mind will allow it!

We so often are self-limiting in our beliefs and our attitudes which inevitably become a self-fulfilling prophecy. If you learn to convert this "stinking thinking" to positive expectation, you will unlock your true potential. A classic illustration of self-limiting thinking on a global scale was the four minute mile. Dating back to the 19th century and halfway through the 20th century, thousands of runners tried to run the mile in under four minutes but not one succeeded. Why? At that time it was popularly believed to be physiologically impossible for a human being to run a mile in under four minutes.

Then in 1954, along came a medical student and athlete named Roger Bannister who made it his goal to achieve the impossible. After months of intense training and with a clearly defined goal pushing him to achieve it, he officially clocked the mile in 3 minutes and 59 seconds. He did it! It was an amazing feat for sure, but what is even more enlightening is the effect it had on the minds of other runners. Suddenly, a seemingly impossible barrier was lifted and despite no one doing it for centuries, many other runners went on to accomplish the milestone in the same year, and one, an Australian named John Landy, did it the very next month. Seeing is believing! Once these athletes realized it could be done, they lifted their own self-limiting beliefs, and their bodies produced the physical capacity and tolerated the pain necessary to achieve their own sub-four minute mile.

Like the runners before Roger Bannister, self-limiting thinking is pervasive in the gym and in life too. All too often we let our internal voice use defeating words like can't, shouldn't, won't, and couldn't instead of empowering words like must, will, and can. If you tell yourself you can't do something then guess what? You can't. Your mind can be your own worst enemy and you have to learn to recognize "stinking thinking" and stop it in its neuro-synaptic tracks. By learning how to stretch yourself, you will accomplish so much more.

"All personal breakthroughs begin with a change in beliefs."
Anthony Robbins

Let me give you a classic example of self-limiting thinking at work in the gym. I had a client named Anne, but her name should have been "Can't" because that's all she would say when it came to exercise. Anne was an attractive woman in her mid-forties who wanted to lose about 30 pounds. She had no functional problems or physical ailments, other than her attitude. When we were doing her first warm-up on the treadmill, she told me "I can't do this for more than three minutes." I wanted to tell her she had enough stored energy on her body to walk for three months straight, but being the consummate professional, I bit my tongue. When we were mapping out her exercise program to accomplish the ambitious goals she had, she told me "I can't exercise more than three times a week." Yet she revealed to me during our initial assessment she had plenty of time for other less beneficial uses of her time like watching TV and bowling a few nights a week. When we were using a leg press machine with a ridiculously light weight, I told her to do 20 repetitions as a warm-up and she stopped at 15 and said "I just can't do anymore."

Now when I say this was ridiculously light, I'm not speaking in macho trainer talk. A child's birthday balloon could have lifted this weight. I felt it was time to teach Anne a lesson about her self-limiting thinking. I asked her "Are you absolutely positive you can't do anymore than 15?" She replied "Yes." I wanted to tell her that my three year old daughter could lift it more than 20 times, but again, being the consummate professional and because I don't have a three year old daughter, I again bit my tongue. Anne loved to talk and pontificate about her extensive opinion on uninteresting subjects (and not workout), so I decided to use her gift of gab as my ally in said lesson.

At the beginning of the next set (at the same weight as before) I asked Anne a good, open-ended "What do you think about..." question to which Anne went on an almost three minute diatribe while she unknowingly performed 47 perfect repetitions with the weight she was "absolutely positive" she could only do 15 times. Again, I will say: Your body can do it if your mind will allow it. I pointed out to Anne her amazing feat of strength and we began to crack the self-limiting shell she was encased in and we had fewer problems with "can't" in our future workouts together.

Beyond the Comfort Zone

By short-circuiting her self-limiting belief system with my question, Anne learned she was much more capable than she thought herself to be. Many of us find ourselves trapped by the confines of our own thoughts.

Are you in the same sinking boat as Anne? If you answered yes, it's time to jump out of that boat and swim to a new way of thinking. Too many people slide into the comfort zone of mediocrity. It's time to move beyond the comfort zone! Working out at a high intensity is way beyond most people's comfort zone. I've had mothers tell me high-intensity training is "worse than child birth." Several of my clients tell me I'm sadomasochistic. I consider this a compliment because if I didn't teach them that this level of exertion was in their realm of possibility, they would never get there. The reality is that most people enjoy the process of stretching themselves to achieve new heights of fitness and strength by pushing through the pain that limited them in the past.

Knowing how to push people to their physical limits and pain threshold helps my clients achieve better results, but more importantly, teaches them they are capable of stretching the boundaries in other areas of their lives too. Maybe it's starting their own company, pursuing a childhood dream, or asking out someone who makes their heart flutter. Maybe it's confronting problem areas in their life or problem relationships. The only way to achieve more is to stretch ourselves beyond our comfort zone.

Where are you now? Are you firmly planted on the metaphorical couch of comfort and in survival mode? Or are you out there exploring new possibilities, learning new skills, and challenging yourself? Like Chuck Yeager who broke the sound barrier by literally pushing the aerodynamic limits of his Bell X-1 aircraft, you too can discover your true potential and capabilities by stretching your own limits. This is what makes America so great and is the secret to our nation's success: Bill Gates walking away from his Harvard education to pursue his crazy ambition in starting Microsoft; Jim Simplot gambling $400 borrowed dollars to start a potato farm, then going on to become the chief supplier of potatoes for McDonalds and other fast food companies with the beloved French fry; and Lance Armstrong propelling himself through his ordeal with cancer and back onto the bike, going on to win a record seven Tour de France victories, pushing human capabilities to new heights. Is there something you can achieve by stepping out of your comfort zone? I believe there is but what *you* believe is far more important.

Live with an attitude of gratitude

People are always on the lookout for happiness and the things that make them happy. Countless books have been written about this quest and people will continue to seek it. In his book titled *The Happiness Prescription* Deepak Chopra outlines 10 keys to happiness which include: living in the present moment, getting rid of toxins and toxic emotions, and learning not to judge others or ourselves. The Dalai Lama, spiritual leader of the Tibetan people and co-author of *The Art of Happiness* says: "I believe that the very purpose of our life is to seek happiness." His approach to happiness includes training the mind, shifting perspective, and developing compassion.

Despite the volume of expertise available on happiness, it somehow seems to elude most people. The irony here is that happiness is not something or someone you seek or obtain, but it simply comes from within. Learn to embrace the everyday miracles and celebrate even the smallest of victories in your life. We live in an amazing country which grants its citizens personal freedom. Ask anybody who has lost it for even a day, and you can better appreciate how valuable freedom truly is. We too often let the trivial details of life weigh us down like an anchor tethered to our spirit. Cut that anchor line and soar to your destiny. If you need to lose weight, get a new job, find someone to love, or move to a new city, then do it without delay. But keep in mind that happiness comes from within and it isn't a destination or the green grass on the other side of the fence.

Most of the time, happiness is staring you in the face with so many things in your life to be grateful for. It only eludes you because you choose to focus on what you don't have instead of all the things you do have. Some of the happiest people in the world are the ones who have every reason to be miserable. They lost their true love in an unexplained accident, have cancer, live in a third world country in a dirt hut, lost their home in a hurricane, or have no worldly possessions, yet they resolve to focus on being thankful for the things they do have — freedom, shelter, friendship, or their health. Retired broadcaster and author Hugh Downs put this succinctly when he said: "A happy person is not a person in a certain set of circumstances, but rather a person with a certain set of attitudes."

If you have your eyesight (and I assume you do if you're reading this book), then you have a lot to be thankful for. There are so many beautiful things to see around us, but all too often we overlook them. Most of the time, the things we are seeking to make us happy or to feel fulfilled are right under our nose. Back during the gold rush days of the 1800's, there was a metallurgist who became renowned for his detailed knowledge of metals, geology, and topography. He was offered a professorship at the university he had attended on the East Coast, but decided instead to head west to lay claim to his fortune in gold, silver, copper, or whatever he could discover. He figured with his vast knowledge and skill he would become rich. He quickly sold his house and left town. It was later discovered that the large and unusual stone on his former property, the very stone he sat on when he signed over the deed to his house, was actually a solid piece of silver worth over one hundred thousand dollars! That is a whole lot of money today, but an extraordinary sum 120 years ago. The fortune he was looking for was right there all along.

The moral of this story is to take a long and good look around before you skip town for greener pastures. Look before you leap, make sure the ship is actually sinking before you abandon it, and most importantly, observe the miracles surrounding you every day in your own life. All too often, we give up on things too easily, especially ourselves. Before you buy a new car, learn to appreciate the one you currently have. And that is especially true regarding your spouse and children, as well as your house, job, friends, clothes, and life itself. Cherish the treasures of the present moment because life is a gift.

HOPE - Give Yourself Something to Believe in

"We must accept finite disappointments but
we must never lose infinite hope."
Dr Martin Luther King, Jr.

We can survive 40 days without food, 4 days without water, 4 minutes without oxygen, but only 4 seconds without hope. You may have read or heard these words (or Dr King's) before which clarify the importance hope has in our lives. I believe hope is the foundation of happiness and without it we are trapped in the bonds of despair. I believe there are six undeniable truths of life which are:

1. We must have faith.
2. We must love our family.
3. We must eat nutritious food.
4. We must get adequate sleep.
5. We must exercise frequently.
6. We must have hope.

How well you embrace these undeniable truths will largely determine the quantity and quality of life you will have. Unfortunately, there are many hopeless people walking around dying a slow death. Living without hope causes the body to age faster, weakens the immune system, makes our cells more prone to cancer, and sucks the energy out of life. This listless and lifeless existence is completely avoidable with hope. For most people, finding a purpose or passion can provide a quick fix. Having purpose in our lives connects us to something or someone and gives us hope. Find purpose in your life no matter how trivial it may seem. Whether it is a job, loving a spouse or child with all your heart, volunteering for a charitable organization, reading to children at your local elementary school, learning a new hobby, coaching a little league team, or even keeping your house clean and tidy, all purpose makes a difference.

A friend of mine named Darrell just returned from New Orleans and I was thrilled to learn from him the Big Easy has bounced back and moved on after the devastation caused by Hurricane Katrina. This natural disaster literally destroyed much of the city known for its parties, Mardi Gras, jazz music, beignets, and Creole attitude. The people relied on hope and vision to accomplish the rebuilding process. Darrell told me about a locally famous singer in New Orleans who attained his celebrity due to his massive size and musical ability. Darrell said "You have to see this guy! I would guess he weighs over 800 pounds." He went on to tell me that it took the man over 15 minutes and the help of three people just to walk on stage and assume the seat where he would stay and play for the next six hours. This guy's musical talent gets lost in our fascination with his largess.

I have to admit I was originally torn by this story. On one hand, I was happy that this gentleman still pursued his musical passion despite the almost insurmountable obstacles he faces just getting on stage. On the other hand, I was deeply saddened by the reality that at some point in his life, he gave up hope. I wanted to know more about him. Was I right? I asked Darrell: "Do you think he just gave up at some point?" Darrell told me that he had a few drinks and conversations with the band between sets which led to the discovery that this extremely talented man had essentially given up any hope of having a functional life. He is resolved to the fact he will die young, but rationalizes it with himself by proclaiming: "At least I'll die doing one of the two things that makes me happy... eating and singing."

This is a classic example of losing hope and giving up on ourselves and unfortunately, he had help. The very people who love him were the ones bringing him the food that's digging his early grave. My intuition tells me these "enablers" struggle with what the right thing to do is and I'm not sure if I, or anyone else, would or could do anything differently, given the same circumstances. We often resolve these internal conflicts by telling ourselves we're doing the right thing because it makes the person happy. Having an impact on someone in this predicament is obviously a tremendous challenge. The goal of losing several hundred pounds of weight would seem unattainable when considered all at once. It would take a lot more effort, patience, and self-discipline to help someone like this musician by getting them help, taking steps to reverse the weight gain, and being patient with their internal struggle. It is never too late to lose weight and there have been countless success stories with extreme weight loss. Even a ten percent weight reduction can have a positive impact on a morbidly obese person's health. You climb the highest mountains the same way you climb the small ones — one step at a time.

"You're going to fall. It's how you get up that defines you."
Dwayne Wade, NBA star

Hope can come in many forms including owning a pet. Scientific studies have proven that pet owners live longer and while many theories exist as to why, I firmly believe cats, dogs, and other pets give us hope and purpose. When you come home from a long day at work, you hope your poodle named Fluffy is waiting for you with her tail wagging and her unyielding enthusiasm to jump in your lap and lick your face. Taking care of a pet can also subconsciously communicate your ability to provide for and nurture another life which gives your existence some critical value.

So owning a pet can be one simple strategy for gaining hope. What are some others? Exercise is one of the best ways to add hope to your life. "How is that Matt?" you may ask. The answer is simple. When you begin and maintain an exercise program, you prove to yourself you have control over one area in your life. One of my workout partners named Justin likes to say: "In the gym two hundred pounds is always two hundred pounds." In other words, you know what to expect. Exercise will extend your functional life and thus gives you a daily purpose. As you reap the healthy rewards, inevitably you gain the hope of a brighter future — one filled with independence, physical ability, good health, and longevity. You can go to the gym with the hope of making new acquaintances and expanding your circle of friends. Exercise can give you the physical ability to try something you've always wanted to do. Having control over your health is very empowering. When you apply the universal principles we've discussed in this book, you will achieve results in any area of your life you so choose.

Remember this: Success breeds success! It is called transference: when one area of your life improves, other areas of your life will start to improve too. I've always believed if you take care of your body, this will take care of your mind, and combined together, they will take care of your heart...body, mind and spirit. By improving your body, mind, and spirit, other areas of your life will start to fall into place. I've seen it time and time again in my own life and my clients' lives. I can't tell you how many times I've seen someone achieve their fitness goals and soon thereafter, they get the pay raise they deserved, get the dream job they've always wanted, find the right person to be in a relationship with, or reconnect with their spouse and other family members. It truly is amazing to witness and is by far the most rewarding part of my job.

Success and hope are available to everyone and I encourage you, if you haven't already, to take personal responsibility for your health. I promise it will lead to gaining personal ownership of your life, your weight, your relationships, and your happiness. Start simple and start today!

> *"Accept responsibility for your life. Know that it is you who will get you where you want to go, no one else."*
> Les Brown

Need change?

Steven Covey, author of *The Seven Habits of Highly Effective People* advises: "Live out your imagination, not your history." Sometimes it takes a crisis situation or a tragic event to initiate change. You see evidence of this with government, large corporations, professional sports teams, great athletes, celebrities, and most importantly, in our personal lives. It shouldn't take a multi-million dollar lawsuit to get a company to do the right thing. It shouldn't take getting lung cancer to get someone to stop smoking. It shouldn't take getting a DUI to get us to stop drinking and driving. It shouldn't take infidelity or the threat of divorce to force couples to invest more time and energy into their marriage. It shouldn't take our kids failing in school for us to realize they deserve our time and attention to help them with their schoolwork. It shouldn't take having colon cancer or getting type 2 diabetes for us to make changes in how and what we eat.

Likewise, it shouldn't take having a heart attack or stroke to inspire us to start exercising. Life can be complicated if we let life control us. With all of the demands placed on us, it is very easy to get caught in the rip tide of modern living and get sucked out into the sea of despair to ultimately drown. You have to learn how to swim across the current before this happens. Like water, human nature will always seek the path of least resistance. We want to seek the easy path. But to get to the top, you have to climb the mountain and exert yourself. The reward is oh so worth it when you get there. Not only is the view better from the top, but you will receive a positive infusion of energy for your accomplishment.

In his book *The Energy Bus*, Jon Gordon explains the importance of having a personal vision. Vision is rule number one in choosing the direction of his metaphorical "energy bus." Choose where you want to go or others will choose it for you, sapping your energy like weeds in a garden. Develop a personal vision statement to serve as your life's compass. This will keep you pointed in the right direction. My personal vision for the past 10 years has been to educate, motivate and inspire people to exercise. Initially this led me into personal training so I could make a difference in a handful of lives. Then I developed and started presenting informational seminars to help hundreds of people. And more recently, my vision has led me to write this book so I can hopefully reach out to thousands of people. That's just one example of how a vision statement can help you navigate your life and help you find your personal destiny. If I accomplished nothing else, I hope you will at the very least keep the vision of personal health at the front and center of your life.

Don't flame out

With your personal vision statement providing the direction, it is just as important to have goals to drive you where you are trying to go. Goals can galvanize and strengthen your desire for accomplishment. Having an intense desire for something or someone can provide a lot of fuel for your motivational fire. If you are a hopeless romantic like me, you probably have experienced the passionate influence and emotional power of meeting the person of your dreams. Suddenly, you can survive on three hours of sleep, be more productive at work, and still have the energy to go out on an exciting date with "the one." Your mind is flooded with positive thoughts and positive expectations, your heart is filled with emotion, and your stomach is filled with butterflies. Having any goal you are truly excited and passionate about can have a similar influence on you too.

If passion is the flame then having a clearly stated goal is the fuel that keeps the flame burning. When you have a powerful goal it is like turning the burners on the stove to high or if you are flying a military fighter jet it is like putting the throttle into afterburner. Just like the fighter jet at full throttle, you will have more energy to propel you forward. If you don't continuously fuel the fire, eventually the flame will go out and it can take time to get the fire lit again. Like the torch lit before each Olympics, it may take you another four years to get the passion flame burning again in your life. In the meantime, you are meandering through life without direction, purpose, or passion and life becomes the "same old drag." Don't let this happen to you. Keep the motivational fire burning with persistent thoughts about what you want to achieve.

Ever start a campfire or light a cozy fire in a fireplace? Initially it takes time to gather the wood and kindling, clear an area, light the fire, fan the flames, and watch it attentively until it is burning bright. To keep it going, you simple throw another log on the fire. Having a burning desire and purpose works the same way. It may initially take you some time to figure out what motivates you and what you are passionate about. But once you do and your flame is lit, keep adding logs to the fire by creating and reviewing passionate goals. You will want goals for each area of your life including: love, relationship, and marital goals; financial goals; spiritual goals; and I hope after reading this book and for the rest of your life, health and fitness goals.

Writing this book was the manifestation of many goals I set. From the content, to the length of the book, and the timelines for getting each chapter done, I had goals for each. And while I saw many of my self-imposed writing deadlines come and go, some with success and most without, I never beat myself up because I kept the larger goal (to write the book) and my personal vision statement (to help motivate people to exercise) front and center in my thoughts. I knew that persistence would eventually payoff and if you are reading this now, then I hope we both would agree that it has. Apply the wisdom of Winston Churchill's timeless words to your own life: "Never give up. Never give up. Never, never, never, never give up."

Goal setting 101: the Garden and the Gardener

Goal setting is a prerequisite to achievement even if you are in the right place at the right time. Even the so-called "lucky ones" had goals to direct their success. The Roman philosopher Seneca said over two thousand years ago: "Luck is what happens when preparation meets opportunity." Bill Gates and Michael Dell left college early in pursuit of a grander and more immediate purpose in their lives and went on to achieve tremendous success. Both men had high goals to guide them to their ultimate destiny. If you want success in any area of your life, you need goals to be your lighthouse to guide you in the right direction. Having powerful goals will direct you to your destination and steer you clear of the dangerous saboteurs who can and will sink your ship.

What do you want out of life? What do you want to accomplish? What burning desire for achievement do you have? Motivational speaker and author John Di Lemme calls this finding your why. Rick Warren, author of *Purpose Driven Life*, calls it finding your purpose. Call it whatever you want, but you must have goals in life to maximize your true potential. Goals should be specific, measurable, timely, and have an emotional connection.

To be an effective goal setter, you need to have a process. I like to equate the process to the garden and the gardener; you being the gardener. The first step in planting a garden is determining what you want to grow, which in this case represents any goal you may have. If you want to grow corn, it wouldn't make sense to plant apple seeds would it? Likewise, if functional health and longevity are two of your desires in life, you wouldn't want to set a goal to become the world's pie-eating champion. Rather, you would want to set a goal or goals related to the attainment of health. So pick your crop or if you have several goals, your garden can have many crops. In my experience, it is best to limit yourself to a few major goals at a time so you can capitalize on the power of focus. If you have too many different goals, your energy may become diluted between them and your results will be diluted too.

Once you know what you want to grow in your garden, the second step is picking the right land to grow it in. Just like you would want to plant your seeds in fertile soil, you want to create a fertile environment for achieving your goals. Negative and cynical friends and family can be like toxic, dead, unproductive soil where nothing will grow. Surround yourself with positive, encouraging, and like-minded people to support you in the good times and help you out of the valley of defeat in the bad times. Just like gardeners may put up a fence around their garden to keep the vermin out, you may have to put up your own wall (or emotional boundaries) to protect yourself from negative outside influences. This may include people close to you who unfortunately are typically the first ones to say: "Put off the gym until tomorrow. What difference is one day gonna make?" One day can turn into two and before you know it, your goal is slipping away from you. Protect your goal from the parasites in your life.

The third important step in your goal setting garden is to till the soil to prepare it for planting. Similarly, achieving any goal requires preparation to get your body and mind ready. This is the time to get a gym membership, find the proper workout attire, buy a heart rate monitor and consult with a personal trainer or experienced exercise buddy. Plan out what you need, what time and days of the week you will devote to your goal, and any other who, when, where, and how so you have everything ready to support you in your quest. Being adequately prepared will remove the likelihood of excuses cropping up (pardon the pun).

Now you are ready to plant the seeds and seedlings which represent the fourth step in starting your garden: creating the ideas and processes necessary to achieve your goal. Great ideas take root with proper nurturing and will help produce a more bountiful harvest. Remember the Law of Attraction we discussed earlier in the chapter: the more you focus your thoughts on what you want, the more good ideas will pop into your head to help you get there. During the germination process, you will also want to remove the weeds of temptation from your garden. Weeds sap vital nutrients and water from the soil and can strangle the life out of an otherwise productive plant. If having chocolate chip cookies in your cupboard is too tempting, get rid of them. If you live across the street from a fast food restaurant you can't seem to avoid, then move. Your life and health are worth it. That doesn't mean you have to pack you're your bags and hire a moving company this very minute, but relocating to a more health-supporting location may (and should) be one of your goals.

Before you will reap the bounty of your goals, you will need to provide your crop or crops adequate water each day (consistency), monitor growth (accountability), and if necessary add some organic fertilizer (mentorship). Like fertilizing the soil can be a catalyst to better farming yields, hiring a personal trainer or working out with a like-minded workout partner can provide you better and faster results in the gym. If you have a financial goal, a good financial advisor can be your fertilizer or if you are getting married, an experienced wedding planner can organize a beautiful wedding more efficiently and with fewer headaches (assuming you are willing to listen to them) than you can. Don't feel like you have to accomplish anything in life on your own. Be willing to solicit help and advice from others.

By following this process, you will eventually harvest the fruits of your goal-setting labors and enjoy the success and self-confidence that comes with it. When you want to start on your next goal or goals, just repeat the process. Pick your new crop, till the soil, add water and fertilizer, keep the weeds in check and then enjoy the harvest. In the next and last chapter of this book I will help you facilitate the process of goal setting to guide your life in the positive direction that exercise and good health can take you. You are well on your way to a longer, healthier, and happier life! Remember you reap what you sow. Happy planting!

Calista
Age: 42
Music Teacher

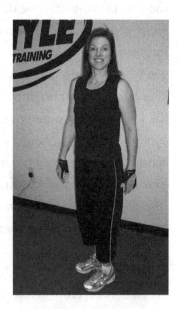

THE FACTS:

- Lost over 29 pounds
- Lowered her body fat by 8%
- Lost 6 inches off her waist
- Gained self-confidence

"It feels great to finally be in shape! I love the fact that I am now a size 8, down from a size 14. I lost about 30 pounds and many inches from my body. I no longer worry about waist bands being too tight and have a lot more self-confidence in my clothes. Most importantly, I have more energy to handle a full-time job and still have enough left over to keep up with my two young children.

I am 42 years old and I have people tell me I look at least 10 years younger than I am. I feel great, I have a positive attitude, I feel confident and I know people look at me in an admiring fashion and I love it. I could not have reached this fitness goal without the help of a personal trainer. Matt O'Brien was instrumental in transforming my body from borderline obesity to a strong, fit and healthy one. If you have never worked out with a personal trainer you have no idea how beneficial it can be. Matt motivates me to do more, lift more, and achieve more than I ever could on my own. He is supportive, encouraging and very knowledgeable about the body, nutrition, and physical training.

Working with a trainer is the catalyst that takes me to a higher exertion level than I ever thought possible. I would never work this hard on my own. Matt also emphasizes the importance of good nutrition with all his clients. Using his nutritional traffic light is a practical solution to staying on task with nutrition but also being able to live a 'normal' life. I eat in the green to stay lean! Try working out with Matt O'Brien one time and you will be hooked as I am."

- Calista Zebley

CHAPTER THIRTEEN

Direct Yourself

"The gateway to lasting success does not swing outward, it opens inward."

> Robin Sharma
> Author of *Discover your Destiny* series

Action Leads the Way to Your Destiny

So far in this book, I hope you have discovered the motivational benefits of good health; learned the educational tenets of exercise, nutrition, and supplementation; and been inspired by some people just like you who have earned the outward and inward rewards of exercise. In the previous chapter, we empowered your mind for positive outcomes and expectations and learned how to harvest the bounty of setting goals. Now it's time to take action and direct ourselves toward getting results. All the knowledge in the world is useless without action. If you are already vigilant about exercise but want to refresh your passion or sharpen your exercise sword a bit, this will still be very useful information. Action, not words, determines your destiny in life.

Thus I ask my glorious readers: Do you want a healthier, happier, longer, and better life? If you answered yes, than simply *decide* you want it! Success in any endeavor starts always with a decision. D.E.C.I.D.E. is my acronym for achieving a lifetime of positive results. Whether it is losing weight, gaining cardiovascular stamina, increasing functional strength, or improving any other area of your life (in addition to your health of course), you must *decide* it is important and take action. Don't let another day go by without taking at least one step, no matter how big or small, in the direction of your hopes and dreams. One of the many hopes I have for this book is that by the end of this chapter, you will have a lifetime resource to help take you wherever you want to go. Are you ready to decide?

D - Destiny   *What is your purpose?*
E - Expectancy   *Have a positive mindset (beliefs create reality)*
C - Commitment   *Go "all-in" and prioritize your life*
I - Inspiration   *Seek out that which inspires you*
D - Discovery   *Pursue a lifetime of learning*
E - Enthusiasm   *Do things you enjoy*

Destiny

Start with your goal or purpose in mind! The first step to take towards any achievement is to decide what you are trying to accomplish. Think seriously about this for a moment. Are you trying to lose weight, get in shape, have more energy, or improve your health? Are you getting ready for a physically active vacation? Do you want to be physically more capable to allow you to play with your children, future children, or grandchildren? Do you want to extend your life expectancy by reducing your risk factors for heart attack, stroke, diabetes, and cancer so you can enjoy more time with your spouse, family, and

> **HELPFUL HINT**
>
> Listen to music which inspires you or moves you emotionally while you write down your goals. I guarantee the goals will be more powerful and music can help you tap into the emotional center of your brain. Personally, I always find "Believe" by Brooks and Dunn and "Lucky Man" by Montgomery Gentry gets me in the goal-writing mood. If you are in a committed relationship, I would recommend "God Bless our Love" by Anne Murray or "I believe in you and me" by The Four Tops. Music is very individualistic, so select what works for you.

friends? Do you want to feel better, sleep better, or fit into smaller clothes? Maybe you want some or all of these things?

Having a clearly thought out and powerful goal will galvanize your efforts and dramatically increase your likelihood of success. I cannot emphasize this enough. It could be the difference between success and failure and since failure is not an option when it comes to incorporating exercise into your life, I encourage you, implore you even, to decide why you are starting an exercise program (or any other goal you have) and what you *will* accomplish. Then absolutely, positively take the time to write it down. This is very, very important!

Derek Jeter, love him or hate him, is a powerful example of goal setting working at the highest level. Growing up he not only dreamed about playing Major League Baseball, he specifically set his sights on playing shortstop for the New York Yankees. In a recent interview he is quoted as saying: "Seriously, I never thought about playing anywhere else." Derek went on to achieve his goal of playing shortstop for the New York Yankees, arguably the most storied and prolific franchise in all of sports, and is also now the team captain and all-time leader in hits. Call it the Law of Attraction. Call it goal setting. Call it whatever you want, but it really works. You attract what you think about most.

Written goals are much more powerful then stated goals, so put a pen to paper for your own good. Write it in your own hand, in ink. Want the abridged version of goal setting 101? If you said no, sorry, cause here it is: Determine your goal or purpose, write it down, commit it to memory, read or repeat it to yourself everyday at least twice, eliminate any doubts, and believe in yourself! You can use the guide below to help structure your goals or simply write down the reason *why* you are starting and *what* you will accomplish. Please do this now on a separate piece of paper or if you prefer, in the space provided below.

My Goal is: _____

_____

_____

The MOST IMPORTANT reason I *will* succeed is: _____

_____

_____

Five compelling reasons for me to exercise:

1. _____

2. _____

3. _____

4. _____

5. _____

Examples: Watch my children / grandchildren grow up; Get my blood pressure down; Be there for my spouse as we age so he / she won't be alone; See my daughter / son get married / graduate / have children; I'm overweight and it's time to do something about it; My doctor told me to get my cholesterol down.

By exercising everyday I will:

1. _____

2. _____

3. _____

4. _____

5. _____

Examples: Lose 25 pounds by Christmas/my 50th birthday/25th anniversary; Lower my total cholesterol by 30 points; Add years to my life; Have more energy; Feel better about myself; Do the breast cancer walk next summer; Get rid of some excess stress in my life; Get my health back.

Now that you have done this, I am going to ask you to take the next step to success. Put your written goals in a location or multiple locations where you can see them everyday. Here are some suggestions: the bathroom mirror, refrigerator door, inside of the front door, work desk, computer monitor, TV remote, dashboard of car, or anywhere else you encounter on a daily basis. You *must* take the time to read your goal or goals at least two times each day. Read them out loud so you can really hear them. You will have to remind yourself to do this. You don't want your written goals to slip into the distant landscape and hectic clutter of your life. Put them front and center in your life everyday and read them!

Personally, I have used goal setting in all areas of my life and especially with my personal health. Every significant accomplishment in my own life was preceded by a written goal to achieve it. I have used goal setting to get me into college. I have used it in competitive sports. I have used it in job interviews and sales calls. Goal setting has put this book in front of you right now. I had to set a goal to make the time to research and write it. I had to set a goal to nurture the relationships and friendships necessary to help me get it in your hands. I made the opportunity to help change peoples' lives for the better the motivational fuel to drive me to get it done.

I've also used goal setting to improve my business, relationships, marriage, and quality of life. I even have a goal to set aside time for relaxation and travel. I schedule it on the calendar and pay for it in advance because having something to look forward to keeps me motivated during the fourteenth hour of a long, tiresome day. In my business, I have to maintain high energy and a positive attitude to help motivate my clients. Nothing helps me more than thinking about an upcoming weekend trip, social event, or even a nice dinner at one of my favorite restaurants. I encourage you to create your goals and to set-up rewards to propel you towards success along the way.

It takes 21 days for something to become a habit (so make exercising for 21 days one of your first goals) and 6 months for something to become a lifestyle. I like to tell prospective clients: Give me a day and

I'll make you feel better. Give me a week and you'll feel and sleep better. Give me a month and you'll be stronger, feel and sleep better, and start to see visible changes. Give me six months and together we'll change your life forever.

If you make the decision to lose some excess weight, begin with a mindset that you are changing your lifestyle in a positive way, rather than telling yourself "I'm going on a diet." Think long term and incorporate one, several, any, or all of my recommendations into your daily life. You can do this gradually or immediately, you decide. Some people thrive on an "all-or-nothing" approach.. Other people resist change fervently and will need more time for gradual and progressive change. Either strategy produces lifelong changes. What is your destiny?

Expectancy

What do you expect out of life? What do you expect out of each day? Do you wake up thankful to be alive and excited about the possibilities for that day? As we discussed at length in the previous chapter, the Law of Attraction dictates the outcomes of your predominant thoughts. Think positive and good things happen. Think negative and bad things happen. Train your mind to have positive expectations and watch the magical power of positive thinking materialize into your life.

This isn't something you can give lip service to. You have to convincingly believe it and your expectations have to be morally sound and realistic. Going to bed believing you will wake-up a supermodel with one million dollars cash and a supermodel of the opposite sex lying next to you would not be realistic (unless you are Tom Brady or Giselle München). Believing you will make lots of money so you can have "look at me now" vengeance on people who ostracized you in high school would not be morally sound. However, having the expectation and belief that you will meet the loving, caring, trusting, honest, and funny man or woman you will spend the rest of your life with could be something worth considering. It worked for me and I've been happily married ever since. Or more relevant to the subject of this book, believing that exercising five days a week will help you lose the excess weight you've gained since high school and as a result, allow you to live a longer and more rewarding life, would be a sound and realistic expectation.

It is critical to have a positive outlook and a healthy perspective with regard to exercise. You must have the mindset that exercise is something you will be doing for the rest of your life and if you pursue this as a goal, eventually you will love exercise and find it difficult to live without. Beliefs create reality and if you believe exercise is going to be a chore or boring then guess what? It will be. If you have the expectancy that you won't lose weight despite all your best efforts in the gym, then you most definitely won't lose weight. Only you know what your innermost thoughts are and you must confront them if they are negative. Steer your thinking in a positive direction, towards what you *will* achieve, and you will lose weight and exercise won't be boring.

Recently I used positive expectancy to match me with a like-minded training partner. I have always been self-disciplined about exercise, but it adds extra excitement, intensity, and motivation when you have someone to suffer with you when you are pushing through those last few painful repetitions of each set. Three months ago (at the time of this writing) I created an expectation in my heart and mind that I would find a reliable, motivating, knowledgeable person who I could work out with. Within a month I met Justin who not only is the best training partner I have ever had, but someone I am now proud to call my friend. When Justin's work schedule wouldn't allow us to workout together as much, I used the same positive expectancy to meet my other training partner Matt. Now on a good day I get to workout with Matt or Justin, but on a great day, we all get to workout together. It all started with positive expectation. Do you expect good things to happen to you?

Commitment

Once you know your destiny and have the expectancy that you will get there, then the next step is commitment. Now I'm not talking about a superficial obligation like "I'll get a gym membership" but rather going "all in" like an aggressive poker player and committing every ounce of your moral fiber to achieving your written goals. This may require a little sacrifice like dedicating some extra time to preparing your foods and making the necessary time and effort for exercise. But in reality it isn't a sacrifice when you consider the likelihood that exercise will help you feel better, look better, and live longer. Exercising for just three hours a week, statistically speaking, can add seven to eleven years to your life. If you are extremely overweight or morbidly obese, exercise can add even more precious time to your life than the eleven years I just mentioned. With those benefits, why wouldn't you want to commit a little time and effort? Like many things in life, you get out of it what you put into it. In Chapter 6, I covered the typical excuses that hold people back. Making a true commitment ignores all excuses! It's ok to make time for yourself and making health a priority in your life will make you a better husband, wife, mother, father, boss, coworker, teacher, student, brother, sister, or friend.

If you are completely new to exercise and have a goal to lose a significant amount of weight, commit to a smaller goal first like losing ten pounds. If you have access to a well-run health club or a community fitness center, take advantage of their fitness services and group fitness classes. Don't be ashamed to explain your situation to the gym staff because you have to be proud of yourself for taking action. Most people will want to help you and can point you in the right direction if you tell them where you are trying to go. I call this: *Putting it out there.* By broadcasting your goal to the world, you add another layer of commitment and empower the universe to help you achieve it. Don't just tell the membership consultant at the gym; tell your friends, coworkers, and family too. This is what I mean by commitment. By telling the people closest to you that you have a goal and you need their help to achieve it, you will dramatically increase your likelihood of success.

If you have a like-minded friend or family member who wants to go through the journey with you, commit to each other by handshake, hug, or written contract that you will support and motivate each other during the process. When I was a young boy growing up, my friends and I used to make "blood-brothers" pacts about things we would do. I'm not suggesting you gouge yourself with a knife and shake bloody hands with someone, but it's important to create a true bond. Commit to when, where, and how long you will meet to exercise. Commit to achieving your mutual goals. Commit to supporting each other with regard to nutrition and healthy eating habits. Commit to the *Ten Commandments of Nutrition*. Commit to not sabotaging each other by making ill-thought food suggestions during moments of weakness.

Everybody has their own strengths and weaknesses so learn to use each others strengths for the collective good of the group. If someone is punctual and reliable with their time, they should be in charge of keeping the scheduled workouts on track. If someone is a good cook, they should be in charge of planning out some healthy and tasty meals. If someone has exceptional skills as a motivator and lots of energy, they should lead the workout sessions and remind the collective group of what you are all going to accomplish. Keep in mind there will always be setbacks along the way so don't give up on each other. We are all human and no one is perfect, particularly the ones who think they are. People will inevitably let you down from time to time. So what, it happens. You have to let it go, not hold grudges, and move on. Be thankful that you have someone to help you and be sure to sincerely thank them from time to time. Keep the destination in mind, but enjoy the journey along the way. Can you commit?

Inspiration

Whether it is listening to or watching recorded Martin Luther King Jr. or John F. Kennedy speeches, reading the Bible, listening to opera, or watching NBC's *The Biggest Loser*, seek out something that inspires you. Life can be repetitive and mundane if you just let it happen. Instead, break out of the well-traveled ruts in the road of life and take the path less traveled. If you haven't found someone or something that inspires you, keep trying. Most people can find inspiration from people who came from a similar set of circumstances and went on to attain success. The *Chicken Soup for the Soul* series has inspired millions of readers over the years with touching stories of human kindness and generosity. Most multi-level direct marketing companies fuel their associates' motivational tanks with success stories they share during meetings and company events. Each month, magazines like *Shape* and *Men's Health* profile inspirational people who have successfully lost weight and kept it off. There is no shortage of inspiration to tap into; you just have to seek it out. With the convenience of the internet, inspiration is now easier than ever to find.

I'm a huge fan of motivational self-help books and I always find inspiration amongst their pages. Just like the positive feelings and self-esteem boost I get whenever I exercise, I get a similar "pump up" from reading books that can help me improve a skill or be a better person. If you enjoy reading, this can be a source of inspiration for you. Daily reading of motivational books is like an intravenous drip of inspiration. Positive energy will course through your body. Likewise, listening to uplifting, joyous music can have an inspirational effect on your day too. Nothing puts a smile on my face faster than when a good song plays on the radio. My wife recently told me that listening to our local Christian radio station always gives her a rush of positive energy and puts her in a great mood. If you are a fan of the arts, make sure you regularly schedule time to go to an art museum; attend the ballet, opera, or symphony; or get tickets to a show like Cirque du Soleil which combines music, dance, and amazing human feats of strength, power, and balance into a cohesive story. Don't underestimate the inspirational power of the arts because most works of art are the manifestation of someone's inspiration.

Many of my weight-loss clients find some inspiration by watching the NBC show *The Biggest Loser*. The rapid and dramatic weight loss achieved by the contestants on the show can remind us of what is humanly possible given the right circumstances. Following the lives and challenges other people face who also struggle with their weight may help us conquer our own enemies in the battle of the bulge. However, I would caution you not to hold yourself to the standard of weight loss achieved on the show. Biggest Loser contestants are living in a controlled environment without the outside distractions of life. They have 24-hour access to a wonderful fitness facility, have expert trainers to work with them virtually every day, have a huge financial incentive to lose weight, and are being watched by their fellow contestants, family members, and millions of people around the world. Put anyone in the same situation and even the most unmotivated person on the planet will find a way to exercise and eat right. That being said, many people have been inspired by the show to make positive changes in their life and for that reason, I tip my hat to all the people who make it happen. What inspires you?

Discovery

I've been fascinated by the anatomy, physiology, and biomechanics of the human body for as long as I can remember. In high school, this fascination led me to take every science class I could. In college, it led me to major in biology and learn about exercise physiology, sports psychology, and human nutrition. After college, I continued to learn about how the human body interacts with the world by reading books and research articles on the topic and also attending related seminars and workshops. Ultimately, my fascination led me to personal training where I have been able to apply my lifetime of discovery into a very rewarding career.

I encourage you to find your own passion and begin to discover more about it. If it isn't obvious at the moment, take some time alone to let your mind wander and often your thoughts will keep coming back to something that interests you. If you have access to a beach then a sunset walk listening to the waves crash on shore can open your mind to discovery. Whatever comes to mind may surprise you or it may be very familiar to you. Many people discover music. Whether it's playing an instrument or singing in a band or the church choir, music has a special connection with our souls. Some people are fascinated with building things or working with wood. The process of creating something beautiful and functional that you can share with others can be a wonderful hobby or even a livelihood if you are truly passionate about it. Sewing, sailing, or sight-seeing, whatever it is you are interested in, there is a ton of information available to help you learn more about it. I say discover your passion and your purpose will be fulfilled.

Pertaining to exercise and your health, you can discover different types of exercise over the course of your life. In your twenties and thirties, competitive sports can be a fun means of exercise and social networking. In your forties and fifties, maybe you discover ocean kayaking, adventure hiking, or triathlons. In your sixties and seventies, ballroom dancing can be a great form of exercise. The possibilities are endless and I encourage you to give many things a try to see if they interest you. Just keep in mind that you should always keep a base of strength training and cardiovascular exercise to keep you strong and fit which will allow you to participate in other forms of exercise throughout your lifetime. What passion in life will you discover?

Enthusiasm

Pick things you enjoy doing not only with regards to exercise, but in all aspects of your life...jobs, relationships, where you live, etc. I've always professed that variety is the spice of life, but some people are obviously happier with familiarity. If you like variety as much as I do, then incorporate programmed changes into your training. Keep strength training, but change your workouts, where you workout, when you workout and who you workout with from time to time. If you enjoy a certain sport or activity, incorporate it into your life and exercise plan. Personally, I have mapped out my own training to include triathlons, skiing, competitive bodybuilding, competitive racquetball, power lifting, golf, and mountain biking in my twenties; fitness and strength training, core conditioning, motocross, spin classes, and Olympic style lifting in my thirties; and going forward with speed training, hiking mountain peaks, auto racing, completing an Ironman triathlon and the NYC marathon, skiing, golf, swimming, and mountain biking during my forties and fifties; then competing in the senior Olympics in my sixties and seventies. I always remind myself that the exertion time I spend sweating in the gym allows me to continue doing the exciting things I enjoy doing outside the gym.

Exercise never needs to be boring. So pick things you enjoy and if need be, hire a strength and conditioning coach or personal trainer to show you how to incorporate sport or activity-specific training into your gym workouts. It makes it more relevant and purposeful, which will tap into your enthusiasm. I have many clients who enjoy snow skiing and snowboarding. So I incorporate exercises that improve strength, balance, joint resilience, endurance, and proprioception. If you know that what you are doing in the gym will help you be a better skier, decrease your likelihood of injury while you are skiing, and allow you to stay on the slopes well into your seventies, than you are more likely to be excited about what you are doing. I have worked with several teenagers who liked surfing but didn't necessarily enjoy coming to the gym. Once I incorporated exercises that would help them be better surfers and explained the relevance of strength, balance, and coordination in their sport, they became fans of exercise and came to the gym more often.

If you find yourself dreading the time spent exercising, then something is wrong and you need a new, different, fresh approach. Exercise must be of sufficient intensity to challenge your muscles and cardiovascular system, but it doesn't have to be dreadful. If you like group activities, use the internet to find local cycling, running, kayaking, or swimming groups or clubs. A friend of mine wanted to run a relay race in New Hampshire (he lives in Florida) and was able to find people to do it with using a simple search on the internet. If you enjoy playing golf, focused sessions on the driving range can be a good source of activity. I have burned as many as 450 calories in an hour hitting golf balls (granted, I'm a little gung ho).

If you like team sports, most communities have youth and adult leagues for softball, baseball, tennis, soccer, flag football, volleyball, and many other sports. Check with your local community fitness centers, health clubs, bicycle stores, and specialty stores pertaining to the sport you're interested in and chances are they will have information on local leagues, teams, and clubs. A word of caution though: if the recreational sport you are interested in typically involves drinking alcoholic beverages and eating calorie-dense foods during or afterwards (bowling comes to mind), then maybe you should choose another activity. Remember, enthusiasm is contagious and if you find something that gets you excited, chances are others around you will get excited too. Where does your enthusiasm lie?

Putting it all together

Now it's time to put it all together and take action!!! By investing the time and mental energy necessary to read this book, you have hopefully filled your brain with enough useful information to motivate, educate, and inspire you to commit to a lifetime of exercise. The bottom line is that all this information will be worthless if you don't apply it in some way. If you have never exercised before, take the first step and start as soon as possible. If you have been exercising regularly, maybe you're ready to take it to the next level by increasing the intensity of your workouts. If you have had personal success with exercise and are passionate about the benefits of exercise, maybe you're ready for a career as a personal trainer or fitness instructor. If exercise has changed your life like it has mine, I hope you will pay it forward and share your success with others. Whatever is right for you and your current situation, take that step.

Sometimes all it takes is a little direction. Like a roadmap can lead us in the right direction to where we want to go, this book can lead anyone who is ready, willing, and able in the right direction towards a longer, healthier, and happier life. I hope I have presented you with a foolproof case that exercise is the true magic pill we all wish we had. It is available to anyone willing to invest the small price of time, energy, and effort. Decide what you want to accomplish and set a goal and timeframe to accomplish it. Commit to yourself to make exercise a priority in your life. If you don't have access to a variety of quality exercise equipment, then join a reputable health club, wellness center, or fitness center. Recruit a like-minded exercise partner or hire a personal trainer to help facilitate results. Get a pedometer and a heart rate monitor to serve as your accountability tools. Create and follow an exercise plan. Create and follow a nutrition plan. Obey the 10 Nutritional Commandments. Take a high quality multivitamin every day. Develop a positive mental attitude by learning to appreciate all the God-given talents, abilities, hopes, and dreams you have. That's it in a nutshell and now you have the tools to move you in the right direction. No more procrastination. No more excuses. The time is now! You have a lifetime of happiness and healthy living to look forward to.

Happiness

Happiness eludes us because it comes from within;
   It doesn't come from things, places, possessions, or people.
Happiness is having persistent patience with others;
   It doesn't celebrate people's failures or limitations.
Happiness is being thankful for everything you have;
   It doesn't lament on what you don't have or what you want to have.
Happiness is knowing when to speak up for what you believe in,
   And also knowing when to remain silent so you can truly hear.
Happiness doesn't come from getting;
   It comes from giving, forgiving, and understanding.
Happiness comes from serving others
   with your time, resources, and whole heart.
Happiness is not a destination;
   It is all around us,
      And it is within us.
      Waiting to be found.

Acknowledgements

The Long and Winding Road

I was listening to David Archeletta sing Paul McCartney's "The Long and Winding Road" and I couldn't help reflecting back on the long and very winding road that has led me to this point in life. It took me a long time and many of life's humbling experiences to learn the value of the journey we are all on. I have survived failed relationships and suffered severe heartbreak. I have been deservingly and undeservingly fired from jobs I've both loved and hated. I have made bad hiring decisions and had to fire people I cared about. I have been in the fortunate position of earning hundreds of thousands of dollars and then went on to lose every last dime of it. I have been through several periods of emotional despair and intellectual paralysis, all while I was sinking in the brutal quagmire of indecision with what to do with my life. I have toiled through 90 hour work weeks and felt the self-defeating toil of not working at all. I have rejoiced in the culinary ecstasy of eating in some of the best restaurants in the world and I have also had to wonder where my next meal was coming from. I have moved over 18 times in my adult life, always seeking something better. Each time I discovered just the scenery, weather, and people are different. I learned that the grass really isn't greener on the other side of the fence.

Through all of this, I have arrived at this very point in my life and have realized the ultimate lesson in life which is to live in the moment. I'm sure you have heard the old adage… "Yesterday is history, tomorrow is a mystery, but today is a gift, the present!" Living our lives in full awareness, consciousness, and appreciation can be positively transforming emotionally, spiritually, mentally, and physically. Taking five minutes on your drive home to think about the wonderful qualities of your spouse can make every evening a loving reunion and most of the bickering and anger in the relationship will miraculously dissolve. When you are driving to work, taking a moment to say "thank you" for the fact that you have a job, can make the work day go by more joyously and help ease the inevitable frustrations which rear their ugly heads throughout the day. Living in the moment with sincere appreciation can also be the difference in feeling fortunate that you were blessed with the gift of life in having children, rather than feeling burdened with the responsibility of raising them.

Applying this strategy has brought happiness to my daily life and helped me find my life's purpose. It helps me remind myself every day of where I have been and how lucky I am to have such a wonderful and supporting family who loves me, my own bed to sleep in, food to cook in the kitchen of my own house, my own car to drive me wherever I want to go, vision to see the beauty which surrounds us each day, a healthy body which allows me to do almost anything I want to do, a sharp mind to process my thoughts, goals, and dreams, and a loving heart to share with all the people in my life.

Most importantly, living life in positive expectation and appreciation has helped me find the woman who exceeds every wish I've ever had in a relationship and who I get to share my experiences with every day, instead of being alone. I used to think my life was a long and *lonely* road, but now I am blessed with the loving relationship we are all deserving and capable of having. So fill up your emotional gas tank with love and appreciation and enjoy the journey down your long and winding road. Stop and smell the roses each day, open your heart to possibility, and live with hope because a small miracle is just around the next bend. Keep your eyes open so you don't miss it!

This book would not have been possible without many small miracles in my own life and I think it is important to acknowledge their contributions to my personal journey. I would like to thank all the research scientists, physiologists, kinesiologists, nutritionists, and psychologists who have dedicated the time, energy, and effort to determining the why's, who's, what's, and how's of the human body.

Having met many of these great people, read their books and research articles, and watched their presentations over the years; I proudly tip my hat to them because of their commitment to scientific study. Without their efforts, the scientific basis of my conclusions would not be possible.

I would like to thank my many teachers for giving me the academic ability to compile research, intellectualize an opinion, and put pen to paper. I'm especially appreciative of Marjorie Paulsen who relentlessly drilled the rules of the English language into my head. If and when I made a mistake, I apologize to her because it would be an oversight on my part. I would like to thank the many coaches for developing my athletic ability and fostering the leadership skills I've used throughout my life. Looking back, I am particularly grateful for Coach Ray Jenks who showed me early in life the value of hard work, sweat, and team commitment and Coach Eugene Blaufarb who taught me how to lead a team and to believe in myself. I would like to thank the military community that I am so proud to have served with and a special thanks to my first commander, Colonel William Burner, who taught me that in order to know and love someone else, you first must know and love yourself.

I graciously thank Lifestyle Family Fitness for providing such an excellent fitness laboratory to work in and I especially thank all my clients who have put up with me over the past 10 years. If you are reading these words, I want you to know I am thankful you gave me the wonderful opportunity to earn a living doing what I love to do. You also unknowingly served as my human guinea pigs as I experimented with different exercise and nutrition protocols. We have had a blast together and I really don't like watching you suffer through one of my grueling, gut-wrenching workouts. Ok, maybe I do just a little bit. Thank you from the bottom of my heart for all your hard work, loyalty, friendship, humor, and wisdom. I have learned so much from all of you.

I thank my brothers, Tim and Brendan, and sisters, Michelle and Megan, for all the fun, love, laughter, and support over the years.

Through all the ups and downs in my life, you have all been there for me and are a constant source of security and friendship. The times when we get together are truly the best of times and it is during those precious moments when I feel like a kid again. I think it is truly special that we all have made the time to rendezvous for family events over the years despite the demands life places on each of us.

I thank my wonderful parents, Anita and Michael, who are the best mom and dad a son could ever ask for. You have both shaped my life by your examples of kindness, goodness, discipline, and love. I am happy with the person I have become. Your encouragement kept me going forward in life even when I didn't want to. You gave me every opportunity in the world and introduced me to the world of opportunity. Like you always said Mom, "life is a great big can of tuna" and I'm glad you gave me such a big appetite for it. Thank you Mom for pushing me when I needed to be pushed, pulling me when I needed to be pulled, and leaving me on my own when I needed to spread my wings and fly. Dad, I would be hard-pressed to find anyone who worked harder than you did when I was growing up. To this day, I don't know how you summoned the energy to work 50-plus hours each week, maintain a 10-acre farm with a Noah's Ark-like two of every animal to feed, plant and maintain gardens and greenhouses, do woodworking, volunteer for our youth baseball and football teams, and manage to keep us all grounded at the same time. I reminded myself of your example whenever I didn't feel like I had the time to get this book done.

Finally, I thank my wonderful wife Hollie for being an angel sent from Heaven to be my constant companion, my best friend, and the love of my life. You have supported me beyond measure with your time getting me ready for each day, your understanding while I was away writing, and your patience with all things involved in getting this project done. Marriage is a team effort and I consider myself so blessed and fortunate to have such a great teammate. Together we can accomplish so much more than I ever could alone. My long and winding road always takes me home to the loving embrace of your arms.

Selected References and Further Reading

Anti-Aging

Buettner, Dan *The Blue Zones*
Washington, DC: National Geographic Society, 2008

Crowley, Chris and Lodge, Henry *Younger Next Year*
New York: Workman Publishing, 2004

Klatz, Ronald and Goldman, Robert *The New Anti-Aging Revolution*
Laguna Beach, CA: Basic Health Publications, 2003

Masley, Steven *Ten Years Younger*
New York: Broadway Books, 2005

Roizen, Michael F. *The Real Age Makeover*
New York: HarperCollins, 2004

Roizen, Michael F. and Oz, Mehmet C. *YOU: Staying Young*
New York: Free Press, 2007

Roizen, Michael F. and Oz, Mehmet C. *YOU: The Owner's Manual*
New York: HarperCollins, 2005

Diabetes

American Diabetes Association *The Complete Guide to Diabetes*
New York: Bantam Dell, 2005

Barnard, Neal D. *Dr Neal Barnard's Program for Reversing Diabetes*
New York: Rodale, 2007

Diet and Nutrition

Agatston, Arthur *The South Beach Diet*
New York: St Martin's Press, 2003

Campbell, T. Colin and Campbell II, Thomas M. *The China Study*
Dallas, TX: BenBella Books, 2006

Eades, Michael and Eades, Mary *Protein Power*
New York: Bantam Books, 1996

Heller, Rachael and Heller, Richard *The Carbohydrate Addicts Diet*
New York: Signet, 1991

Helmering, Doris and Hales, Dianne *Think Thin Be Thin*
New York: Broadway Books, 2005

Pratt, Steven and Matthew, Kathy *Superfoods: Fourteen Foods that Will Change Your Life*
New York: HarperCollins, 2004

Rolls, Barbara *The Volumetrics Eating Plan*
New York: HarperCollins, 2005

Schlosser, Eric *Fast Food Nation*
New York: Houghton Mifflin Company, 2001, 2002

Sheats, Cliff *Lean Bodies*
New York: Warner Books, 1992, 1995

Strand, Ray D. *BioNutrition*
Norwell, MA: Health Concepts Publishing, 2009

Wansink, Brian *Mindless Eating*
New York: Bantam Books, 2006

Wolcott, William and Fahey, Trish *The Metabolic Typing Diet*
New York: Broadway Books, 2000

Exercise
Aerobics and Fitness Association of America *Fitness: Theory & Practice*
Julie van Roden, managing editor (4th Edition); Sherman Oaks, CA:
AFAA, 2002

American College of Sports Medicine *ACSM's Guidelines for Exercise Testing and Prescription*
Mitchell H. Whaley, senior editor (7th Edition); Indianapolis, IN:
ACSM, 2006

McGovern, Artie *The Secret of Keeping Fit: An Easy and Sure Way to Better Health*
New York: Simon and Schuster, 1935

National Strength and Conditioning Association *The Essentials of Strength and Conditioning*
Thomas R Baechle, Roger W. Earle, editors(2nd Edition); Human
Kinetics, 2000

Phillips, Bill *Body for Life*
New York: HarperCollins, 1999

Verstegen, Mark and Williams, Pete   *Core Performance*
New York: Rodale, 2004

Health and Wellness

Esselstyn, Jr. Caldwell B. *Prevent and Reverse Heart Disease*
New York: The Penguin Group, 2007

Goldberg, Linn and Elliot, Diane *The Healing Power of Exercise*
Hoboken, NJ: John Wiley & Sons, 2000

McDougall, John A. *The McDougall Program: 12 Days to Dynamic Health*
New York: The Penguin Group, 1990

Ornish, Dean *Dr Dean Ornish's Program for Reversing Heart Disease*
New York: Ivy Books, 1990

Self-Help

Canfield, Jack *The Success Principles*
New York: HarperCollins, 2005

Carnegie, Dale *How to Win Friends & Influence People*
New York: First Pocket Books, 1936, 1982

Dalai Lama and Cutler, Howard *The Art of Happiness*
New York: Riverhead Books, 1998

Gordon, Jon *The Energy Bus*
Hoboken, NJ: John Wiley & Sons, 2007

Niven, David *The 100 Simple Secrets of Happy People*
New York: HarperCollins, 2000

Peale, Norman Vincent *The Power of Positive Thinking*
New York: Fawcett Crest, 1952

Robbins, Anthony *Awaken the Giant Within*
New York: Fireside, 1991

Ruiz, Don Miguel *The Four Agreements*
San Rafael, CA: Amber-Allen Publishing, 1997

Sharma, Robin *Discover Your Destiny with the Monk Who Sold His Ferrari*
New York: HarperCollins, 2004

Tolle, Eckhart *The Power of Now*
Novato, CA: New World Library, 1999

Vitamins and Supplementation
Firshein, Richard *The Nutraceutical Revolution*
New York: Riverhead Books, 1998

Hendler, Sheldon Saul *PDR for Nutritional Supplements 2nd Edition*
Physicians Desk Reference, 2008

Ivy, John and Portman, Robert *Nutrient Timing*
Laguna Beach, CA: Basic Health Publications, 2004

Mindell, Earl and Mundis, Hester *Earl Mindell's New Vitamin Bible*
New York: Warner Books, 2004

Reader's Digest *The Healing Power of Vitamins, Minerals, and Herbs*
Pleasantville, NY: The Reader's Digest Association, 1999

ABOUT THE AUTHOR

Matt O'Brien is a lifelong teacher, coach, and motivator who is passionate about helping others attain a healthy mind and body through proper exercise, nutrition, and dietary supplementation. Matt began personal training professionally in 1997 in New York City and has trained corporate executives, television personalities, high fashion models, competitive athletes, and lots of "real world" people seeking results. Matt earned his Bachelor of Science degree from the US Air Force Academy (1991) and is a Certified Strength and Conditioning Specialist (CSCS). He currently is working on his next book *The Fast 40* and resides in the Tampa Bay area of Florida with his wife Hollie and son Keegan.